Translational Research Methods for Diabetes, Obesity and Cardiometabolic Drug Development

Andrew J. Krentz • Lutz Heinemann
Marcus Hompesch
Editors

Translational Research Methods for Diabetes, Obesity and Cardiometabolic Drug Development

A Focus on Early Phase Clinical Studies

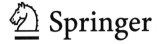

Editors
Andrew J. Krentz, MD, FRCP
Profil Institute for Clinical Research
Chula Vista, CA
USA

Marcus Hompesch, MD
Profil Institute for Clinical Research
Chula Vista, CA
USA

Lutz Heinemann, PhD
Profil Institute for Clinical Research
Chula Vista, CA
USA

ISBN 978-1-4471-4919-4   ISBN 978-1-4471-4920-0 (eBook)
DOI 10.1007/978-1-4471-4920-0
Springer London Heidelberg New York Dordrecht

Library of Congress Control Number: 2014956922

© Springer-Verlag London 2015
This work is subject to copyright. All rights are reserved by the Publisher, whether the whole or part of the material is concerned, specifically the rights of translation, reprinting, reuse of illustrations, recitation, broadcasting, reproduction on microfilms or in any other physical way, and transmission or information storage and retrieval, electronic adaptation, computer software, or by similar or dissimilar methodology now known or hereafter developed. Exempted from this legal reservation are brief excerpts in connection with reviews or scholarly analysis or material supplied specifically for the purpose of being entered and executed on a computer system, for exclusive use by the purchaser of the work. Duplication of this publication or parts thereof is permitted only under the provisions of the Copyright Law of the Publisher's location, in its current version, and permission for use must always be obtained from Springer. Permissions for use may be obtained through RightsLink at the Copyright Clearance Center. Violations are liable to prosecution under the respective Copyright Law.
The use of general descriptive names, registered names, trademarks, service marks, etc. in this publication does not imply, even in the absence of a specific statement, that such names are exempt from the relevant protective laws and regulations and therefore free for general use.
While the advice and information in this book are believed to be true and accurate at the date of publication, neither the authors nor the editors nor the publisher can accept any legal responsibility for any errors or omissions that may be made. The publisher makes no warranty, express or implied, with respect to the material contained herein.

Printed on acid-free paper

Springer is part of Springer Science+Business Media (www.springer.com)

Foreword

This book provides an important contribution to the literature on the scientific basis of drug development and clinical trials in the general field of metabolism. There is a worldwide epidemic of obesity, type 2 diabetes, and associated cardiometabolic diseases, which have collectively emerged as one of the greatest public health problems we face. Consequently, there is a huge unmet medical need for improved therapeutic options. This has created the opportunity and incentive to test a number of new potential drugs for these disorders. Given the high level of interest in drug development in this field, this book focuses exclusively on early phase (phase 1 and 2) clinical studies, rather than later-stage phase 3 development. As such, the chapters in this book discuss a variety of current methodologies in metabolic research, which focus on proof of mechanism, early indicators of efficacy, biomarkers, and safety. A key goal of these early phase studies is to learn as quickly as possible whether a potential drug candidate works through the expected mechanism with the desired degree of efficacy. This provides for earlier "go/no go" decisions, allowing biopharmaceutical companies to focus their resources on the most promising projects.

By using the latest in vivo methodologies to measure physiologic variables such as insulin secretion, insulin sensitivity, thermogenesis, metabolomics, and a variety of other outputs, a great deal can be learned in the initial stages of drug testing, which has not been possible in the past. Thus, thoughtfully designed proof-of-mechanism studies are highly feasible and make current discussions and resource allocations in metabolic drug development far more efficient and informative.

The editors of this book, Andrew J. Krentz, MD, Lutz Heinemann, PhD, and Marcus Hompesch, MD, are all highly experienced experts in academic research and drug development, and they have recruited an expanded list of world leaders in metabolic research to cover a range of topics. Each chapter in part one chapter focuses on a specific approach or methodology, representing the leading edge of knowledge in clinical research and early-stage drug development. To maintain uniformity, each chapter in the first part of the book is organized in a comparable format, which greatly enhances its accessibility and usefulness to the reader. This includes an up-to-date summary of the latest scientific knowledge concerning each topic, coupled with practical information as to how the various methodologies can be best employed. The second part of the book considers emerging investigative approaches, regulatory and practical issues of early phase cardiometabolic drug development.

The intended readership includes industry-based scientists who are involved in the design and interpretation of first-in-human efficacy and proof-of-mechanism studies, as well as academic physicians engaged in metabolic research. This book should also be useful to a broader audience, including students and fellows who are just beginning or contemplating a career in this field.

San Diego, USA   Jerrold M. Olefsky, MD

Preface

This book is offered as a contribution to the complex quest for safe and effective new drugs for the burgeoning global challenge of diabetes, obesity, and associated disorders. In creating the textbook, we hope to help fill what we perceive to be a gap in the scientific literature. Specifically, the focus is firmly on early phase (i.e., phase 1 and 2) safety, efficacy, and proof-of-mechanism studies of relevant new therapies.

As editors, we combine backgrounds anchored in the academic diabetes research environment with extensive experience of the professionalism of the biopharmaceutical industry. We hope that this dual – and, in our view, complementary – perspective is evident in our choice of topics. The primary format is detailed reviews and critiques of the available methods along with illustrations of their use using examples derived from the literature.

We are delighted to be joined in this venture by many renowned clinical investigators drawn from leading academic institutions and scientific service providers in the USA and Europe. We thank the contributors for their shared enthusiasm in providing chapters each of which we believe stands as a self-contained state-of-the-art review. In addition, where relevant we have provided signposts that connect relevant sections of the book.

The need to "fail early in appropriate subjects" has become a guiding principle in the development of new molecular entities for diabetes and obesity. In large part, this pressure reflects the more stringent regulatory environment that was a response to recent high-profile safety concerns of approved drugs. A new challenge facing the biopharmaceutical industry is fulfilling the requirements for approval of biosimilar insulins, the pitfalls of which have already been demonstrated. For novel diabetes therapies, there is an increasing realization that blood glucose lowering to a similar degree to available therapies is no longer sufficient. This realism recognizes the existence of an already crowded therapeutic arena that faces ever-increasing restrictions imposed by payers faced with cost-benefit decisions.

We anticipate that the primary readership of the book will be industry-based clinical scientists involved in the design and interpretation of first-in-human efficacy and proof-of-mechanism studies. We hope that academic physicians engaged in clinical metabolic research will also find the book of value. While we have assumed a high level of knowledge among readers, we have tried to provide relevant background science concerning the etiopathogenesis of diabetes that informs the selection of the most appropriate investigative methods. In addition to core methods for determining insulin action, time-action profiles of insulin formulations, body composition, etc., we review the ethics of early phase clinical research in diabetes and obesity, notably the move toward "first-in-patient" studies that is increasingly accepted. The potential application of emerging disciplines such as the omics technologies and complex modelling techniques to diabetes drug development is also considered.

Many clinicians, while familiar with the later stages of drug development, i.e., phases 3 and 4, may be rather less conversant with the aims of first-in-human and proof-of-concept studies. Being mindful of this potential disconnection, we have tried to bridge from the highly regulated early phase clinical research space to integrate new glucose-lowering drugs into clinical practice. For example, how does an improvement of X% of whole-body insulin sensitivity translate into glucose-lowering efficacy? What "added value" do patients and prescribers want from a new diabetes drug, and conversely, what unwanted effects must be avoided? Perhaps a more developed dialogue between clinicians and clinical scientists would be of value when contemplating the future of diabetes therapies.

We wish to thank Diane Lamsback, Emma Sinclair, and Rebecca Owen of Springer for their unstinting assistance and support.

Chula Vista, CA, USA Andrew J. Krentz, MD, FRCP
Fall 2014 Lutz Heinemann, PhD
Marcus Hompesch, MD

Contents

Part I Review of Clinical Investigation Methodologies

1. **Methods for Quantifying Insulin Sensitivity and Determining Insulin Time-Action Profiles** 3
   Andrew J. Krentz, Lutz Heinemann, and Marcus Hompesch

2. **Assessment of β-Cell Function** 45
   Andrew J. Krentz, Lutz Heinemann, and Marcus Hompesch

3. **Isotopic Tracers for the Measurement of Metabolic Flux Rates** 71
   Carine Beysen, Marc K. Hellerstein, and Scott M. Turner

4. **Imaging Techniques for the Assessment of Ectopic Fat in Liver and Skeletal Muscle** 99
   Gavin Hamilton, Michael S. Middleton, Elhamy R. Heba, and Claude B. Sirlin

5. **Positron-Emission Tomography and Computed Tomography Measurement of Brown Fat Thermal Activation: Key Tools for Developing Novel Pharmacotherapeutics for Obesity and Diabetes** 121
   Monte S. Buchsbaum and Alex DeCastro

6. **Assessment of Body Composition** 139
   Mark Punyanitya and Paul R. Clark

7. **Measurement of Energy Expenditure** 169
   Klaas R. Westerterp

8. **Omics: Potential Role in Early-Phase Drug Development** 189
   Harald Grallert, Carola S. Marzi, Stefanie M. Hauck, and Christian Gieger

Part II Emerging and Complementary Research Methods; Ethical and Regulatory Considerations

9. **Early Phase Metabolic Research with Reference to Special Populations** 225
   Linda A. Morrow and Andrew J. Krentz

10 **Quantitative Approaches in Translational Research: An Overview**.. 243
    Puneet Gaitonde, Shannon A. Miller, Mirjam N. Trame, and Stephan Schmidt

11 **Computational Modelling of Energy Metabolism and Body Composition Dynamics**........................ 265
    Kevin D. Hall

12 **Regulatory Considerations for Early Clinical Development of Drugs for Diabetes, Obesity, and Cardiometabolic Disorders**........................ 283
    G. Alexander Fleming

Index... 305

Contributors

Carine Beysen, PhD KineMed, Inc., Emeryville, CA, USA

Monte S. Buchsbaum, MD Department of Psychiatry and Radiology, University of California, San Diego, San Diego, CA, USA

Paul R. Clark, PhD(Dist), BE(Hons) MagnePath Pty. Ltd., Perth, Australia

Alex DeCastro, MS Department of Psychiatry, University of California, San Diego, San Diego, CA, USA

G. Alexander Fleming, BS, MD Kinexum Services LLC, Harpers Ferry, WV, USA

Puneet Gaitonde, PhD Department of Pharmaceutics, College of Pharmacy, University of Florida, Orlando, FL, USA

Christian Gieger, PhD Research Unit of Molecular Epidemiology, Institute of Genetic Epidemiology, Helmholtz Zentrum München, German Research Center for Environmental Health (GmbH), Neuherberg, Germany

Harald Grallert, PhD Research Unit of Molecular Epidemiology, Institute of Epidemiology II, Helmholtz Zentrum München, German Research Center for Evironmental Health (GmbH), Neuherberg, Germany

Kevin D. Hall, PhD Laboratory of Biological Modeling, National Institute of Diabetes and Digestive and Kidney Diseases, National Institutes of Health, Bethesda, MD, USA

Gavin Hamilton, PhD Department of Radiology, University of California, San Diego, San Diego, CA, USA

Stefanie M. Hauck, PhD Research Unit Protein Science, Helmholtz Zentrum München, German Research Center for Environmental Health (GmbH), Neuherberg, Germany

Elhamy R. Heba, MD Department of Radiology, University of California, San Diego, San Diego, CA, USA

Lutz Heinemann, PhD Profil Institute for Clinical Research, Chula Vista, CA, USA

Marc K. Hellerstein, MD, PhD KineMed, Inc., Emeryville, CA, USA

Marcus Hompesch, MD Profil Institute for Clinical Research,
Chula Vista, CA, USA

Andrew J. Krentz, MD, FRCP Profil Institute for Clinical Research,
Chula Vista, CA, USA

Carola S. Marzi, PhD, MPH Research Unit of Molecular Epidemiology,
Institute of Epidemiology II, Helmholtz Zentrum München, German
Research Center for Evironmental Health (GmbH), Neuherberg, Germany

Michael S. Middleton, MD, PhD Department of Radiology,
University of California, San Diego, San Diego, CA, USA

Shannon A. Miller, PharmD, BCACP Department of Pharmacotherapy
and Translational Research, College of Pharmacy,
University of Florida, Orlando, FL, USA

Linda A. Morrow, MD Profil Institute for Clinical Research,
Chula Vista, CA, USA

Mark Punyanitya, MA, MS Image Reading Center, Inc.,
New York, NY, USA

Stephan Schmidt, PhD Department of Pharmaceutics,
College of Pharmacy, University of Florida, Orlando, FL, USA

Claude B. Sirlin, MD Department of Radiology,
University of California, San Diego, San Diego, CA, USA

Mirjam N. Trame, PharmD, PhD Department of Pharmaceutics,
College of Pharmacy, University of Florida, Orlando, FL, USA

Scott M. Turner, PhD KineMed, Inc., Emeryville, CA, USA

Klaas R. Westerterp, PhD Department of Human Biology,
Maastricht University, Maastricht, The Netherlands

Part I
Review of Clinical Investigation Methodologies

Methods for Quantifying Insulin Sensitivity and Determining Insulin Time-Action Profiles

Andrew J. Krentz, Lutz Heinemann, and Marcus Hompesch

Keywords
Insulin resistance • Glucose clamp technique • Time-action profiles of insulin • Oral glucose tolerance test • Intravenous glucose tolerance test

Summary

Background

Impaired insulin action is a prominent metabolic feature in obese subjects and patients with type 2 diabetes as well as many cardiovascular disorders. Reducing obesity through non-pharmacological or pharmacological interventions improves insulin sensitivity. Drugs that directly improve insulin sensitivity, e.g. thiazolidinediones, are widely used in the treatment of type 2 diabetes. Accurate measurement of insulin action is required to evaluate new drugs with insulin-sensitizing properties.

Determining the time-action profiles of insulin formulations provides important pharmacodynamic information that guides use in clinical practice. Novel insulin delivery systems, e.g. inhaled insulin, adjunctive measures to alter insulin action, and biosimilar insulins, require quantitative assessment of pharmacodynamic properties.

Key Methods

Assessment of Insulin Sensitivity
Methods for measuring insulin action may be classified according to whether the feedback loop between the islet β-cells and insulin-sensitive target tissues is maintained (closed-loop) or interrupted through pharmacological manipulation (open loop).

A.J. Krentz, MD, FRCP (✉) • L. Heinemann, PhD • M. Hompesch, MD
Profil Institute for Clinical Research,
Chula Vista, CA, USA
e-mail: andrew.krentz@profilinstitute.com;
lutz.heinemann@profilinstitute.com;
marcus.hompesch@profilinstitute.com

Closed-Loop Methods

	Method	Measurement	Advantages	Disadvantages	Value in drug development decisions
Fasting serum insulin and glucose; mathematic models include HOMA-IR[a] and QUICKI[b]	Venous serum insulin and plasma glucose are measured in blood samples drawn after an 8–12 h overnight fast	Insulin sensitivity (%S)	Technically simple; relatively inexpensive; provides an indication of insulin sensitivity in relation to hepatic glucose metabolism	Indirect assessment of insulin action; only assesses metabolism in basal (non-stimulated) state; insulin resistance may be underestimated in the presence of hyperglycaemia	May provide useful exploratory data in early-phase studies; results should be confirmed with a dynamic test
Frequently sampled intravenous glucose tolerance test (FSIVGTT)	Glucose, insulin and C-peptide responses to an intravenous bolus of glucose; minimal model analysis of	Minimal model yields insulin-sensitivity index (S_I) and glucose effectiveness (S_G)	Provides dynamic data; widely used in clinical metabolic research	Indirect integrated assessment of glucose metabolism; questionable relevance to normal physiology	Limited value
Mixed-meal tolerance test (MMTT)	Plasma glucose and serum insulin responses at defined intervals to a standardized meal	Area under the curve (AUC) for insulin; mathematical models of insulin and glucose responses (e.g., Matsuda index; Stumvoll index)	Provides data relevant to normal physiology; flexible, i.e. nutrient components can be adjusted; assesses integrity of incretin axis	Indirect assessment of insulin action; issues of intra-individual and between-individual variability; affected by gastric emptying rate	May be of value in providing early signal of effects of drugs on insulin action
Oral glucose tolerance test (OGTT)	Glucose, insulin and/or C-peptide responses to 75 g oral glucose	AUC for insulin; mathematical models of insulin and glucose responses (e.g. Matsuda index; Stumvoll index	Simple; reference methods for diagnosing diabetes and impaired glucose tolerance; vast scientific literature	Indirect assessment of insulin action; intra-individual and between-individual variability; β-cell response to secretagogues other than glucose not assessed; affected by gastric emptying rate	May be of value in providing early signal of effects of drugs on insulin action
Insulin tolerance test (ITT)	Response of blood glucose to an intravenous bolus of glucose	Glucose disposal rate (K_{ITT})	Technically simple	Risk of hypoglycaemia; cannot partition between insulin-mediated glucose disposal and suppression of hepatic glucose production	Limited role in diabetes drug development

[a] Homeostasis model assessment
[b] Quantitative insulin-sensitivity check

Open-Loop Methods

	Method	Measurement	Advantages	Disadvantages	Value in drug development decisions
Insulin suppression test (IST)	Somatostatin is infused to suppress endogenous insulin secretion; insulin and glucose are infused to achieve steady-state plasma glucose	Steady-state plasma glucose (SSPG)	Reproducible steady-state method which eliminates endogenous insulin secretion and assesses insulin-mediated glucose disposal	Indirect assessment of insulin action on glucose metabolism; labour-intensive; relatively inflexible; hepatic insulin sensitivity cannot be determined	Limited value
Insulin-sensitivity clamp (two-step hyperinsulinaemic-euglycaemic clamp)	Insulin is infused to provide steady-state hyperinsulinaemia at predetermined insulin concentration; variable rate glucose is infused to maintain plasma glucose at euglycaemia	Glucose disposal rate (M); M/I; insulin-sensitivity index (SI$_{clamp}$)	Direct measure of insulin-mediated glucose disposal; reproducible; low coefficient of variation; may be readily combined with complementary techniques, e.g. isotopic determination of glucose turnover, indirect calorimetry; automatic clamps using the Biostator offer advantages over manual clamps	Labour intensive; requires skilled technical staff	Generally regarded as the reference method for determining insulin sensitivity

Determination of Pharmacodynamic Properties of Insulin Formulations

	Method	Measurement	Advantages	Disadvantages	Value in drug development decisions
Time-action profile – glucose clamp (euglycaemic clamp)	Insulin is administered by subcutaneous injection/inhalation, etc.; hypertonic glucose is infused intravenously at a variable rate to maintain plasma glucose at euglycaemia	Maximal glucose infusion rate (GIR$_{max}$); time to GIR$_{max}$ (t_{max}); area under the curve (AUC$_{0-T}$)	Yields simultaneous detailed pharmacodynamic and pharmacokinetic data	Labour intensive; requires skilled technical staff; assessment of ultra-long acting insulins has limitations	Clamp-derived time-action profiles for insulin and biosimilar insulins are required by US and European regulators for market approval of new insulins

Conclusions

Of the available methods for quantifying insulin action, the euglycaemic glucose clamp technique is widely regarded as the reference method. The hyperinsulinaemic-euglycaemic glucose clamp provides robust and reproducible measures of insulin sensitivity. When combined with isotopic determination of glucose turnover, the sensitivity of hepatic glucose metabolism to insulin can also be quantified. The glucose clamp technique is highly adaptable and may be complemented by methods such as indirect calorimetry to measure substrate oxidation or tissue biopsy of fat or muscle to examine enzyme activity in the stimulated state.

The euglycaemic/isoglycaemic glucose clamp technique is used extensively to assess the time-action profiles of insulin preparations. Glucose clamp studies are resource-intensive. All variants of the glucose clamp technique, including automated clamps, are to some extent operator dependent and require experienced technical staff to ensure accurate and reproducible data.

Introduction

Insulin is a pivotal hormone controlling critical energy functions including regulation of glucose and lipid metabolism at cellular, tissue, and whole-body level. Impaired action of insulin, i.e. insulin resistance, is a well-documented feature of many physiological and pathological states (Table 1.1) [1–4]. These range from temporary subclinical decrements in insulin action to rare genetic syndromes of severe insulin resistance requiring innovative pharmacotherapeutic approaches [5]. From a global public health perspective, excess adiposity is the most common form of acquired insulin resistance. Impaired insulin action is a major modifiable factor in the pathogenesis of glucose intolerance and type 2 diabetes and is closely associated with the adverse profile of risk factors for cardiovascular disease [6].

Insulin Physiology and Metabolic Regulation

Hepatocytes, skeletal myocytes, and white adipocytes are regarded as classic insulin-responsive tissues [7]. Most cells express surface insulin receptors. Insulin regulates glucose metabolism both through direct actions [8] and in part by influencing interorgan crosstalk pathways including the synthesis and secretion of fat-derived adipocytokines (Table 1.2) [9]. Insulin signalling in the brain influences energy balance and peripheral glucose metabolism [10]. Other nonclassic target tissues for insulin include the heart [11], skeleton [12], brown adipocytes [13], and ovaries [14]. The metabolic function of these organs may be favourably or unfavourably affected by insulin-sensitizing drugs [15]. The range of physiological actions of insulin has expanded beyond regulation of carbohydrates and other macronutrients to include antioxidant, anti-inflammatory, and vascular effects (Table 1.3) [16, 17].

Table 1.1 Physiological and pathological states associated with whole-body insulin resistance

Physiological states
  Adolescence
  Pregnancy (2nd and 3rd trimesters)
  Luteal phase of the menstrual cycle
  Postmenopause[a]
  Ageing[a]
Common pathological conditions
  Obesity[b]
  Glucose intolerance
  Type 2 diabetes
  Metabolic syndrome[c]
  Sedentary lifestyle (vs. regular physical activity)
  Non-alcoholic fatty liver disease/steatohepatitis

Modified from Krentz [4]
[a]The evidence for direct effects of these physiological processes on insulin sensitivity is inconsistent. Changes in body composition and other factors may, at least in part, explain the reduced insulin action reported in some studies
[b]Includes lesser degrees of overweight. Abdominal adiposity is more closely associated with whole-body insulin resistance than gynecoid subcutaneous fat deposition. Ethnicity is an important modifier of the metabolic effects of adiposity; non-white populations including East and South Asians develop adverse cardiometabolic profiles at lower levels of body mass index compared with counterparts of white European ancestry. Ectopic fat in skeletal muscle and liver are closely correlated with impaired whole-body insulin action. Ectopic fat may also be deposited in the pancreas and the heart and vascular system with detrimental effects on organ function
[c]Various definitions of the metabolic syndrome have been proposed. The main features are abdominal adiposity, glucose intolerance, hypertriglyceridaemia, low levels of high-density lipoprotein cholesterol, hypertension in variable combinations and in association with insulin resistance, and hyperinsulinaemia

Cellular Insulin Signalling

In peripheral tissues, e.g. muscle and fat, insulin must leave the intravascular compartment and traverse the interstitial space before interacting with cellular insulin receptors [18]. The

Table 1.2 Classic metabolic actions of insulin

	Direct effects	Indirect effects
Skeletal muscle[a]	↑Glucose uptake ↑Glucose oxidation ↑ Glycogen synthesis	↓ NEFA availability and oxidation
Liver	↓ Glucose output ↓ Glycogenolysis ↓ Gluconeogenesis ↑ Glycogen synthesis ↑ Glycolysis ↑ Lipogenesis	↓ NEFA availability and oxidation
Adipose tissue	↑ Glucose uptake ↑ Lipogenesis	↓ Lipolysis Regulation of adipocytokines

Adapted from Konrad et al. [8]
[a]Cardiomyocytes are also regulated by insulin

Table 1.3 Nonclassic actions of insulin

Antioxidant
↓ Reactive oxygen species
Anti-inflammatory
↓ NFκB ↓ C-reactive protein
Antithrombotic
↓ Tissue factor ↓ platelet activation
Pro-fibrinolytic
↓ Plasminogen activator inhibitor-1
Vasodilatory
NO-mediated improvements in endothelial function
Large vessel compliance
Lipid regulation
↓ Hepatic production of very-low-density lipoproteins
Sympathetic nervous system
↑ Activation
Anti-atherosclerotic actions
Apo E null mouse, IRS-1 null mouse

Adapted from Refs. [16, 17]

insulin receptor is a transmembrane heterodimer comprising two α- and two β-subunits (Fig. 1.1). Binding to the α-subunit induces a conformational change resulting in release of the inhibitory effect of the α-subunit and autophosphorylation of tyrosine residues in the β-subunit [19]. Insulin receptor tyrosine kinase phosphorylates and recruits substrate adaptors such as the insulin receptor substrate (IRS) family of proteins. This initiates molecular events that result in translocation of the facilitative glucose transporter (GLUT4) from the cytosolic vesicles to the cell membrane [20, 21]. Fusion of GLUT4 with the cell membrane transports glucose into the cell where it is phosphorylated to glucose-6-phosphate. A post-binding cascade of phosphorylation/dephosphorylation reactions leads to activation of key enzymes including glycogen synthase and pyruvate dehydrogenase. In the presence of hyperinsulinaemia, glucose-6-phosphate is mainly (approximately 70 %) polymerized to form glycogen; the remainder enters the glycolytic pathway and is either oxidized or converted to lactate [22].

Insulin is a potent growth factor that exerts transcriptional effects on cell growth and differentiation [23], via the mitogen-activated protein (MAP) kinase pathway [24]. Other actions of insulin include regulation of protein metabolism [25] and aspects of cellular ion transport [26].

Insulin Resistance

Insulin resistance may be defined as a state in which physiological concentrations of insulin produce a less than normal biological response [27]. The assessment of insulin sensitivity in clinical practice is recognized as being problematic. Accurate quantification of insulin action is possible only within a specialized clinical research setting. While obesity is closely associated with insulin resistance, body mass index (BMI) is a relatively unreliable indicator of whole-body insulin sensitivity (essentially the inverse of insulin resistance) [28]. Visceral adiposity, which is often accompanied by chronic low-grade systemic inflammation and alterations in cytokine physiology, is more closely associated with insulin resistance and risk factors for cardiometabolic diseases (see below) [29]. Clinically useful biomarkers for insulin resistance remain underdeveloped [30].

Cardiometabolic Consequences of Insulin Resistance

Insulin resistance is strongly implicated in the pathogenesis of hyperglycaemia, dyslipidaemia, and vascular disease [31–33]. It is estimated that

Fig. 1.1 (**a**) Insulin signal transduction system in individuals with normal glucose tolerance. NOS, nitric oxide synthase. (**b**) In patients with type 2 diabetes, insulin signalling is impaired at the level of insulin receptor substrate (IRS)-1 leading to decreased glucose transport/phosphorylation/metabolism and impaired nitric oxide synthase activation/endothelial function. At the same time, insulin signalling through the mitogen-activated protein (MAP) kinase pathway is normally sensitive to insulin. The compensatory hyperinsulinaemia due to insulin resistance in the IRS-1/phosphatidylinositol-3 (PI-3) kinase pathway results in excessive stimulation of the former pathway, which is involved in inflammation, cell proliferation, and atherogenesis. *SHC* Src homology collagen (With kind permission from Springer Science + Business Media: DeFronzo RA. 2010. [46])

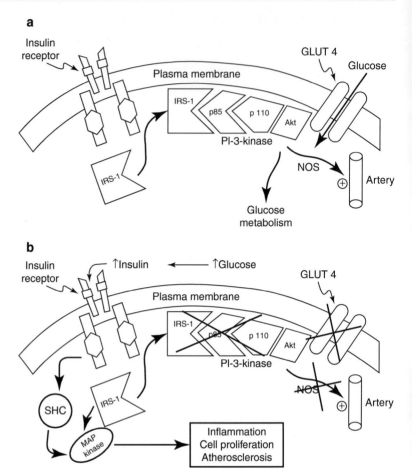

approximately 30 % of the variability in insulin-mediated glucose uptake is accounted for by BMI, with factors such as physical activity levels and genetic influences contributing to the remainder of the variance [34]. Ectopic fat deposition, which may occur in the liver, skeletal muscle, the myocardium, and the pancreas, is associated with organ dysfunction and decreased insulin action both locally and more systemically [32, 35].

The leading cause of premature mortality in patients with diabetes is cardiovascular disease [36]. The metabolic syndrome (also known as the insulin resistance syndrome) encompasses the major obesity-associated clinical risk factors for atherothrombotic vascular disease, i.e. central adiposity, hyperglycaemia, dyslipidaemia (hypertriglyceridaemia or low levels of high-density lipoprotein cholesterol), and hypertension [37]. At the cellular molecular level, maintained insulin stimulation of the MAP kinase pathway by hyperinsulinaemia has been proposed as a pathway to atherosclerosis activation of inflammatory pathways (see Fig. 1.1) [38].

Insulin Resistance in the Pathogenesis of Type 2 Diabetes

Using quantitative techniques the majority of subjects with impaired glucose tolerance and patients with type 2 diabetes are insulin resistant, together with 25 % of otherwise apparently healthy normoglycaemic individuals [1, 39]. According to a widely accepted model, islet β-cells respond to reduced insulin signalling in target tissues with an appropriate increase in secretion of the hormone [39, 40]. If the rise in insulin production is less than the amount required for full metabolic compensation, glucose intolerance develops; progressive β-cell failure leads to degrees of glucose intolerance that may culminate in type 2 diabetes [39, 41].

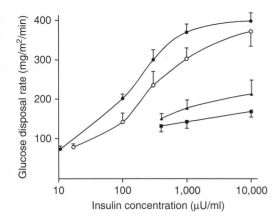

Fig. 1.2 Mean dose-response curves for control subjects (*solid circles*), subjects with impaired glucose tolerance (*open circles*), and nonobese (*solid triangles*) and obese (*solid squares*) subjects with type 2 diabetes. Hyperinsulinaemic-euglycaemic clamps were performed at multiple circulating insulin levels. The dose-response curve for the subjects with impaired glucose tolerance is shifted to the right relative to the health controls. This decrease in insulin sensitivity has been interpreted as consistent with a defect at the level of the insulin receptor. The subjects with type 2 diabetes show a more profound impairment of insulin-mediated glucose disposal. Not only is the shift to the right more pronounced, there is also a decrease in maximal insulin action, i.e. reduced insulin responsiveness. This is considered to be indicative of defects in the insulin signalling pathway distal to the interaction of insulin with its receptor (Data from Kolterman et al. [43] with permission) To convert μU/mL to pmol/L, multiply by 6.0

In widely cited early study, Jerrold Olefsky, Orville Kolterman, and colleagues used the hyperinsulinaemic-euglycaemic glucose clamp technique to construct dose-response curves for insulin action across a range of insulin concentrations in subjects with obesity with or without type 2 diabetes. Defective insulin-mediated glucose disposal was most marked in the more insulin-resistant, hyperinsulinaemic obese subjects [42]. In less insulin-resistant nondiabetic obese individuals [42] and in subjects with impaired glucose tolerance [43], there was a rightward shift in the whole-body glucose disposal curve indicative of decreased insulin sensitivity. This was considered to be consistent with a defect in insulin action at the level of the insulin receptor (Fig. 1.2) [27, 42, 43]. In patients with type 2 diabetes, an additional defect was evident with an inability to achieve maximal response even in the presence of very high insulin concentrations (see Fig. 1.2) [42, 43]. The latter observation is characteristic of type 2 diabetes and is considered to be consistent with impaired insulin signalling distal to the interaction of the hormone with its receptor [43].

Post-binding intracellular defects in insulin action that have been described in type 2 diabetes include impaired transmembrane glucose transport, reduced glucose phosphorylation, lower rates of glucose oxidation, and reduced glycogen synthesis [22]. Defective insulin action, compounded by impaired physiological suppression of glucagon secretion [44], leads to fasting and postprandial hyperglycaemia [45]. In health, hepatic glucose production is appropriately suppressed by hyperinsulinaemia following a meal. Higher insulin levels are required to suppress glucose output by the liver in the presence of insulin resistance [43]. In subjects with type 2 diabetes, rates of postprandial glucose release into the circulation are increased. This glucose originates partly from endogenous sources, i.e. liver and kidney, due to a combination of increased glycogenolysis and gluconeogenesis, in concert with decreased splanchnic glucose uptake [45]. In absolute terms postprandial glucose disposal by skeletal muscle is not significantly impaired relative to nondiabetic subjects as a consequence of the mass action effect of hyperglycaemia [45]. However, the metabolic clearance rate of glucose, which takes prevailing hyperglycaemia into account, is reduced. In patients with type 2 diabetes, impaired insulin-mediated glucose disposal is associated with reduced non-oxidative metabolism, i.e. glycogen synthesis, in skeletal muscle [46].

Insulin Sensitivity: A Therapeutic Target in Type 2 Diabetes and Cardiovascular Disease

Improving insulin sensitivity through weight reduction and physical exercise remains the cornerstone of management of type 2 diabetes [47]. However, lifestyle modifications alone rarely provide adequate metabolic control and glucose-lowering medications are usually required [48,

49]. Insulin sensitizers are effective glucose-lowering agents [50]. The biguanide metformin, which lowers blood glucose primarily by improving hepatic insulin action, is widely regarded as the drug of choice [49, 51]. In the Diabetes Prevention Program, metformin reduced progression from glucose intolerance to type 2 diabetes in high-risk obese subjects [52]. Protection against the development of diabetes has also been reported with for thiazolidinediones [53].

Insulin-sensitizing drugs may be of value in preventing cardiovascular events [54, 55]. However, some investigators consider that this evidence supporting this assertion remains less than conclusive [56, 57]. The controversy surrounding the reported increase in myocardial infarction with rosiglitazone highlighted the potential for molecule-specific adverse effects even within a class of glucose-lowering agents [58, 59]. Safety concerns have led to discontinuation of the development other insulin-sensitizers including tesaglitazar [60] and muraglitazar in 2006 [61] and aleglitazar in 2013 [62]. Better understanding of peroxisome proliferator-activated receptor (PPAR-γ) signalling may help reduce or eliminate adverse effects of fluid retention, weight gain, congestive cardiac failure, and skeletal fractures [15, 63]. The identification of novel mechanisms of insulin resistance, e.g. adipose tissue inflammation [64], has opened the door to new therapeutic approaches [65].

Principles of Insulin Therapy

Exogenous insulin is used in the treatment of all patients with type 1 diabetes and in a substantial proportion of patients with type 2 diabetes [66]. In the latter population, insulin is usually deferred until other glucose-lowering strategies have proved insufficient [67]. Many technical advances in purity, pharmacokinetics, and delivery systems have been achieved since the introduction of insulin into clinical practice in 1922 (see below; Tables 1.4 and 1.5). Nonetheless, optimal insulin replacement remains a formidable therapeutic challenge. During the 1980s the advent of recombinant DNA technology permitted the creation of insulin analogues with improved pharmacokinetic (PK) properties [68]. This advance facilitated the use of so-called basal-bolus intensive insulin regimens that aim to reproduce the complex and finely tuned physiological pattern of insulin secretion [69–71]. Rapid-acting insulin analogues (e.g. insulin aspart, insulin lispro, insulin glulisine) [72] and analogues with prolonged action (e.g. insulin

Table 1.4 Chronological evolution of insulin therapy

Animal insulin
Beef
Pork
Highly purified insulins
Monocomponent insulin
Human insulin
Recombinant DNA technology
High-strength insulin
U500 human insulin
U300 insulin glargine
Insulin analogues
Rapid acting
Long acting
Ultra-long acting
Inhaled insulin
Exubera®
Afrezza®
Biosimilar insulins
'Smart' insulins, i.e. glucose-responsive
Premixed combinations with glucagon-like peptide-1 agonists, e.g., Ideg Lira (insulin degludec + liraglutide)

Table 1.5 Modified insulin preparations with altered pharmacokinetics

Isophane
Neutral protamine hagedorn
Lente
Semi-lente
Lente
Ultralente
Protamine zinc insulin
Modified analogue (retarded action)
Pegylatation
Fc- carrier
Absorption enhancers (accelerated action)
Hyaluronidase
EDTA[a] destabilization of insulin hexamers

[a]Ethylenediaminetetraacetic acid

glargine, insulin detemir, insulin degludec) are now well established in clinical practice [73]. More recently, ultra-rapid-acting insulin formulations, injectable, e.g. hyaluronidase [74, 75], VIAject® [75, 76], and inhaled [77, 78], have been evaluated; in June 2014 the FDA approved the first inhaled human insulin (Afrezza®) since Exubera in 2006 [79]. The quest for a viable orally delivered insulin continues to drive clinical research activity [80]. In parallel, basal insulin analogues with ultra-long durations of action with potential for once-weekly administration are being developed [81].

Type 1 Diabetes

Modern intensive insulin regimens aim to sustain near-normal blood-glucose profiles, including low postprandial glycaemic excursions [70]. On a day-to-day basis, the risk of acute metabolic decompensation, i.e. hyperglycaemia and diabetic ketoacidosis, resulting from insufficient insulin must be balanced against the risk of hypoglycaemia. The latter, which is the main limiting factor to achieving glycaemic goals, occurs when insulin action is in excess of physiological requirements. The quest for insulin preparations and regimens that further improve this risk-benefit equation remains a research priority. Much effort continues to be directed towards the creation of a closed-loop 'artificial pancreas' [82]. Glucose-responsive insulins that aim to match insulin availability to ambient glucose levels are also under investigation [83]. Pramlintide, glucagon-like peptide (GLP)-1 agonists, dipeptidyl peptidase (DPP)-4 inhibitors, and leptin have been explored as adjunctive therapies.

Type 2 Diabetes

In patients with type 2 diabetes other glucose-lowering agents are often used in combination with insulin with the aim of attenuating unwanted aspects of insulin therapy [84, 85]. The risk of severe hypoglycaemic events is generally lower than in patients with type 1 diabetes [86]. This risk increases over time as β-cell function progressively declines and physiological counter-regulatory responses to hypoglycaemia become impaired [86]. Weight gain is a frequent and unwanted effect of insulin therapy. With greater degrees of obesity, daily insulin requirements may become cumbersome. Use of high concentration insulin preparations reduces the required volume of insulin [87]. While U500 insulin is unmodified soluble human insulin, its pharmacokinetics resemble those of an intermediate-duration insulin [88].

Measurement of Insulin Action in Humans

In clinical studies during the 1930s using an oral glucose challenge with a concomitant injection of insulin, Professor Sir Harold Himsworth of London University made a series of classic scientific observations that continue to inform current views of quantifying insulin action [89]. Himsworth divided diabetes into insulin-sensitive and insulin-insensitive subtypes, effectively pre-empting the modern diagnostic categories of type 1 and type 2 diabetes [90].

A major step forward came several decades later with the development of a method to measure insulin in the circulation [91], an achievement for which Rosalyn Yalow and Solomon Berson were awarded the Nobel Prize in medicine. It rapidly became clear that obesity and glucose intolerance were conditions characterized by elevated systemic insulin concentrations [92]. This led John Karam and Gerold Grodsky to speculate about antagonism of insulin action from an excess of nonesterified fatty-acid levels in muscle. By this time Professor Sir Philip Randle and colleagues at the University of Cambridge had described the glucose-fatty-acid cycle in rat myocardial and skeletal myocytes [93]. Kenneth Zierler and David Rabinowitz examined the dose-response effects of intrabrachial insulin infusion on glucose, fatty acids, and potassium metabolism in elegant isolated forearm experiments [94].

During the 1970s techniques for quantifying insulin action at the whole-body level, most notably the hyperinsulinaemic euglycaemic glucose clamp, were devised and implemented (see below) [95]. The 1980s was a decade of many notable advances concerning insulin receptor binding and intracellular signal transduction [96, 97]. Using techniques such as indirect calorimetry, isotopic tracers, and tissue biopsy, the details of defective insulin action in obesity, diabetes, and related cardiometabolic disorders became ever clearer [2].

The 1990s saw the introduction of the thiazolidinediones, a therapeutic advance that was later to have a profound and enduring impact on safety requirements for glucose-lowering agents [58, 98, 99]. In the 1980s and 1990s, the glucose clamp technique was also used to systematically evaluate time-action profiles of novel insulin formulations [100].

Table 1.6 Investigative techniques for the assessment of insulin action in man

Closed-loop assessment of basal metabolism
Fasting insulin
Homeostasis model assessment (HOMA)
Closed-loop dynamic tests
(a) Endogenous insulin
Oral glucose tolerance test, e.g., Matsuda index
Intravenous glucose tolerance test with minimal model assessment
(b) Exogenous insulin
Insulin tolerance test
Open-loop steady-state tests
Insulin suppression test
Hyperinsulinaemic-euglycaemic clamp

Classification of Methods for Measuring Insulin Sensitivity

Methods in current use for quantifying insulin action may be classified according to whether metabolism is studied at levels of insulin relevant to normal physiology or at pharmacological concentrations of the hormone. An alternative classification considers whether the feedback loop between the β-cells and insulin-sensitive tissues remains intact or is interrupted by pharmacological intervention (Table 1.6) [4]. Methods may also be subdivided into either whether they are basal or dynamic tests or whether they involve an experimental steady state of hyperinsulinaemia.

All of the commonly used methods focus primarily on the assessment of glucose metabolism. In the context of developing new drugs for diabetes, this approach is, of course, entirely appropriate. However, the complex dynamic interconnections that exist between carbohydrate, lipid, and protein metabolism support consideration of a broader perspective [101]. We propose that such an approach might prove useful in diabetes drug development. For example, in animal models the fibrate class of lipid-modifying drugs improve glucose metabolism via effects on PPAR-α receptors [102]. In 2008 the bile-acid sequestrant colesevelam was licensed by the US Food and Drug Administration (FDA) for the adjunctive treatment of hyperglycaemia in patients with type 2 diabetes. While the glucose-lowering mechanisms of this lipid-modifying agent have yet to be clarified, improved hepatic insulin sensitivity has been reported [103]. Selective cannabinoid receptor agonists [104, 105] and novel PPAR-γ agonists [106] have effects on multiple facets of intermediary metabolism that may contribute to their glucose-lowering actions.

Minimizing Confounding Factors in Studies of Insulin Sensitivity

When designing clinical studies evaluating novel insulin-sensitizing drugs or insulin preparations, confounding factors that may impact insulin sensitivity should be carefully considered (Table 1.7). Subjects should be maintained on a stable diet with constant exercise levels and should be free of acute illness or a history of recent hospitalization. These factors, if not held constant as far as possible, may contribute to day-to-day variability in insulin sensitivity thereby reducing the statistical power of the study. Admission to the clinical facility a day or two ahead of glucose clamp study days is recommended in order to stabilize diet, exercise, and sleep patterns [100, 107]. A practical consideration is the residual effect of prior treatment with drugs affecting glucose metabolism or body weight. In countries with well-developed healthcare systems, it may be difficult to recruit drug-naïve patients with type

Table 1.7 Factors that may influence insulin sensitivity of relevance to metabolic studies of insulin action

Ethnicity (e.g., East and South Asians may be insulin resistant even in the absence of generalized obesity)
Body weight should be stable (within 5–10 %) in the weeks preceding a metabolic study. For in-house studies, care must be taken to maintain body weight
Family history of type 2 diabetes may be associated with greater degrees of insulin resistance
Personal history of glucose intolerance (e.g., gestational diabetes; an insulin-resistant state carrying a high risk of progression to permanent type 2 diabetes)
Recent intercurrent illness (moderate inflammatory response and/or tissue damage/repair are associated with reduced insulin sensitivity via release of cytokines)
History of recent (within 6–8 weeks of study) major surgery (includes minimally invasive procedures requiring a general anaesthetic)
Current or recent history of malignant disease
Polycystic ovary syndrome (relatively common among women of reproductive age)
Male hypogonadism
Impaired function of major organs, i.e. heart, liver, kidney – see Table 1.1
Medications; many drugs may affect insulin sensitivity and glucose tolerance
Diet – calorie consumption, macronutrient composition, and micronutrient intake may each independently influence insulin sensitivity
Recent acute physical exertion (avoid rigorous exercise for >24 h prior to metabolic studies)
Alcohol consumption (U-shaped association with insulin resistance; excess alcohol consumption may aggravate hypertriglyceridaemia; avoid alcohol for 24 h prior to study)
Tobacco (use associated with insulin resistance; smoking activates sympathetic nervous system activity)
Caffeine (high caffeine consumption may acutely reduce insulin sensitivity; in contrast, habitual coffee consumption is protective against the development of type 2 diabetes)
Disorders associated with antagonism of insulin action, e.g., hyperthyroidism, hypothyroidism, hyperprolactinaemia
Rare inherited or acquitted syndromes, e.g., lipoatrophic diabetes, insulin receptor antibody syndromes

2 diabetes since metformin is recommended at an early stage after diagnosis [49]. Monotherapy may be withheld from suitable patients with type 2 diabetes in preparation for early-phase studies of an experimental diabetes drug (see Chap. 9). For thiazolidinediones [108] and glucagon-like peptide (GLP)-1 receptor agonists [109] which have sustained effects on insulin sensitivity and/or body weight, a sufficient period of withdrawal is recommended to ensure a new steady state.

Closed-Loop Assessments
Tests of Basal Insulin Sensitivity
Fasting Insulin Levels

In the fasting state hyperinsulinaemia in the presence of normo- or hyperglycaemia is indicative of insulin resistance. Homeostasis model assessment (HOMA) is a mathematical model that estimates insulin sensitivity as a percentage of a normal population based on fasting serum insulin and blood-glucose concentrations.

HOMA-IR

This test was originally described by David Matthews and colleagues at the University of Oxford [110]. Both the original HOMA approach and the updated version (HOMA2) [111] assume the presence of a feedback loop between the liver and β-cells. HOMA-IR is the reciprocal of %S (100/%S).

$$\text{HOMA-IR} = G_b \times I_b / k$$

G_b and I_b are, respectively, basal (fasting) glucose (in mmol/L) and insulin (in mU/L) with $k = 22.5$.

Since physiological insulin secretion from the β-cells is pulsatile, the mean of three samples taken at 5 min intervals to compute HOMA may be more accurate than a single sample. In practice a single measurement is often used and for large sample sizes, this compromise provides comparable data [112]. Since insulin action is not measured directly, HOMA-IR may be more appropriately considered a surrogate of insulin resistance.

A similar approach, the quantitative insulin-sensitivity check (QUICKI), is the reciprocal of the logarithm of HOMA-IR with k assigned a value of 1 [113]. In this model, logarithmic transformation accounts for the nonnormal distribution of fasting serum insulin concentrations.

HOMA has been compared with a variety of investigative methods for assessing insulin sensitivity, including the glucose clamp [112], albeit with varying conclusions [114]. It has been proposed that HOMA-IR provides information that is primarily relevant to basal hepatic glucose metabolism. Thus, if insulin-stimulated glucose uptake in skeletal muscle is of interest, consideration should be given to using a technique that raises circulating insulin concentrations. The insulin-glucose HOMA model cannot be used to assess β-cell function in patients taking exogenous insulin.

HOMA-IR is technically straightforward, quantitative, and relatively inexpensive. Accuracy is dependent in part on the precision of the insulin assay as well as the type of sample, i.e. serum vs. plasma [115]. The absence of an international standardized insulin assay [116] precludes use of HOMA-IR to define universal cut-off points for insulin resistance. For subjects without diabetes, the correlation between HOMA-IR and fasting insulin concentration is close to unity [117]. HOMA-IR is well suited to large-scale studies where it is perhaps most appropriately positioned [118]. The relatively high intra-individual variability of HOMA-IR renders the index less suitable for determining the impact of an intervention on insulin sensitivity in early-phase studies in patients with type 2 diabetes [119]. The correlations between HOMA and a more sophisticated measure of insulin-mediated glucose uptake were less good in normal weight individuals than in overweight or obese subjects (correlation coefficients 0.36, 0.55, and 0.60, respectively [117]. Similar (inverse) trends were observed for QUICKI [117].

HOMA-IR may be of value as an exploratory endpoint in interventional studies where a change in insulin sensitivity is postulated. For example, a study of the effects of niacin/laropiprant in women with ovary syndrome showed an impairment of glucose regulation despite beneficial effects on blood lipid profiles. The adverse effect on glucose metabolism was accompanied by an increase in HOMA-IR (3.8 vs. 2.2; $p=0.02$) indicating reduced insulin sensitivity [120]. In a meta-analysis of non-diabetic patients, angiotensin receptor blockers improved HOMA-IR relative to calcium channel blockers for a similar degree of blood pressure lowering [121]. These effects on insulin sensitivity may be of relevance to the hierarchy of risk of new-onset type 2 diabetes associated with the use of different classes of antihypertensive agents [122].

Closed-Loop Dynamic Tests

An oral glucose or mixed-meal challenge can be used to provide indirect or surrogate information about insulin resistance under more physiological conditions. In both scenarios, the release of endogenous insulin is stimulated by intestinally absorbed glucose in part via the activation of the incretin system [123]. In the situation wherein fasting and/or postprandial hyperglycaemia are present, the degree of hyperinsulinaemia will underestimate the level of insulin resistance. If compensatory endogenous insulin secretion were to be restored, e.g. by use of a classic insulin secretagogue drug, such as a sulphonylurea, then the resulting hyperinsulinaemia would return blood-glucose levels towards normality. In the case of sulphonylureas, the dynamics of insulin secretion are not normalized in an important sense; insulin secretion is not regulated by prevailing glucose concentrations [50]. Sulphonylureas will stimulate insulin secretion even when plasma glucose is normal with a well-recognized risk of hypoglycaemia. The risk varies according to the sulphonylurea [124]. The risk of inappropriate hyperinsulinaemia is largely avoided with glucagon-like peptide (GLP)-1 agonists and dipeptidyl peptidase (DPP)-4 inhibitors [50, 125]. This recently introduced class of incretin mimetics promotes insulin secretion only in the presence of hyperglycaemia [125].

Intravenous Glucose Tolerance Test

This technique, in which the caveat concerning impaired β-cell function also applies, has been widely applied in clinical metabolic research. A bolus of glucose (0.3 g/kg) is administered via an indwelling venous catheter after an overnight fast. Venous blood is sampled frequently from the contralateral arm for insulin and glucose over a period of 3 h [126]. The peak, and subsequent decline, in blood glucose reflects both the insulin response and whole-body insulin sensitivity. Modifications of the frequently sampled intravenous glucose tolerance test (FSIVGTT) include co-administration of tolbutamide to enhance insulin secretion [127] or a bolus of exogenous insulin (0.5 U/kg) [18]. Richard Bergman and colleagues advanced the analysis of data derived from the FSIVGTT and modified FSIVGTT with the introduction of the so-called minimal model [128, 129]. The insulin-sensitivity index, S_I, is calculated from two differential equations. S_I, which reflects composite insulin action on muscle and adipose tissue, reportedly correlates well with the M-value obtained using the hyperinsulinaemic-euglycaemic glucose clamp technique, at least in relatively insulin-sensitive and glucose-tolerant subjects [130]. In addition, the minimal model permits an assessment of the ability of glucose to promote its own disappearance from the circulation (and inhibit its endogenous appearance) independently of insulin; this value is known as glucose effectiveness or S_G [131]. The FSIVGTT avoids potential variations in gastric emptying that may affect the metabolic response to an oral glucose challenge in patients with diabetic autonomic neuropathy [132]. However, this advantage comes at the expense of losing the contribution of the powerful incretin effect on insulin secretion [133].

Concerns have been expressed about aspects of the validity of the minimal model and its limited correlation with more direct methods for assessing insulin action [134–136]. Nonetheless, using the theoretical framework of the minimal model, Michael Schwartz and colleagues at the University of Washington, USA have recently proposed the development of novel diabetes therapies that target a putative brain-centred glucoregulatory system modulating insulin-independent mechanisms (S_G) [137].

Oral and Mixed Meal Tolerance Tests

The oral route of glucose delivery is self-evidently more physiological than an intravenous glucose infusion. However, the oral glucose tolerance test (OGTT) cannot be regarded as a physiological stimulus, even though this is sometimes implied in the literature. The OGTT is recognized as having relatively low day-to-day reproducibility [138]. Factors contributing to intra-individual variability include inconstant rates of glucose absorption and splanchnic glucose uptake, variations in gastric emptying including gastroparesis due to autonomic neuropathy in some patients [139], and the modulating effects of gut-derived incretin hormones A longer-term influence on glucose tolerance is the macronutrient composition of the diet, e.g. percentage of calories derived from carbohydrate vs. fat and the proportion of monounsaturated fat [140]. Less well-documented dietary factors include micronutrient status [141] and the influence of the intestinal microbiome [142].

The 75 g OGTT is widely used in clinical practice to confirm diagnostic categories of glucose intolerance and type 2 diabetes [143]. After overnight fast, venous blood samples for glucose and insulin concentrations are taken at baseline and then every 30 min until 120 min following a standard oral glucose load (75 g); in a mixed meal tolerance test a standardized meal or meal substitute, e.g. Ensure®, may be used for clinical research purposes. The diagnosis of impaired glucose intolerance and diabetes are based solely on the baseline and 120 min blood-glucose levels [143]. Note that the classification limits differ according to the sample used, e.g. venous plasma vs. whole blood. Glucose should be dissolved in water so that the maximum glucose concentration in the beverage is 25 g per 100 mL. The drink, which may be made more palatable with a non-calorie flavour additive, should be consumed within 5 min with the subject sitting quietly throughout the test. For children, the glucose load is calculated according to body weight, i.e. 1.75 g per kg of weight to a maximum of 75 g. It has long been recognized that dietary carbohydrate restriction in the days preceding an OGTT may impair glucose tolerance. Accordingly, 100–150 g/day carbohydrates should be consumed as part of the diet for 3 days prior to the scheduled OGTT. In parentheses, the clinical impact of carbohydrate intake on insulin action is illustrated by the benefits of oral carbohydrate loading on surgical outcomes [144].

The OGTT (and meal tolerance test) mimics the glucose and insulin dynamics of physiological conditions more closely than the insulin suppression test, FSIVGTT, or hyperinsulinaemic-euglycaemic glucose clamp. Several insulin-sensitivity indices based on the OGTT are available. These include the Matsuda index [145] and the Stumvoll index [146]. The latter has been validated against the glucose clamp technique in subjects with a range of metabolic states and is widely regarded as a reliable indicator of insulin sensitivity. Others include the $OGIS_{120}$ index of Mari et al. [147] and an oral glucose minimal model enabling measurement of insulin sensitivity that has been developed and validated against multi-tracer and hyperinsulinaemic-euglycaemic glucose clamp protocols [136, 148]. In general, these indices of insulin sensitivity are more accurate in nondiabetic individuals with normal β-cell function.

Moving beyond measures of insulin and glucose, Beysen et al. developed the deuterated-glucose disposal test (^{2}H-GDT). The stable isotope [6,6-^{2}H$_2$]glucose is administered in a 75 g oral glucose load in order to determine whole-body glycolysis. Glycolytic disposal of the deuterated glucose generates ^{2}H$_2$O from which an index of insulin sensitivity is calculated using the insulin exposure resulting from the glucose challenge [149]. The investigators report close correlations with measures of insulin resistance using the hyperinsulinaemic-euglycaemic glucose clamp and the insulin suppression test (see below) across a range of insulin sensitivities [149].

The rise in blood glucose following oral loading is determined in part by the degree of suppression of hepatic glucose production in addition to the absorption and disposal of the oral glucose load [150]. Radiolabelled tracers may be used to ascertain the metabolic fate of an intestinal glucose load and quantify the contribution of endogenous glucose production to the post-challenge blood-glucose concentration. The merits of the various tracer options, which involve use of two or three ingested and infused tracers, have recently been reviewed [151]. As an example of the application of tracer methodology in a proof-of-mechanism study, Polidori et al. used a mixed-meal tolerance test with a dual-tracer (^{3}H-glucose, ^{14}C-glucose) method to examine the effects of canagliflozin, a sodium-glucose cotransporter (SGLT)-2 inhibitor which also has activity at the intestinal SGLT-1 receptor. Canagliflozin reduced postprandial plasma glucose and insulin levels in healthy subjects by increasing urinary glucose excretion (via renal SGLT-2 inhibition) and by delaying the rate of appearance of oral glucose (R_aO), the latter being attributed to intestinal SGLT-1 inhibition [152]. In this study, plasma insulin level was reduced as a secondary consequence of reduced intestinal glucose absorption [153]. This study provides an illustration of the well-recognized phenomenon whereby an improvement in insulin sensitivity, indicated by lower insulin levels in conjunction with improved post-challenge glucose tolerance, may occur secondary to a reduction in hyperglycaemia achieved by other means. This is an important general point that should be borne in mind since any intervention that lowers blood glucose such as dietary modifications or exercise, and a range of non-insulin-sensitizing drugs, can reduce insulin resistance by relieving the negative metabolic impact of hyperglycaemia i.e. glucotoxicity [48]. Determining whether a drug exerts a primary insulin-sensitizing effect requires direct evidence of improved insulin action using appropriate investigative techniques. Of these, the hyperinsulinaemic-euglycaemic glucose clamp is regarded as reference method (see below).

Insulin Tolerance Test (ITT)

This involves an intravenous injection of a bolus of exogenous insulin (typically 0.1 U/kg) in the fasting state. The response of blood glucose reflects the combined effects of the injected insulin on hepatic and peripheral insulin-sensitive tissues. Due to the dynamic rise and subsequent fall in serum insulin concentrations, the contribution to the decline in blood glucose by reduced hepatic glucose production and insulin-stimulated glucose uptake, respectively, will vary during the test according to relative dose-response characteristics (Fig. 1.3). An insulin-sensitivity index may be calculated from the ratio of the change in blood glucose to the

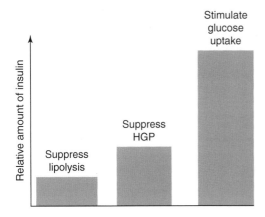

Fig. 1.3 Approximate relative amounts of insulin required for maximal effects on major metabolic processes in vivo. *HGP* hepatic glucose production

basal glucose concentration. The glucose disposal rate (K_{ITT}) may be calculated from the slope of the regression line of the logarithm of blood glucose against time during the first 3–15 min [154]. The ITT has important limitations, notably the risk of inducing hypoglycaemia. Clinical hypoglycaemia is usually unpleasant and is potentially hazardous in certain subjects, e.g. patients with ischaemic heart disease. Furthermore, the release of the counterregulatory hormones, primarily glucagon and catecholamines antagonizes the actions of insulin confounding the test results. A mean coefficient of variation of 30 % for the ITT was reported in a study using 0.05 U/kg insulin healthy volunteers [154]. However, better reproducibility has been reported using the same insulin dose by other investigators [155]. The ITT is not widely used in clinical metabolic research nor is the technique regarded as meeting the requirements for drug development studies.

Open-Loop Methods

Insulin Suppression Test (IST)

This method, introduced by Gerald Reaven and colleagues at Stanford University, USA in 1970, was the first to offer a direct measurement of insulin action in human subjects [136, 156]. In its original inception, an intravenous infusion of adrenaline (epinephrine) was used to suppress endogenous insulin secretion. The non-selective β-adrenergic blocker propranolol was co-infused to counter the metabolic and haemodynamic effects of the adrenaline. However, complete blockade of the adrenergic receptors could not be guaranteed and the hazard of cardiac arrhythmias led to a modification of the approach by which to interrupt the glucose-β-cell feedback loop [157]. After an overnight fast, an intravenous infusion of somatostatin or the somatostatin analogue octreotide [158] is used to suppress the endogenous secretion of insulin and glucagon from the pancreatic β- and α-cells, respectively [158]. Simultaneous infusions of insulin (25 mU/m²/min) and glucose (240 mg/m²/min) are delivered for 3 h. Blood samples for the determination of glucose and insulin are drawn from the contralateral arm every 30 min for 2.5 h and then at 10 min intervals to 180 min. Under these controlled conditions, the steady-state plasma glucose (SSPG) concentration between 150 and 180 min reflects the net effect of the achieved hyperinsulinaemia on insulin-sensitive tissues. Since SSPG is inversely related to insulin sensitivity, it is predicted that the SSPG concentration will be higher in more insulin-resistant subjects. Assumptions inherent in the interpretation of the IST include the complete suppression of endogenous insulin, glucagon and growth hormone secretion (which is also suppressed by somatostatin), reproducible direct effects of somatostatin on splanchnic blood flow and peripheral glucose metabolism, and attainment of steady-state hyperinsulinaemia. While the IST has been used extensively in clinical metabolic research, it has not been widely applied in diabetes drug development.

Insulin-Sensitivity Clamp

This technique, usually known as *hyperinsulinaemic-euglycaemic glucose clamp*, is widely regarded as the 'gold standard' among methods for quantifying insulin action. However, while this accolade attests to advantages that the technique has over some of the alternatives, it should not be taken to imply that the glucose clamp technique offers unique insights into insulin action that more fundamentally reflect human physiology. The hyperinsulinaemic-euglycaemic glucose clamp technique is a pharmacological perturbation of homeostatic metabolic mechanisms that provides quantifiable and reproducible data with which to test hypotheses concerning the role of insulin resistance in human disease.

The hyperinsulinaemic-euglycaemic glucose clamp establishes a temporary state of sustained hyperinsulinaemia. This permits quantification of a key aspect of glucose metabolism, i.e. insulin-mediated glucose disposal. One of the advantages of the glucose clamp technique is that it be can be readily adapted to provide a broader perspective of human metabolism, including assessments of hepatic glucose production and lipolysis. When selecting target insulin levels it should be noted that the inhibitory effect of insulin on hepatic glucose production requires lower plasma insulin concentrations than those required to maximally stimulate glucose uptake in skeletal muscle (Fig. 1.3) [129, 159, 160]. In a one-step hyperinsulinaemic-euglycaemic glucose clamp study performed in healthy volunteers, Rizza et al. observed half-maximal suppression of hepatic glucose production (determined using [3-^{3}H]glucose as a tracer) at a mean (±standard deviation) plasma insulin concentration of 174±12 pmol/L (29±2 mU/L). In contrast, the insulin concentration required for half-maximal stimulation of glucose utilization was nearly twice as high at 330±36 pmol/L (55±7 mU/L) [161]. Maximal glucose utilization occurred at pharmacological insulin concentrations of 1,320–4,200 pmol/L (220–700 mU/L). Other groups have reported similar findings. As discussed above, impaired insulin-mediated suppression of hepatic glucose production, i.e. hepatic insulin resistance, is the main driver of pathological states of fasting hyperglycaemia. Accordingly, assessment of liver glucose output is of interest in the context of the development of new diabetes drugs.

Following an overnight fast, plasma glucose concentrations are maintained entirely from endogenous sources. The liver and the kidney are the only organs in the human body with sufficient gluconeogenic enzyme activity and glucose-6-phosphatase to release glucose into the circulation via gluconeogenesis. Glucose production by the liver accounts for approximately 80 % with renal glucose production accounting for the remainder [162, 163].

When the insulin sensitivity of glucose metabolism is impaired, other defects are detectable using appropriate techniques [164, 165]. Lipolysis is very sensitive to inhibition by insulin, with only small increments above fasting levels being sufficient to restrain hydrolysis of triglycerides (see Fig. 1.3) [160, 164, 165]. Circulating levels of nonesterified ('free') fatty acids are often elevated in subjects with obesity, impaired glucose tolerance, and in patients with type 2 diabetes and fail to suppress normally in response to insulin [164]. These defects are indicative of insulin resistance within adipocytes.

Two-Step Hyperinsulinaemic-Euglycaemic Glucose Clamp

This variant can be used to assess direct suppression of fatty acids by insulin and other hormones, e.g. insulin-like growth factor)-1, at low and high insulin concentrations [166]. The multistep hyperinsulinaemic glucose clamp technique may also be combined with isotopic determination of glycerol turnover to provide an alternative measure of lipolysis [167]. The glucose clamp technique is suitable for pairing with various complementary methods that permit insulin action to be studied under controlled conditions at whole-body, regional, or tissue level (Table 1.8). For example, the hyperinsulinaemic-

Table 1.8 Examples of complementary investigative methods that may be combined with the hyperinsulinaemic-euglycaemic clamp technique

Method	Measure of interest
Isotopic glucose tracer	Glucose turnover (Ra_G, Rd_G)
Indirect calorimetry	Substrate oxidation
Magnetic resonance spectroscopy	Intramyocellular lipid; hepatic lipid content
Positron emission tomography	Regional brain/heart glucose metabolism
Venous occlusion plethysmography	Endothelial function
Isotopic glycerol tracer	Lipolysis
Tissue biopsy (muscle, fat)	Insulin-responsive enzyme expression
Microdialysis	Adipose tissue substrate metabolism

euglycaemic glucose clamp may be performed in conjunction with indirect calorimetry to quantify substrate oxidation. While combining these two methods is conceptually intriguing and if done properly might can generate useful data, it has to be pointed out that managing this sophisticated experimental setup is demanding and requires a high level of expertise and experience. Using this approach, a study of pioglitazone in insulin-resistant women with polycystic ovary syndrome demonstrated that increases in circulating levels of the insulin-sensitizing cytokine adiponectin correlated closely with improvements in glucose and lipid oxidation as well as inversely with changes in fasting fatty acid concentrations [168]. The investigators considered that their observations provided support for the hypothesis that improvements in multiple aspects of insulin sensitivity with pioglitazone were at least partly explained by an increase in adiponectin levels [168].

The flexibility of the glucose clamp readily permits the design of studies in which multiple target glucose levels can be achieved. This approach has been used, for example, to test new glucose sensors [169].

Hypoglycaemic Glucose Clamp

This technique, which does not quantify insulin action, is widely used to assess counterregulatory hormone responses under standardized conditions of experimental hypoglycaemia [170]. This design variation of the glucose clamp will usually be based on administering individualized intravenous insulin infusions that will be titrated to the point of achieving a predefined hypoglycaemic blood glucose target, or if designed as a stepwise hypoglycaemic glucose clamp, to achieve and maintain for a certain period of time, e.g. 30 min, several euglycaemic and hypoglycaemic target levels in sequence, e.g. 7, 5, 4, and 3 mmol/L. At each target level blood samples to assess variables of interest, e.g. counterregulatory hormones, incretins, can be collected. At the end of the lowest clamp target level, the intravenous insulin infusion is terminated and the time to spontaneous recovery to euglycaemic blood-glucose levels can be captured as an additional outcome variable.

Islet Cell Clamp

In this variant of the clamp approach, somatostatin or octreotide is infused to suppress endogenous insulin secretion [171]. Target steady-state circulating insulin and glucagon levels may be achieved by appropriate intravenous infusions of theses hormones. Growth hormone, secretion of which from the pituitary is also suppressed by somatostatin, is replaced at basal levels. The islet cell (also known as the pancreatic) clamp can be combined with the hyperglycaemic glucose clamp technique thereby being of particular value for assessing urinary glucose excretion [172].

In another variant, Tonelli et al used the islet cell clamp to investigate the effects of pioglitazone on glucose kinetics in patients with type 2 diabetes during low and high insulin infusion rates at euglycaemia [173]. While endogenous glucose production was suppressed by pioglitazone at both levels of hyperinsulinaemia glucose disposal was increased only during the high insulin infusion rate.

Hyperglycaemic Glucose Clamp

This technique is primarily a method used to evaluate endogenous insulin secretion. However, it can be also be used to measure insulin sensitivity [136] and to assess urinary glucose excretion [95, 172]. A variable quantity of hyperosmolar glucose is infused intravenously to establish predefined levels or a single level of hyperglycaemia, for periods of time during which blood or urine samples are collected in order to determine endogenous insulin secretion or urinary glucose excretion, respectively. The amounts of intravenous glucose needed to establish predefined levels of hyperglycaemia can vary widely between individuals according to insulin sensitivity and the ability of hyperglycaemia per se to enhance glucose uptake [174]. The method, when applied in healthy subjects, also has very practical limitations in that above certain hyperglycaemic target levels, e.g. 10–11 mmol/L or higher, the volume of intravenous glucose needed to establish and then maintain the target level can be excessive due to the ever-increasing concentrations of insulin stimulated by the hyperglycaemia.

The versatility of the glucose clamp technique is illustrated by a recent study in which a pancreatic and stepped hyperglycaemic glucose clamp (plasma glucose range 5.5–30.5 mmol/L) were combined to characterise major components of renal glucose reabsorption in response to dapagliflozin in healthy subjects and patients with type 2 diabetes [172]. Patients with type 2 diabetes ($n=12$) and matched healthy subjects ($n=12$) were studied at baseline and after 7 days of treatment with dapagliflozin. A pharmacodynamic model was developed to describe the major components of renal glucose reabsorption for both groups and then used to estimate these parameters from individual glucose titration curves. At baseline, the patients with diabetes had elevated maximum renal glucose reabsorptive capacity (Tm_G), splay (the rounding of the glucose reabsorption curve), and renal threshold compared with controls. Dapagliflozin reduced the Tm_G and splay in both groups. The most significant effect of dapagliflozin was a reduction of the renal threshold for glucose excretion in the patients with type 2 diabetes and the controls. It was concluded that dapagliflozin increases urinary glucose excretion in patients with type 2 diabetes by reducing the Tm_G and the threshold at which glucose is excreted in the urine [172].

Experimental Procedure for the Hyperinsulinaemic-Euglycaemic Glucose Clamp

This glucose clamp method, whether comprising a single step or two steps of steady-state hyperinsulinaemia, is conducted in the morning after an overnight fast. An arm vein is cannulated for the infusion of insulin and glucose. In the contralateral forearm, another cannula is placed for sampling, the hand being enclosed in a thermostat-controlled warming unit at approximately 55 °C to open arteriovenous channels and so provide 'arterialized' blood that approximates the arterial supply; this avoids the reduction in plasma glucose due to extraction during the passage of blood through insulin-sensitive tissues and so avoids potential overestimation of insulin action [134]. However, hand warming may induce peripheral vasodilatation resulting in a rise in heart rate and changes in blood pressure [175]. Soluble insulin or a rapid-acting insulin analogue is infused using a precision pump at a rate calculated to elevate serum insulin concentration from basal levels to a pre-defined target within the euglycaemic range, i.e. to approximately 4–5 mmol/L. A typical insulin infusion dose is 1.0 mU/kg/min (6 pmol/kg/min) or 40 mU/min/m^2 body surface area (0.24 nmol/min/m^2). Insulin doses based on surface area are preferred for obese subjects (body mass index >30 kg/m^2) in order to avoid over-insulinization [134]. Infusing insulin at a rate of 1 mU/kg/min generally provides plasma insulin levels in the high physiological range, albeit with wide variations reported in the literature (see below). Adsorption of insulin to the plastic surfaces of the infusion tubing can be avoided by adding 2 mL of the subject's blood to the insulin/saline solution used for infusion [176].

The response of the key outcome measure, i.e. glucose disposal rate (also known as the M-value), is approximately linear over the physiological range of plasma insulin concentrations (see Fig. 1.2). It has been suggested that very high doses of insulin, i.e. producing pharmacological serum insulin concentrations of 200 mU/L (1,200 pmol/L) or more, carry the risk of saturating the physiological clearance of insulin leading to unpredictable hyperinsulinaemia. However, dose-response effects have been described using doses as high as 5.0 U/kg/min in insulin-resistant subjects [177]. Some centres advocate the use a primed-continuous infusion of insulin to achieve the desired level of hyperinsulinaemia more rapidly, accepting a temporary overshoot above target for this advantage.

Manual vs. Automated Glucose Clamp

During the glucose clamps plasma, glucose is monitored online at intervals ranging from 1 to 10 min. For the purposes of a hyperinsulinaemic glucose clamp, a precise and accurate glucose oxidase or hexokinase reference method which meets requisite quality control standards is required [178]. In response to hyperinsulinaemia, glucose starts to decline as hepatic glucose production is inhibited and, at higher insulin concentrations, glucose uptake is stimulated. Glucose (20 % v/v) is therefore infused intravenously to maintain the arterialized blood glucose constant at the target level. In an isoglycaemic glucose clamp, a pre-existing level of plasma glucose for the individual is selected as the target. In patients with diabetes, blood-glucose levels may be normalized overnight before the studies by a variable rate low-dose intravenous insulin infusion [179]. This approach is valuable for standardizing the baseline metabolic state prior to the clamp in studies in which a therapeutic intervention is tested. While published algorithms for calculating glucose infusion rates during clamps are available [95], many investigators prefer to rely on their own judgment – the so-called manual clamp.

An alternative to the manual clamp is provided by the automated clamp using the Biostator® glucose-controlled insulin infusion system (Life Science Instruments, Elkhart, IN, USA; Fig. 1.4). The Biostator was originally developed as an extracorporeal artificial pancreas [180, 181] but failed to fulfil its clinical potential due to degradation of insulin by the mechanical pump [182]. The device was repositioned for clinical metabolic research as an automated method for performing glucose clamps [183, 184]. In brief, the Biostator senses plasma glucose every minute and adjusts an intravenous infusion of glucose according to an algorithm originally described by Clemens et al. [185]. A double-lumen venous catheter is used for continuous glucose measurement: one tube administers saline-heparin solution at a constant rate and is then mixed and returned with the blood that is withdrawn at an equal rate via the other (inner) lumen. The Biostator algorithm takes the current measurement of blood glucose and the variations in glucose levels during preceding minutes into consideration. In addition to its application in the setting of the hyperinsulinaemic-euglycaemic glucose clamp, the Biostator has been used extensively to determine time-action profiles of glucose-lowering drugs (see below) [186]. Blood glucose is measured continuously by a glucose oxidase sensor. This permits rapid alterations of the glucose infusion rates. However, periodic recalibration of the glucose measurement is required using an external reference method due to inherent drift of the glucose sensor, which is in constant contact with sampled blood. Advantages of the Biostator compared to a manual euglycaemic glucose clamp include relatively small blood volume requirements for measurement of glucose and minute-by-minute adjustment of glucose infusion rates. Perhaps the most compelling advantage that the Biostator offers is the removal of risk of any unconscious bias on the part of the clamp operator [186]. The cost of automated clamps compared to manual clamps is higher only if consumable materials are considered, mainly arising from the expense of glucose sensor membranes and other materials, e.g. the double-lumen sampling catheter. Balanced against these costs are the better quality of the clamp data (=smaller swings of glycaemia around the target values, expressed as the coefficient of variation (CV) of glycaemia), which is unbiased by a human operator, and the fact that a single human operator can manage more than one automated glucose clamp in parallel. Biostator devices have to be carefully maintained and require expertise in application. Second-generation proprietary automated glucose clamp technology is now available that allows an even tighter management of the target glucose concentration to CVs of <5 % and provides results immediately ready for data processing.

Experimental Conditions

If strictly defined, a steady state of glucose infusion will typically not be achieved during a typical 120 min hyperinsulinaemic-euglycaemic glucose clamp procedure [187]. With hyperinsulinaemia extending beyond this time, insulin-mediated glucose uptake continues to rise [188, 189]. However, for practical purposes data from the final 30–60 min of a 2–4 h glucose clamp study are generally accepted as being sufficiently stable for the determination of insulin-mediated glucose uptake [134, 176]. A more rigorous approach is to define steady state as a CV in blood glucose of <5 % [135].

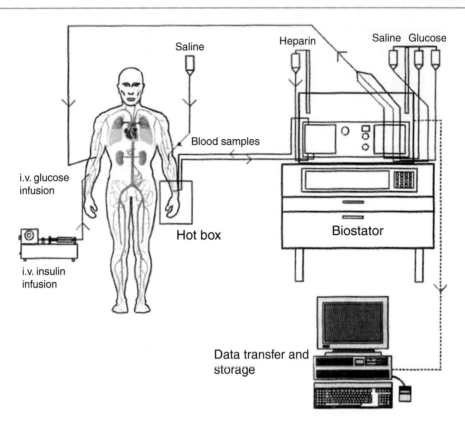

Fig. 1.4 Euglycaemic glucose clamp technique using a Biostator. The subject's left hand is in a heated box maintained at an air temperature of 55 °C. Blood supplemented with heparin is continuously pumped from the hand vein to the Biostator. The intravenous glucose infusion delivered into the forearm of the contralateral arm is continuously adjusted to the current blood-glucose concentration according to an algorithm. Saline solution is continuously infused with a low flow rate in order to keep the venous access patent. Intravenous insulin is infused into the vein of the same arm. In the 2-step hyperinsulinaemic-euglycaemic clamp, insulin concentrations are achieved that are appropriate to assess hepatic insulin sensitivity (step 1) and insulin-mediated glucose uptake (step 2). In the euglycaemic clamp variant test, insulin is administered by subcutaneous injection. A constant low-dose infusion of insulin may also be administered, as necessary, in order to establish similar baseline glucose concentrations. In the euglycaemic clamp variant, insulin may also be infused to suppress endogenous insulin production in healthy subjects. Blood samples for blood-glucose determinations and subsequent hormone measurements are drawn from a cubital vein of the left arm at regular intervals. The results printed by the Biostator are, at the same time, stored in a computer for subsequent data analysis (Reprinted with permission from Heinemann and Anderson [100])

Since inhibition of hepatic glucose production is insulin-dependent full suppression must be achieved in order to provide a reliable estimate of insulin-mediated glucose disposal. For healthy insulin-sensitive subjects, this assumption will often be valid. However, for insulin-resistant subjects complete suppression of hepatic glucose production cannot be assumed and should be confirmed using an isotopic tracer. Under the conditions of a hyperinsulinaemic-euglycaemic glucose clamp using 1 mU/kg/min of insulin infusion rate or more, the majority (approximately 85–90 %) of the glucose infused to maintain plasma glucose at target is accounted for by uptake and metabolism in skeletal muscle with adipose tissue largely accounting for the remainder. The mean glucose infusion rate (GIR) under these circumstances represents the integrated insulin-mediated glucose uptake. While theoretical considerations favour normalization of the M-value by kg fat-free mass rather than per kg body weight for within-subject comparisons, correction by body weight is a more practical and widely used approach [134].

Insulin-Sensitivity Measures Derived from the Hyperinsulinaemic-Euglycaemic Glucose Clamp

Insulin sensitivity as measured by the glucose clamp technique can be expressed in a variety of ways (see below and Table 1.9). Division of the M-value by the prevailing mean serum/plasma insulin concentration (M/I) accounts for minor differences in insulin levels between clamps, albeit at the expense of potentially introducing additional variability [129]. The metabolic clearance rate of glucose during steady state is calculated by dividing M by the mean plasma glucose concentration. However, metabolic clearance rate of glucose is not independent of blood glucose [190]. Since glucose clearance is dependent upon blood glucose concentration as well as circulating insulin levels, comparison of insulin sensitivity between groups of subjects clamped at markedly different target glucose levels should be done only with caution. A variant of the clamp technique that involves two steps of hyperinsulinaemia above basal (fasting) levels avoids these issues. This approach has also the advantage over single-step glucose clamps of permitting insulin-dependent glucose uptake to be determined [191]. During the clamp, two periods of 120 min serial intravenous insulin infusion rates are applied at rates of 0.5 mU/kg/min and 2.0 mU/kg/min (infusion rates might differ according to the level of insulin resistance of the subjects studied). Step 1 provides an elevation of circulating insulin concentrations suitable for determining the suppression of hepatic glucose production, whereas step 2 attains levels of hyperinsulinaemia that ensures stimulation of glucose uptake. The last 30 min of each insulin infusion phase is regarded as having reached a steady state. Glucose (20 % v/v) is infused intravenously to maintain arterialized venous blood glucose constant at the target level. Blood samples for the determination of plasma glucose and serum insulin are drawn at 0, 90, 100, 110, and 120 min in period 1 and at 90, 100, 110, and 120 min in period 2. The procedure is readily combined with an isotopic tracer, e.g. [6,6-^{2}H$_2$] glucose tracer, permitting the suppression of hepatic glucose production from baseline to be determined during each step. The following primary endpoint, the quotient of augmentation of M/I between periods is calculated as follows:

$$SI_{clamp} = \text{Insulin sensitivity index}$$

$$= \frac{\text{mean}(GIR)_{Period2} - \text{mean}(GIR)_{Period1}}{\left[\text{mean}(I)_{Period2} - \text{mean}(I)_{Period1}\right] \times \left[\text{mean}(BG)_{Periods1\&2}\right]}$$

GIR = glucose infusion rate and BG = blood glucose. SI_{clamp} should be corrected for body surface area (or weight) and is expressed in mL/(min × m²) per pmol/L. The increment in glucose uptake between step 1 and step 2 must be attributable to insulin-dependent mechanisms since non-insulin-mediated glucose uptake will be unchanged [191].

In addition to determining the effects of new insulin-sensitizing drugs, the adverse effect of other commonly used drugs, e.g. corticosteroids, β-adrenergic blockers (especially non-selective), and high-dose thiazide diuretics, on insulin sensitivity can also be quantified using the hyperinsulinaemic euglycaemic clamp technique. Using this approach (step 1, insulin infusion = 0.5 mU/kg/min or 20 mU/m²/min; step 2, insulin infusion = 2.0 mU/kg/min or 80 mU/m²/min), the effect of 1 week of treatment with low doses of the synthetic corticosteroid prednisone on insulin sensitivity in healthy nonobese men (n = 17) was evaluated [192]. The coefficient of variation of the clamp glucose concentrations was 2.9–3.7 %. In response to 25 mg prednisone daily, all

Table 1.9 Insulin-sensitivity indexes derived from the two-step hyperinsulinaemic-euglycaemic clamp

M	Whole-body glucose metabolism at steady state	mg/kg/min
MCR	Metabolic clearance rate of glucose	mL/kg/min
M/I	Glucose metabolism divided by mean steady-state insulin concentration	(mg/kg/min)/pmol/L
SI_{clamp}	Insulin-sensitivity index calculated from 2-step clamp	mL/(min × m²) per pmol/L

Notes: kg = fat-free mass; results may also be normalized to body surface area or to alternative measures of metabolically active tissue, e.g. resting energy expenditure indices of insulin sensitivity were significantly impaired in step 2 of the clamp: whole-body glucose disposal (M) was reduced by 33 %, MCR by 32 %, and M/I by 31 % compared to placebo ($p<0.001$). The corresponding values for 10 mg prednisone were 15, 14, and 13 % ($p<0.03$). Insulin-sensitivity index (see above) was reduced in a clinically relevant degree by both doses, i.e. 35.3 % ($p<0.01$) and 23.5 % ($p<0.05$) for the 25 and 10 mg doses of prednisone, respectively. This study confirmed that even short courses of prednisone at clinically relevant but relatively low doses impair insulin action in healthy volunteers in dose-dependent fashion.

Application of the Hyperinsulinaemic-Euglycaemic Glucose Clamp in Drug Development

Since its inception more than four decades ago, application of the hyperinsulinaemic glucose clamp has generated an extensive scientific literature, much of which is concerned with the evaluation of therapeutic interventions. An example of the enduring utility of the hyperinsulinaemic glucose clamp is provided by a recent study which combined the technique with measurement of endogenous glucose production using 3-^{3}H-glucose in male patients with type 2 diabetes treated for 14 days with another SGLT-2 inhibitor dapagliflozin [193]. After 14 days of dapagliflozin, whole-body glucose disposal during the hyperinsulinaemic glucose clamp increased ($p<0.05$) to 5.7±0.4 mg/kg/min and remained unchanged in placebo-treated subjects (4.2±0.5 mg/kg/min). The improvement in muscle insulin sensitivity is congruent with the glucose toxicity hypothesis. However, lowering plasma glucose concentrations by increasing urinary glucose excretion was associated with a paradoxical increase in endogenous glucose production $p<0.05$ vs. placebo). The increase in endogenous glucose production was almost identical to the amount of glucose excreted in the urine in the dapagliflozin-treated subjects. An increase in the fasting level of the counterregulatory hormone glucagon was also observed. This study points first, to the need to use sensitive investigative techniques in proof-of-mechanism studies and second, to the fact that novel diabetes drugs may be associated with unanticipated metabolic effects, in this instance elevated endogenous glucose production blunting the glucose-lowering effect of dapagliflozin. In a study of another drug in this class, empagliflozin, in patients with type 2 diabetes, Ferrannini et al. noted a similar increase in endogenous glucose production that detracted from the therapeutic effects of the SGLT-2 inhibitor on plasma glucose. As would be expected, plasma insulin declined in response to the lowering of blood glucose, whereas plasma glucagon levels increased [194].

Disadvantages of the Glucose Clamp Technique

In all its variants the glucose clamp technique is labour- and resource-intensive. Well-trained and experienced personnel are necessary to ensure reliable and reproducible results. A study of healthy volunteers in whom hyperinsulinaemic glucose clamps were repeated on three separate days reported an intra-individual CV of approximately 6 % [195]. Factors such as differences in subject population, methodology, technical expertise, and statistical analysis may account for differences between studies, some of which have reported higher CVs [196]. The glucose clamps technique is more robust when used in the context of a crossover design because of intrasubject variation in M which is evident even among apparently healthy subjects of the same sex [175].

Some reported disadvantages of the glucose clamp technique may reflect extraneous factors. For example, even when similar insulin doses have been used, wide variations in achieved hyperinsulinaemic plateaus have been reported between studies [129]. Factors that may be relevant to these discrepancies include body weight and body composition, differences in insulin assays between studies, and variable degrees of fasting hyperinsulinaemia and insulin clearance in certain metabolic states, e.g. decreased clearance in patients with renal impairment [197]. Glucose clamps are generally safe and well tolerated. Hypoglycaemia during the period after termination of the clamp is avoidable with appropriate precautions. Clinically relevant hypokalaemia resulting from the hyperinsulinaemia is rare in healthy subjects. The risk of hypokalaemia, which is usually transient, can be countered by appropriate infusion of potassium chloride although this is not our practice [198]. In a study using the two-step hyperinsulinaemic-euglycaemic clamp study in healthy volunteers, preventing the decline in potassium through intravenous supplementation with potassium chloride did not influence SI_{clamp} [198].

In addition to several caveats and assumptions that have already been discussed, perhaps the most important limitation of the hyperinsulinaemic glucose clamp technique is an inherent consequence of the strength of the approach, i.e. interruption of the physiological feedback between glucose and insulin. The method quantifies aspects of integrated glucose metabolism under non-physiological conditions, i.e. sustained hyperinsulinaemia. The insulin levels attained in a glucose clamp study exceed the normal maximal excursions of insulin in response to meals. Thus, the relevance of the data derived from the technique to day-to-day glucose metabolism in patients with diabetes cannot be assumed. This said, it is possible to predict the glucose-lowering effect of a novel insulin-sensitizing drug from hyperinsulinaemic glucose clamps with some confidence. For example, thiazolidinediones are an effective therapeutic option for patients with type 2 diabetes. In clinical practice, a realistic expectation would be a decline in glycated haemoglobin A_{1c} averaging approximately 1 %, with a range of 0.5–1.5 % (indicative of the variable response to therapy that characterizes all glucose-lowering drugs) [199]. This improvement in glycaemic control reflects reported improvements in clamp-measured glucose disposal of approximately 20–50 % [200–202]. This knowledge provides a useful benchmark against which new agents may be compared. Accordingly, a novel insulin sensitizer that produced an improvement of only 10–15 % in insulin sensitivity might not be a viable proposition.

Choice of Test for Quantifying Insulin Sensitivity

Key points to be considered when choosing a test of insulin action in the context of a new insulin sensitizer, aside from limitations that may be imposed by funding and resource issues, include the target population and the predicted efficacy and mechanism of action of the drug in question. A proof-of-concept study for a novel insulin sensitizer requires that the subjects to be studied have degrees of insulin resistance that will permit a therapeutic signal to be identified [203]. Having defined a suitable study population, this objective could be met using a surrogate measure of insulin action such as the oral glucose tolerance test (see above). However, robust evidence of improved insulin sensitivity relies on the hyperinsulinaemic-euglycaemic glucose clamp. Note that for drugs such as nuclear receptor agonists, maximum efficacy is generally not observed until approximately 6 weeks of therapy [108].

The sample size will be influenced by factors such as the study design, e.g. crossover studies generally have a higher statistical power than parallel-group studies, and the expected heterogeneity within the study population. The latter problem is inherent to all studies in patients with type 2 diabetes given the widely varying interindividual degrees of both insulin resistance and insulin deficiency.

Early identification of safety or efficacy concerns has become an accepted strategy in diabetes drug development [204]. Within this paradigm, ascertaining the effects of a novel insulin-sensitizing agent on surrogate markers of vascular integrity, e.g. endothelial function, during early-phase studies may be of value [205]. However, while certain drugs may have favourable actions on cardiovascular risk profiles and the vasculature [206], these have not always translated into clinical benefits.

Methods for Determining the Time-Action Profile of Insulin and Other Glucose-Lowering Drugs

Safe and effective clinical application of insulin therapy relies on knowledge of the time-course of action of all insulin formulations (and other blood-glucose-lowering agents) [100]. Methods used to evaluate the time-action profile can be divided into indirect and direct methods.

Indirect Methods

Radio-Labelled Insulin
The absorption of insulin from a subcutaneous depot can be estimated by labelling the test product with the gamma ray-emitting isotope ^{125}I and measuring the decay in radioactivity using an external scintillation counter placed above the skin area in which the insulin was injected [207].

Gerritzen's Test
Subjects receive low doses of insulin in a single ascending dose (SAD) study design [208]. The test product is administered by subcutaneous injection and complex carbohydrates are consumed at regular intervals to prevent hypoglycaemia. This permits assessment of pharmacokinetics but can provide at best an approximate indication of pharmacodynamics [208]. An approximation of the end of insulin action becomes evident when carbohydrate is no longer required to support blood-glucose levels. Davidson et al. assessed the acute response of severely insulin-resistant obese subjects to U500 insulin. A dose of 100 units was administered by subcutaneous injection to fasting, hyperglycaemic individuals and the decline in blood glucose over several hours was observed until normoglycaemia was achieved, at which point the subjects were provided with a meal [209]. This technically simple clinical study provided limited pharmacokinetic data concerning onset of action together with nonstandardized glucodynamic data. However, due to the pragmatic study design neither observation was independent of the effects of endogenous insulin action [209].

Direct Methods

Euglycaemic Glucose Clamp
The only reliable method for acquiring robust data concerning the pharmacodynamic properties of insulin preparations or sulphonylureas (which act by stimulating endogenous insulin secretion) is the euglycaemic glucose clamp [100, 210]. This technique is a variant of the glucose clamp in which glucose is infused intravenously at a variable rate as needed to maintain blood glucose at euglycaemia following the administration of, e.g. an insulin preparation (Fig. 1.5). Most often this will be a subcutaneous injection of the test insulin, but the technique is adaptable for determining time-action profiles of insulin delivered by other routes, e.g. pulmonary application or other agents that lower blood glucose [211]. The euglycaemic glucose clamp represents the most direct quantitative approach to measure glucose metabolism and is a key method for assessing the pharmacodynamics of new drugs for diabetes therapy, as mandated by both the European [212] and US [213] regulatory authorities:

- The European Medicines Agency (EMA) guidance states: 'Pharmacodynamic data are of primary importance to demonstrate therapeutic equivalence or differences between insulin preparations, including their use in mixture. Data on the time-action profiles using the euglycaemic clamp technique should be available, providing data based on the glucose infusion rate and the exogenous insulin serum concentration' [212].
- The Food and Drug Administration (FDA) states 'In the case of a new insulin with perhaps unique pharmacokinetic characteristics dictating a specific method of use (i.e. dosing interval, timing relative to meals), efficacy can be assumed based on pharmacodynamic (e.g. clamp) studies' [213].

Insulin Pharmacokinetics and Pharmacodynamics

The pharmacokinetics of a drug describes its concentration, along with those of its metabolites, in the body over time. In the case of novel insulin

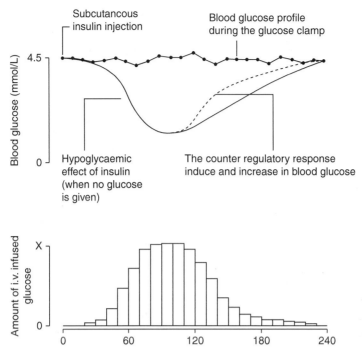

Fig. 1.5 Principle of the euglycaemic glucose clamp technique. After subcutaneous insulin injection, the blood-glucose concentration decreases as hepatic glucose production is inhibited and, at higher insulin concentrations, glucose uptake by muscle and fat is stimulated. After some time, the metabolic activity of the administered insulin decreases, and the blood-glucose level rises again. When the blood-glucose level falls below the threshold at which a hormone secretion causing the blood-glucose level to rise again is elicited (counterregulation), the blood-glucose level increases more rapidly than one would expect from the action profile of the insulin preparation (*dashed curve*). When a decrease of the blood glucose level is prevented by a variable rate intravenous glucose infusion, i.e. the blood-glucose level is kept almost constant at baseline or a given target level (*solid line with dots*), the amount of glucose infused reflects the metabolic activity of the injected insulin at a given point of time. Plotting the glucose requirement over time reflects the time-action profile of the insulin preparation (Reprinted with permission from Heinemann and Anderson [100])

analogues, appropriate analogue-specific assays must be used to reliably measure the molecules in question [214]. For example, insulin glargine is rapidly metabolized into its two main active metabolites: M1 (Gly^{A21}) and M2 (Gly^{A21}, des-Thr^{B30}) with the M1 metabolite accounting for approximately 90 % of the circulating levels following subcutaneous injection [215].

The time-course of action of a glucose-lowering drug is determined by key steps including absorption, distribution, biotransformation, and elimination. The pharmacodynamic properties of a drug describe the biological effects induced over time. In the case of insulin, the primary effect of interest is the blood-glucose-lowering effect. While pharmacodynamic studies using the euglycaemic glucose clamp technique have sought to estimate the time-action profiles of all insulin preparations, differences in methodologies between different research groups and study sites make between-study comparisons difficult. For example, studies of time to peak action of short-acting insulin preparations after subcutaneous administration have produced varying estimates [100]. Similarly, inconsistencies between studies of time-action profiles for long-acting insulin analogues have been observed [216].

When considering the insulin dose to be used in an euglycaemic glucose clamp study, it should be noted that a basal insulin given at an optimal dose for the individual would not require any exogenous glucose infusion at all since hepatic glucose production would be restrained precisely to maintain euglycaemia. The apparent duration of action of an insulin formulation as assessed using the euglycaemic glucose clamp technique may be influenced by several factors, such as definitions of onset and end of action of insulin action (Table 1.10). In recognition of these issues, a standardized approach to the study of the time-action profiles of novel insulin preparations and administration technologies has been proposed (Table 1.11) [100].

First-in-human studies of a new insulin may be performed at appropriate doses initially in healthy volunteers with careful monitoring of blood glucose over a time period anticipated to encompass the time-course of action with a suitable safety margin. In clamp studies of healthy volunteers, endogenous insulin production should be suppressed either by a continuous low-dose exogenous insulin infusion or by maintaining the blood glucose slightly below the usual fasting level for the individual [100]. Patients with type 1 diabetes are an especially suitable study population for insulin time-action profile studies since endogenous insulin production is effectively absent (Table 1.12) [100]. In fact, recent studies have shown that many patients with type 1 diabetes of long duration continue to secrete insulin, albeit at very low concentrations that are unlikely to interfere with the results of a glucose clamp study [217, 218]. For the purposes of clinical research, insulin deficiency can be confirmed at screening by measuring stimulated serum C-peptide [219]. Conversely, when the objective is to ensure the presence of sufficient residual β-cell function, e.g. in the evaluation of a new insulin secretagogue or insulin-sensitizing agent for type 2 diabetes, a lower threshold for C-peptide should be defined since endogenous insulin secretion declines over time [220]. In patients treated with subcutaneous insulin care should be taken to ensure that no carry-over effect from the subject's usual basal insulin contaminates the glucose clamp. This

Table 1.10 Factors that may affect calculation of time-action profiles of insulin as assessed using the euglycaemic glucose clamp technique

Blood-glucose and insulin levels prior to injection of insulin
Endogenous insulin secretion
Insulin dose (higher doses extend insulin action)
Definitions used to identify onset and end of action
Insulin sensitivity

Adapted from Swinnen et al. [216]

Table 1.11 Proposals for a standardized approach to insulin time-action profile studies using the euglycaemic glucose clamp technique

Studies should use a double-blind design as far as possible
Automated glucose clamps using the Biostator may have advantages over manual clamps:
Minimal (first-generation Biostator) or no net blood loss (second-generation Biostator) for glucose sampling
Avoidance of unconscious bias by operator
Frequent measurements of blood glucose, i.e. every minute, are appropriate for rapid-acting insulin
Doses used in clamp studies should be relevant to the clinical application of the insulin
Site and mode of subcutaneous injection should be standardized using syringes with minimal dead space
Blood-glucose target must be identical in all experiments
Subjects should be studied in the fasting state having avoided excessive exercise, caffeine, and alcohol
Studies in patients with diabetes should provide for a sufficiently long equilibration period, that is, blood glucose should be carefully titrated to the target blood-glucose level and maintained at that level for several hours prior to dosing with any study drug
The clock time of the study should be identical for all experiments, e.g. 0800 h, in recognition of chronobiological cycles that may affect insulin sensitivity, e.g. the dawn phenomenon

Reprinted with permission from Heinemann and Anderson [100]

Table 1.12 Study design considerations in insulin analogue time-action profile studies: selection of study population

Type 1 diabetes
Advantage of having no/negligible endogenous insulin secretion
Type 2 diabetes
Largest clinically relevant population. However, variable endogenous insulin secretion may confound results
Healthy volunteers
Endogenous insulin secretion should be suppressed by either (a) clamping at a target blood-glucose concentration below fasting levels or (b) continuous intravenous administration of an appropriate dose of insulin

requires that long-acting insulin analogues are withdrawn and replaced by multiple injections of short-acting insulin well in advance of a glucose clamp study day (see Chap. 9).

Glucose Clamp Parameters

When considering time-action profiles of different insulin formulations, various summary measures may be calculated to characterize the profiles. GIR_{max} denotes the time point at which the maximal glucose infusion rate is reached (Fig. 1.6) [100]. It should be noted that C_{max} for serum insulin levels (pharmacokinetics) and GIR_{max} (pharmacodynamics) are not equivalent due to the hysteresis between the peak insulin concentration and the subsequent effect on glucose metabolism [18, 100]. Thus, full description of the time-action profile of an insulin formulation requires that comprehensive pharmacokinetic and pharmacodynamic data be jointly considered [100]. For insulin preparations with a duration of action >24 h, an important additional consideration is the assessment of pharmacokinetics and pharmacodynamics at steady state using a clinically relevant dose, i.e. the test insulin is applied several days in a row to establish steady-state circulating insulin levels [216].

Statistical techniques such as LOESS (from 'LOcal regrESSion') can reduce the inherent noise in GIR data generated by the time constants of the Biostator and the autoregressive properties of the Clemens algorithm used in the Biostator [186, 221]. Note that for long-acting insulin analogues or formulations designed to avoid peak activity, the concept of GIR_{max} does not readily apply. However, the scientific literature contains somewhat discrepant views about the presence or absence of a peak of glucose-lowering action of insulin glargine and other aspects of the time-action profile of this commonly used basal insulin analogue [216]. Determining the end of action may be problematic for an insulin with a prolonged duration of action [100].

Indeed, with the advent of ultra-long-acting insulin preparations, the value of assessing onset and end of action in single-dose glucose clamps is open to question. In addition to the total area under the curve ($AUC_{0-\infty}$), the AUC for various time intervals (ACU_{0-T}) may be of interest; these can be calculated using the trapezoidal rule [100]. An important practical consideration that impacts the assessment of time-action profiles of ultra-long-acting insulins is the upper limit of duration for a single-clamp experiment, which is ~36–40 h. In this scenario a more complex study design may be required. For example, guided by preclinical and first-in-human clinical data, a euglycaemic glucose clamp might be timed to coincide with the expected onset of glucose-lowering action. Hompesch et al. applied this approach to study a novel ultra-long-acting insulin HM12460A (human insulin is fused via a non-peptidyl connector to a non-glycosylated Fc immunoglobulin carrier) [222]. Additional clamps may be performed with the aim of quantifying the pharmacodynamic properties of the insulin formulation during the plateau phase and subsequently the waning of the glucose-lowering action. This study design would require that each subject has multiple glucose clamps to capture onset, plateau, and end of action, e.g. three glucose clamps with a period of tightly managed glucose metabolism and diet between each glucose clamp assessment. Alternatively the key elements of the time-action profile can be studied in multiple study participants with the aim of providing a composite picture of onset, plateau, and end of action. Summary pharmacokinetic measures typically obtained from time-action profile clamps include C_{basal} (basal concentration), C_{max} (maximal concentration), T_{max} (time at which maximal concentration is attained), early $t_{50\%}$, and late $t_{50\%}$ (time at which the early and late halves of the peak concentrations, respectively, are attained). In studies in which a basal infusion of insulin is used to suppress endogenous insulin secretion in healthy volunteers, the basal insulin concentration must be subtracted, either directly or after fitting a mathematical function.

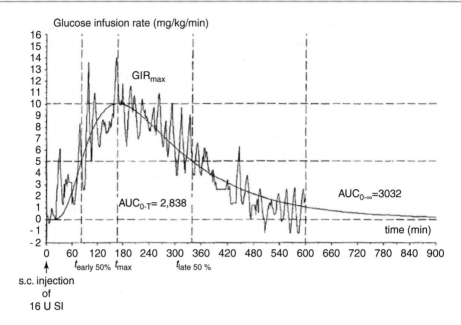

Fig. 1.6 Time-action profile of soluble insulin (SI) with certain summary measures. GIR_{max} represents the maximal glucose infusion rate (GIR) required to maintain the blood-glucose concentration at the desired target value, considering the variations of the original values during the experiments. The time point after subcutaneous (s.c.) injection at which GIR_{max} was achieved is described by t_{max}. The time points at which 50 % of the GIR_{max} occur before (early $t_{50\%}$) and after (late $t_{50\%}$) the GIR_{max} determine the rate of increase/decrease of action. The area under the action profile (AUC) can be calculated either for the entire action profile, i.e. until the latter returns to the zero line ($AUC_{0\text{-}\infty}$), or just for the period of the experiment or for shorter intervals ($AUC_{0\text{-}T}$) (Reprinted with permission from Heinemann and Anderson [100])

Position of Time-Action Profiles in the Clinical Development of Novel Insulin Formulations

Rapid-Acting and Ultra-Rapid-Acting Insulins

As mentioned above, rapid-acting insulin analogues [72] and novel ultrafast insulin formulations designed to accelerate insulin absorption – thereby achieving a more rapid peak than conventional soluble insulin formulations – have been developed. For example, it was shown that the co-administration of hyaluronidase to insulin lispro or soluble human insulin produced earlier and higher peak insulin concentrations and improved postprandial glycaemic control in patients with type 1 [74] and type 2 diabetes [75]. In a double-blind six-way crossover euglycaemic glucose clamp study, co-injection of recombinant hyaluronidase with the rapid-acting insulin analogues aspart, glulisine, and lispro provided accelerated insulin exposure producing an ultra-rapid time-action profile with a faster onset and shorter duration of insulin action in each case [223].

Long-Acting Insulin Formulations

In healthy subjects, endogenous insulin secretion between meals and during the nights controls hepatic glucose production and restrains adipocyte lipolysis in the fasting state while maintaining glucose supply to the brain and other organs. Replacement of these low insulin requirements by means of long-acting insulin formulations has made tremendous progress in the last decades. Isophane insulin (see Table 1.5) has well-recognized pharmacokinetic limitations that detract from use as a basal insulin [224]. These include variable rates of absorption from the subcutaneous depot, relatively high inter- and intra-individual variation, a discernible peak in insulin concentration 3–6 h after injection, and a less than 24 h duration of action. When given before bed, the risk of nocturnal hypoglycaemia rises as doses are increased with the aim of controlling fasting blood-glucose concentrations. To

counter these shortcomings, long-acting insulin analogues have been developed. Strategies used to protract the action of insulin have included:
- Modification of the insulin molecule to achieve lower solubility at physiological pH, e.g. insulin glargine [215].
- Addition of a fatty-acid chain to the insulin molecule that binds to albumin forming a depot from which the insulin analogue is subsequently slowly released, e.g. insulin detemir, or building up of long chains of insulin hexamers, e.g. insulin degludec [225, 226]. Insulin degludec has a half-life of about 25 h [227] with a very flat action profile and a duration of action in excess of exceeding 40 h.
- Attachment of polyethylene glycol to insulin (pegylation), e.g. LY2605541 (insulin peglispro) [228]. Comparative studies in healthy volunteers using the euglycaemic glucose clamp demonstrated the absence of a similar peak of action with insulin glargine [229, 230].

The aim is to develop insulins with improved pharmacokinetics properties that translate into clinical advantages. In a phase 3 open-label study in which insulin glargine was compared with neutral protamine Hagedorn (NPH) as pre-bed insulin added to oral glucose-lowering therapy in 756 patients with type 2 diabetes, both groups achieved good glycaemic control (fasting plasma glucose 6.5 vs. 6.7 mmol/L for glargine and NPH, respectively) [231]. However, the frequency of documented nocturnal hypoglycaemia was 25 % lower for insulin glargine than for NPH ($p<0.05$). A reduced risk of hypoglycaemia with insulin glargine compared with NPH insulin for similar levels of glycaemic control was also observed in subjects with type 1 diabetes [232].

In a single centre, subject and investigator-blinded, parallel, randomized, two-arm, 4-period study of intrasubject pharmacodynamic variability, Ocheltree et al. compared a single subcutaneous injection of the investigational drug insulin lispro protamine suspension with insulin glargine. Patients with type 1 diabetes were admitted to a clinical research institute and received a variable rate intravenous infusion of soluble human insulin for at least 4 h prior to the administration of the study insulin in order to attain a target plasma glucose level of 5 mmol/L. The intravenous insulin was discontinued approximately 15 min prior to the injection of 0.6 U/kg insulin lispro protamine or insulin glargine. The time-action profiles of the two insulin preparations were quantified in 24 h euglycaemic glucose clamps using the Biostator. While the GIR-time profile for insulin glargine was flatter than for lispro protamine suspension, this was associated with lower intrasubject pharmacodynamic variability [221]. The implication of these findings is that lispro protamine suspension might provide more reproducible day-to-day metabolic control in this population. As noted above, injection of hyaluronidase, which increasing the dispersion and absorption of subcutaneously administered drugs, has been shown to alter the pharmacokinetics of rapid-acting insulin analogues to provide an ultra-rapid time-action profile, e.g. fast on and fast off insulin action [223]. In a double-blind euglycaemic glucose clamp study, Morrow et al. studied the effect of co-administration of 5 µg/mL recombinant human hyaluronidase (rHuPH20) on the intrasubject variability of insulin lispro or recombinant human insulin in healthy adults [233]. Compared to insulin lispro alone, rHuPH20 significantly reduced the variability of insulin pharmacokinetics and reduced early exposure intrasubject variability with human insulin (Fig. 1.7) [233]. Lower within-subject variability in aspects of the pharmacokinetics and pharmacodynamics of insulin detemir compared with both NPH and insulin glargine has been reported in patients with type 1 diabetes [234]. Potential clinical benefits of novel insulins may be tempered by unwanted effects. For example, it has been suggested that hepato-selective insulin analogues may have a relative weight-sparing effect [73]. Studies of LY2605541 in dogs have suggested a preferential effect on hepatocytes. The hepatic sinusoidal endothelium has large fenestrations that theoretically might allow greater transport of LY2605541 to hepatocytes than to muscle and fat [235]. However, adverse effects including minor elevations in hepatic aminotransferases and triglycerides along with adverse changes in other components of the lipid profile have been reported [235].

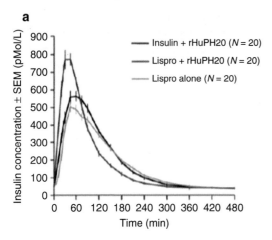
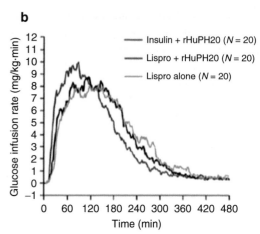

Fig. 1.7 (a) Serum insulin levels and (b) glucose infusion rate values over an 8 h period following subcutaneous administration of human insulin + recombinant human hyaluronidase (rHuPH20) and lispro + rHuPH20 compared with lispro alone in healthy adults studied in a double-blind randomized sequence of six euglycaemic clamps. Plasma glucose was clamped at a level 10 % below baseline glucose concentration using a Biostator. Data are mean ± standard error of the mean (SEM). Intrasubject variability with lispro was significantly reduced ($p<0.0001$) by co-injection of rHuPH20 for pharmacokinetic (PK) parameters (t_{max}, $t_{50\%}$) related to early insulin exposure. The coefficient of variability (CV%) in the percentage of glucose infused during the first 4 h period was significantly ($p<0.05$) lower for lispro + rHuPH20. For most other glucodynamic parameters, intrasubject variability was numerically lower after co-injection of for lispro + rHuPH20 compared with lispro alone. Thus, glucodynamic parameters showed a reduction in variability corresponding to the PK results, but owing to the intrinsically greater variability in the former measures in general, the differences were not statistically significant (Reproduced with permission from Morrow et al. [233])

In the case of insulin analogues, molecules that are not encountered in nature, the issue of altered post-binding signalling has come under scrutiny. In a study of licensed insulin analogues, three rapid-acting analogues showed molecular and biological effects that were considered to be similar but not identical to human insulin. In contrast, the prolonged-duration analogues insulin glargine and insulin determir activated extracellular signal-regulated kinase (ERK) more strongly than human insulin via both the insulin receptor and the insulin-like growth factor (IFG)-1 receptor [236]. Thus, this cell model suggested that long-acting insulin analogues activate the mitogenic signalling pathway to cause increased cell proliferation more effectively than human insulin. However, a caveat of this study is the aforementioned metabolism of insulin glargine to the M1 and M2 active metabolites which were not examined. The potential for enhanced mitotic activity of insulin and insulin analogues (insulin glargine in particular) has been a topic of enormous clinical interest in recent years [237]. However, the FDA and EMA have concluded that there is no evidence of an increased risk of cancer with insulin glargine. The Outcomes Reduction with an Initial Glargine Intervention (ORIGIN) trial of insulin glargine in 12,537 subjects with glucose intolerance or patients with type 2 diabetes over a median of 6.2 years showed no excess of cancers compared to standard care (hazard ratio, 1.00; 95 % confidence interval 0.88–1.13; $p=0.97$) [238, 239]. Based on their structural differences, in can be hypothesized that each insulin analogue may in principle trigger a specific signalling 'signature' when interacting with the insulin or IGF receptor, e.g. the activation of kinases may occur in a different sequence. Therefore, every new insulin analogue should be thoroughly profiled in terms of its safety, in particular its mitogenic and mutagenic potential. In light of the possibility of analogue-specific signalling cascades, the recent discussion about insulin degludec triggered by the FDA's non-favourable assessment of this analogue's cardiovascular safety profile [240] should lead to more research on how differences in downstream insulin signalling may contribute to secondary effects, e.g. in the vasculature or via cardiovascular risk profiles.

Biosimilar Insulins

With the expiry of the patent protection on most of the rapid-acting and long-acting insulin analogues, other pharmaceutical companies have an opportunity to manufacture such insulins and try to get them approved as 'biosimilar insulins' [241]. A number of companies are currently active in this endeavour [242, 243]. Biosimilar insulins are available in some countries outside the European Union. and USA, including 'copies' of insulin glargine, insulin lispro, and insulin aspart. To date, no biosimilar insulins have been approved by the FDA. The FDA has recently issued guideline for biosimilars, but until 2020 these are not of relevance for biosimilar insulins. Until this date they are regarded as drugs. In December 2013 Eli Lilly and Boehringer Ingelheim announced that the FDA had accepted their New Drug Application (NDA) for LY2963016 (a insulin glargine formulation). The company has performed a full clinical development of LY2963016 as a novel insulin. However, an automatic 30-month stay of approval commenced when Sanofi (the originator of insulin glargine) issued a lawsuit against Lilly alleging patent infringements. In Europe, LY2963016 was filed through the EMA's biosimilar pathway, and in June 2014 the EMA's Committee for Medicinal Products for Human Use (CHMP) issued a positive opinion recommending approval for LY2963016 for the treatment of patients with type 1 and type 2 diabetes. Accordingly, this insulin is set to become the first biosimilar insulin approved in the European Union.

The regulatory requirements for approval of biosimilar insulins include adequate evaluation of the pharmacodynamic properties of these insulins and their immunogenicity [244]. The rigorous requirements of the US and European regulatory authorities towards biosimilars reflect the complex nature of these biopharmaceutical products as well as the proprietary manufacturing process [243, 245]. (Pre)clinical studies required by the EMA include in vitro pharmacodynamic evaluation (=performance of glucose clamps, in vitro affinity bioassays, and assays for binding to insulin and insulin-like growth factor-1 receptors). The glucose clamp study should include at least one single-dose crossover study design to be performed in patients with type 1 diabetes. The regulatory environment for biologics, and in particular for biosimilar insulins, remains heterogeneous from a global perspective. In many countries regulation either is nonexistent or does not provide for robust guidance. The EMA has developed a useful set of guidance documents that outline the mandatory elements required in a submission package. The EMA guidance on recombinant human insulin and insulin analogues considers the design of glucose clamp studies and approaches to pharmacokinetic and pharmacodynamic data analysis and interpretation as well as safety studies, the latter focusing on immunogenicity [246]. Using the EMA guidance as a reasonable reference point seems appropriate. Thus, successfully bringing a biosimilar insulin to these markets represents a higher hurdle than in the case of a generic diabetes drug. The demonstration of compatibility of a biosimilar with administration devices is an additional consideration [242].

Concerns have been raised about the aforementioned lack of more rigorous regulations or regulations in principle for approval and pharmacovigilance of biosimilar insulins in countries outside Europe and the USA (see below) [247]. It has been proposed that every biosimilar insulin and insulin analogue should be assessed in well-defined globally harmonized preclinical and clinical studies followed by post-marketing pharmacovigilance programmes [247]. In recognition of a need for globally acceptable standardization, the World Health Organization (WHO) issued guidance for biosimilars in 2009 [245]. The crucial role of the euglycaemic glucose clamp in the evaluation of the pharmacodynamics of a biosimilar insulin is clear [243]. The EMA's CHMP has stated that the sensitivity to detect differences between insulin products is higher for euglycaemic clamp pharmacodynamic studies than for clinical efficacy trials; the latter are considered supportive in this context. The FDA also issued a series of guidance documents directed towards follow-on biologics (the FDA's preferred term for biosimilars) [245, 248]. Mechanistically-related pharmacodynamic assays that are relevant to clinical outcomes and adequate assessment of clinical immunogenicity are included in this guidance [249]. The FDA requires that the sponsor of a proposed product, e.g. biosimilar insulin, must include in its submission information demonstrating that 'there are no clinically meaningful differences between the biological product and the reference product in terms of the safety, purity and potency of the product' [249].

Biosimilar Approval: A Case Study

The failure of the first European biosimilar insulin application in 2007 provides some important lessons [243]. Data from euglycaemic glucose clamps for three biosimilar human insulin preparations (a soluble unmodified version, an isophane product, and a 30:70 premixed formulation) were considered to have failed to demonstrate equivalent blood-glucose-lowering effect compared to the reference products [243, 247]. Unacceptable departures from the reference products in aspects of both the pharmacokinetic and the pharmacodynamic properties were evident for the three biosimilars, along with concerns of waning efficacy over time and inadequate assessment of immunogenicity. Other points of concern included the un-blinded design of the glucose clamp studies and questions concerning the clinical relevance of the primary endpoint presented for the euglycaemic glucose clamps [243]. This case study illustrates the potential for formulations containing products with identical amino acid sequences (primary protein structures) to deviate from the comparator [244].

Reference Product Considerations

A broader issue of relevance to the design of insulin glargine bioequivalence studies that needs to be considered is the high day-to-day variability of the reference product [250] even though insulin glargine has been promoted as an analogue with a more reproducible pharmacodynamics than its predecessors [215, 224]. Larger sample sizes are required to ensure bioequivalence in studies involving long-acting insulin analogues compared with rapid-acting insulin analogues which tend to have more reproducible pharmacokinetic and pharmacodynamic profiles.

Summary and Conclusions

Insulin Sensitivity

Insulin-sensitizing drugs have an important role in the treatment of patients with type 2 diabetes. Accordingly, accurate quantification of insulin action is an important aspect of early-phase development of novel agents purported to improve insulin action. In this endeavour, the hyperinsulinaemic-euglycaemic glucose clamp is a reproducible and adaptable research technique which permits assessment not only of insulin-mediated glucose disposal but also the sensitivity of hepatic glucose production and other relevant aspects of metabolism, e.g. suppression of lipolysis by insulin, substrate oxidation. The flexibility of the hyperinsulinaemic-euglycaemic clamp, and its capacity for use alongside complementary in vivo research techniques, has assured its place as the reference method for measuring insulin action in humans.

Insulin Time-Action Profiles

Characterizing the pharmacodynamic properties of novel insulin formulations is a prerequisite for their safe and effective application in clinical practice. The euglycaemic glucose clamp, by virtue of its versatility and accuracy, is the technique of choice for determining time-action profiles of new insulin products. The pharmacokinetic and pharmacodynamic characteristics of insulin delivered by nonclassic routes, e.g. via the pulmonary system, and the time-action profiles of other classes of blood-glucose-lowering agents are also amenable to assessment using glucose clamp methodology. The euglycaemic clamp has a pivotal role in the requirements of the EMA and FDA for market approval of biosimilar insulins.

References

1. Reaven GM. Banting lecture 1988. Role of insulin resistance in human disease. Diabetes. 1988;37(12):1595–607.
2. DeFronzo RA, Ferrannini E. Insulin resistance. A multifaceted syndrome responsible for NIDDM, obesity, hypertension, dyslipidemia, and atherosclerotic cardiovascular disease. Diabetes Care. 1991;14(3):173–94.
3. Krentz AJ. Insulin resistance. Br Med J. 1996;313(7069):1385–9.
4. Krentz AJ. Insulin resistance: a clinical handbook. 2002. Oxford: Blackwell Science; 2002.
5. Semple RK, Savage DB, Cochran EK, Gorden P, O'Rahilly S. Genetic syndromes of severe insulin resistance. Endocr Rev. 2011;32(4):498–514.
6. Eckel RH, Grundy SM, Zimmet PZ. The metabolic syndrome. Lancet. 2005;365(9468):1415–28.
7. White MF. Insulin signaling in health and disease. Science. 2003;302(5651):1710–1.
8. Konrad D, Rudich A, Klip A. Insulin-mediated regulation of glucose metabolism. In: Kumar S, O'Rahilly S, editors. Insulin resistance: insulin action and its disturbances in disease. Oxford: Wiley; 2005.
9. Rajala MW, Scherer PE. Minireview: the adipocyte – at the crossroads of energy homeostasis, inflammation, and atherosclerosis. Endocrinology. 2003;144(9):3765–73.
10. Schwartz MW, Porte Jr D. Diabetes, obesity, and the brain. Science. 2005;307(5708):375–9.
11. Bertrand L, Horman S, Beauloye C, Vanoverschelde JL. Insulin signalling in the heart. Cardiovasc Res. 2008;79(2):238–48.
12. Klein GL. Insulin and bone: recent developments. World J Diabetes. 2014;5(1):14–6.
13. Orava J, Nuutila P, Lidell ME, Oikonen V, Noponen T, Viljanen T, et al. Different metabolic responses of human brown adipose tissue to activation by cold and insulin. Cell Metab. 2011;14(2):272–9.
14. Diamanti-Kandarakis E, Dunaif A. Insulin resistance and the polycystic ovary syndrome revisited: an update on mechanisms and implications. Endocr Rev. 2012;33(6):981–1030.
15. Ahmadian M, Suh JM, Hah N, Liddle C, Atkins AR, Downes M, et al. PPARgamma signaling and metabolism: the good, the bad and the future. Nat Med. 2013;19(5):557–66.
16. Yki-Jarvinen H, Westerbacka J. Vascular actions of insulin in obesity. Int J Obes Relat Metab Disord. 2000;24 Suppl 2:S25–8.
17. Dandona P, Aljada A, Chaudhuri A, Mohanty P, Garg R. Metabolic syndrome: a comprehensive perspective based on interactions between obesity, diabetes, and inflammation. Circulation. 2005;111(11):1448–54.
18. Bergman RN. Lilly lecture 1989. Toward physiological understanding of glucose tolerance. Minimal-model approach. Diabetes. 1989;38(12):1512–27.
19. Czech MP, Corvera S. Signaling mechanisms that regulate glucose transport. J Biol Chem. 1999;274(4):1865–8.
20. Chang L, Chiang SH, Saltiel AR. Insulin signaling and the regulation of glucose transport. Mol Med. 2004;10(7–12):65–71.
21. Huang S, Czech MP. The GLUT4 glucose transporter. Cell Metab. 2007;5(4):237–52.
22. Abdul-Ghani MA, DeFronzo RA. Pathogenesis of insulin resistance in skeletal muscle. J Biomed Biotechnol. 2010;2010:476279.
23. Straus DS. Effects of insulin on cellular growth and proliferation. Life Sci. 1981;29(21):2131–9.
24. Wang CC, Goalstone ML, Draznin B. Molecular mechanisms of insulin resistance that impact cardiovascular biology. Diabetes. 2004;53(11):2735–40.
25. Fujita S, Rasmussen BB, Cadenas JG, Grady JJ, Volpi E. Effect of insulin on human skeletal muscle protein synthesis is modulated by insulin-induced changes in muscle blood flow and amino acid availability. Am J Physiol Endocrinol Metab. 2006;291(4):E745–54.
26. Andres R, Baltzan MA, Cader G, Zierler KL. Effect of insulin on carbohydrate metabolism and on potassium in the forearm of man. J Clin Invest. 1962;41:108–15.
27. Kahn CR. Insulin resistance, insulin insensitivity, and insulin unresponsiveness: a necessary distinction. Metabolism. 1978;27(12 Suppl 2):1893–902.
28. McLaughlin T, Allison G, Abbasi F, Lamendola C, Reaven G. Prevalence of insulin resistance and associated cardiovascular disease risk factors among normal weight, overweight, and obese individuals. Metabolism. 2004;53(4):495–9.
29. Alexopoulos N, Katritsis D, Raggi P. Visceral adipose tissue as a source of inflammation and promoter of atherosclerosis. Atherosclerosis. 2014;233(1):104–12.
30. Roberts LD, Koulman A, Griffine JL. Towards metabolic biomarkers of insulin resistance and type 2 diabetes: progress from the metabolome. Lancet Diabetes Endocrinol. 2013;2:65–75.
31. Kahn SE, Hull RL, Utzschneider KM. Mechanisms linking obesity to insulin resistance and type 2 diabetes. Nature. 2006;444(7121):840–6.
32. Szendroedi J, Roden M. Ectopic lipids and organ function. Curr Opin Lipidol. 2009;20(1):50–6.
33. Ye J. Mechanisms of insulin resistance in obesity. Front Med. 2013;7(1):14–24.
34. Reaven G, Abbasi F, McLaughlin T. Obesity, insulin resistance, and cardiovascular disease. Recent Prog Horm Res. 2004;59:207–23.
35. Samuel VT, Shulman GI. Mechanisms for insulin resistance: common threads and missing links. Cell. 2012;148(5):852–71.
36. Ryden L, Mellbin L. Glucose perturbations and cardiovascular risk: challenges and opportunities. Diab Vasc Dis Res. 2012;9(3):170–6.
37. Grundy SM. Metabolic syndrome: connecting and reconciling cardiovascular and diabetes worlds. J Am Coll Cardiol. 2006;47(6):1093–100.
38. Cusi K, Maezono K, Osman A, Pendergrass M, Patti ME, Pratipanawatr T, et al. Insulin resistance dif-

ferentially affects the PI 3-kinase- and MAP kinase-mediated signaling in human muscle. J Clin Invest. 2000;105(3):311–20.
39. Reaven GM. Role of insulin resistance in the pathophysiology of non-insulin dependent diabetes mellitus. Diabetes Metab Rev. 1993;9 Suppl 1:5S–12.
40. Kahn SE, Cooper ME, Prato SD. Pathophysiology and treatment of type 2 diabetes: perspectives on the past, present, and future. Lancet. 2013;383:1068–83.
41. Kahn SE. The relative contributions of insulin resistance and beta-cell dysfunction to the pathophysiology of type 2 diabetes. Diabetologia. 2003;46(1):3–19.
42. Kolterman OG, Insel J, Saekow M, Olefsky JM. Mechanisms of insulin resistance in human obesity: evidence for receptor and postreceptor defects. J Clin Invest. 1980;65(6):1272–84.
43. Kolterman OG, Gray RS, Griffin J, Burstein P, Insel J, Scarlett JA, et al. Receptor and postreceptor defects contribute to the insulin resistance in noninsulin-dependent diabetes mellitus. J Clin Invest. 1981;68(4):957–69.
44. Mitrakou A, Kelley D, Mokan M, Veneman T, Pangburn T, Reilly J, et al. Role of reduced suppression of glucose production and diminished early insulin release in impaired glucose tolerance. N Engl J Med. 1992;326(1):22–9.
45. Meyer C, Woerle HJ, Dostou JM, Welle SL, Gerich JE. Abnormal renal, hepatic, and muscle glucose metabolism following glucose ingestion in type 2 diabetes. Am J Physiol Endocrinol Metab. 2004;287(6):E1049–56.
46. DeFronzo RA. Insulin resistance, lipotoxicity, type 2 diabetes and atherosclerosis: the missing links. The Claude Bernard Lecture 2009. Diabetologia. 2010;53(7):1270–87.
47. Taylor R. Type 2 diabetes: etiology and reversibility. Diabetes Care. 2013;36(4):1047–55.
48. Stumvoll M, Goldstein BJ, van Haeften TW. Type 2 diabetes: principles of pathogenesis and therapy. Lancet. 2005;365(9467):1333–46.
49. Inzucchi SE, Bergenstal RM, Buse JB, Diamant M, Ferrannini E, Nauck M, et al. Management of hyperglycemia in type 2 diabetes: a patient-centered approach: position statement of the American Diabetes Association (ADA) and the European Association for the Study of Diabetes (EASD). Diabetes Care. 2012;35(6):1364–79.
50. Krentz AJ, Bailey CJ. Oral antidiabetic agents: current role in type 2 diabetes mellitus. Drugs. 2005;65(3):385–411.
51. Bailey CJ, Turner RC. Metformin. N Engl J Med. 1996;334(9):574–9.
52. Knowler WC, Barrett-Connor E, Fowler SE, et al. Reduction in the incidence of type 2 diabetes with lifestyle intervention or metformin. N Engl J Med. 2002;346(6):393–403.
53. Krentz A. Thiazolidinediones: effects on the development and progression of type 2 diabetes and associated vascular complications. Diabetes Metab Res Rev. 2009;25(2):112–26.
54. Muniyappa R, Sowers JR. Role of insulin resistance in endothelial dysfunction. Rev Endocr Metab Disord. 2013;14(1):5–12.
55. UK Prospective Diabetes Study (UKPDS) Group. Effect of intensive blood-glucose control with metformin on complications in overweight patients with type 2 diabetes (UKPDS 34). Lancet. 1998;352(9131):854–65.
56. Dormandy JA, Charbonnel B, Eckland DJ, Erdmann E, Massi-Benedetti M, Moules IK, et al. Secondary prevention of macrovascular events in patients with type 2 diabetes in the PROactive study (PROspective pioglitAzone Clinical Trial In macroVascular Events): a randomised controlled trial. Lancet. 2005;366(9493):1279–89.
57. Lamanna C, Monami M, Marchionni N, Mannucci E. Effect of metformin on cardiovascular events and mortality: a meta-analysis of randomized clinical trials. Diabetes Obes Metab. 2011;13(3):221–8.
58. Nissen SE, Wolski K. Effect of rosiglitazone on the risk of myocardial infarction and death from cardiovascular causes. N Engl J Med. 2007;356(24):2457–71.
59. Krentz AJ. Rosiglitazone: trials, tribulations and termination. Drugs. 2011;71(2):123–30.
60. Bailey CJ. Learning from tesaglitazar. Diab Vasc Dis Res. 2007;4(3):161–2.
61. Nissen SE, Wolski K, Topol EJ. Effect of muraglitazar on death and major adverse cardiovascular events in patients with type 2 diabetes mellitus. JAMA. 2005;294(20):2581–6.
62. Younk LM, Uhl L, Davis SN. Pharmacokinetics, efficacy and safety of aleglitazar for the treatment of type 2 diabetes with high cardiovascular risk. Expert Opin Drug Metab Toxicol. 2011;7(6):753–63.
63. Colca JR, Tanis SP, McDonald WG, Kletzien RF. Insulin sensitizers in 2013: new insights for the development of novel therapeutic agents to treat metabolic diseases. Expert Opin Investig Drugs. 2014;23(1):1–7.
64. Olefsky JM, Glass CK. Macrophages, inflammation, and insulin resistance. Annu Rev Physiol. 2010;72:219–46.
65. Esser N, Legrand-Poels S, Piette J, Scheen AJ, Paquot N. Inflammation as a link between obesity, metabolic syndrome and type 2 diabetes. Diabetes Res Clin Pract. 2014;105:141–50.
66. Bliss M. The history of insulin. Diabetes Care. 1993;16 Suppl 3:4–7.
67. Evans A, Krentz AJ. Benefits and risks of transfer from oral agents to insulin in type 2 diabetes mellitus. Drug Saf. 1999;21(1):7–22.
68. Vajo Z, Fawcett J, Duckworth WC. Recombinant DNA technology in the treatment of diabetes: insulin analogs. Endocr Rev. 2001;22(5):706–17.
69. Hirsch IB. Intensifying insulin therapy in patients with type 2 diabetes mellitus. Am J Med. 2005;118(Suppl 5A):21S–6.
70. Switzer SM, Moser EG, Rockler BE, Garg SK. Intensive insulin therapy in patients with type 1 diabetes mellitus. Endocrinol Metab Clin North Am. 2012;41(1):89–104.
71. Owens DR. Stepwise intensification of insulin therapy in type 2 diabetes management – exploring the

concept of the basal-plus approach in clinical practice. Diabet Med. 2013;30(3):276–88.
72. Home PD. The pharmacokinetics and pharmacodynamics of rapid-acting insulin analogues and their clinical consequences. Diabetes Obes Metab. 2012;14(9):780–8.
73. Sheldon B, Russell-Jones D, Wright J. Insulin analogues: an example of applied medical science. Diabetes Obes Metab. 2009;11(1):5–19.
74. Hompesch M, Muchmore DB, Morrow L, Vaughn DE. Accelerated insulin pharmacokinetics and improved postprandial glycemic control in patients with type 1 diabetes after coadministration of prandial insulins with hyaluronidase. Diabetes Care. 2011;34(3):666–8.
75. Hompesch M, Muchmore DB, Morrow L, Ludington E, Vaughn DE. Improved postprandial glycemic control in patients with type 2 diabetes from subcutaneous injection of insulin lispro with hyaluronidase. Diabetes Technol Ther. 2012;14(3):218–24.
76. Heinemann L, Nosek L, Flacke F, Albus K, Krasner A, Pichotta P, et al. U-100, pH-Neutral formulation of VIAject((R)): faster onset of action than insulin lispro in patients with type 1 diabetes. Diabetes Obes Metab. 2012;14(3):222–7.
77. Heinemann L. New ways of insulin delivery. Int J Clin Pract Suppl. 2011;170:31–46.
78. Boss AH, Petrucci R, Lorber D. Coverage of prandial insulin requirements by means of an ultra-rapid-acting inhaled insulin. J Diabetes Sci Technol. 2012;6(4):773–9.
79. FDA approves Afrezza to treat diabetes. [Cited June 2014]; Available from: http://www.fda.gov/newsevents/newsroom/pressannouncements/ucm403122.htm.
80. Fonte P, Araujo F, Reis S, Sarmento B. Oral insulin delivery: how far are we? J Diabetes Sci Technol. 2013;7(2):520–31.
81. Hompesch M, Morrow L, Watkins E, Roepstorff C, Thomsen HF, Haahr H. Pharmacokinetic and pharmacodynamic responses of insulin degludec in African American, white, and Hispanic/Latino patients with type 2 diabetes mellitus. Clin Ther. 2014;36(4):507–15.
82. Thabit H, Hovorka R. Closed-loop insulin delivery in type 1 diabetes. Endocrinol Metab Clin North Am. 2012;41(1):105–17.
83. Pandyarajan V, Weiss MA. Design of non-standard insulin analogs for the treatment of diabetes mellitus. Curr Diab Rep. 2012;12(6):697–704.
84. Garber AJ, Abrahamson MJ, Barzilay JI, Blonde L, Bloomgarden ZT, Bush MA, et al. AACE comprehensive diabetes management algorithm 2013. Endocr Pract. 2013;19(2):327–36.
85. Ahren B. Insulin plus incretin: a glucose-lowering strategy for type 2-diabetes. World J Diabetes. 2014;5(1):40–51.
86. Heller SR. Hypoglycaemia in type 2 diabetes. Diabetes Res Clin Pract. 2008;82 Suppl 2:S108–11.
87. Reutrakul S, Wroblewski K, Brown RL. Clinical use of U-500 regular insulin: review and meta-analysis. J Diabetes Sci Technol. 2012;6(2):412–20.
88. de la Pena A, Riddle M, Morrow LA, Jiang HH, Linnebjerg H, Scott A, et al. Pharmacokinetics and pharmacodynamics of high-dose human regular U-500 insulin versus human regular U-100 insulin in healthy obese subjects. Diabetes Care. 2011;34(12):2496–501.
89. Krentz AJ, Hitman GA. Sir Harold Himsworth and insulin insensitivity 75 years on. Diabet Med. 2011;28(12):1435.
90. Himsworth HP. Diabetes mellitus: a differentiation into insulin-sensitive and insulin-insentive subtypes. Lancet. 1936;1:127–30.
91. Kahn CR, Roth J. Berson, Yalow, and the JCI: the agony and the ecstasy. J Clin Invest. 2004;114(8):1051–4.
92. Karam JH, Grodsky GM, Forsham PH. Insulin secretion in obesity: pseudodiabetes? Am J Clin Nutr. 1968;21(12):1445–54.
93. Randle PJ, Garland PB, Hales CN, Newsholme EA. The glucose fatty-acid cycle. Its role in insulin sensitivity and the metabolic disturbances of diabetes mellitus. Lancet. 1963;1(7285):785–9.
94. Zierler KL, Rabinowitz D. Effect of very small concentrations of insulin on forearm metabolism. Persistence of its action on potassium and free fatty acids without its effect on glucose. J Clin Invest. 1964;43:950–62.
95. DeFronzo RA, Tobin JD, Andres R. Glucose clamp technique: a method for quantifying insulin secretion and resistance. Am J Physiol. 1979;237(3):E214–23.
96. Kahn CR, White MF. The insulin receptor and the molecular mechanism of insulin action. J Clin Invest. 1988;82(4):1151–6.
97. Czech MP, Klarlund JK, Yagaloff KA, Bradford AP, Lewis RE. Insulin receptor signaling. Activation of multiple serine kinases. J Biol Chem. 1988;263(23):11017–20.
98. Krentz AJ, Bailey CJ, Melander A. Thiazolidinediones for type 2 diabetes. New agents reduce insulin resistance but need long term clinical trials. BMJ. 2000;321(7256):252–3.
99. Hiatt WR, Kaul S, Smith RJ. The cardiovascular safety of diabetes drugs–insights from the rosiglitazone experience. N Engl J Med. 2013;369(14):1285–7.
100. Heinemann L, Anderson Jr JH. Measurement of insulin absorption and insulin action. Diabetes Technol Ther. 2004;6(5):698–718.
101. Alberti KG. Blood metabolites in the diagnosis and treatment of diabetes mellitus. Postgrad Med J. 1973;49 Suppl 7:955–63.
102. Guerre-Millo M, Gervois P, Raspe E, Madsen L, Poulain P, Derudas B, et al. Peroxisome proliferator-activated receptor alpha activators improve insulin sensitivity and reduce adiposity. J Biol Chem. 2000;275(22):16638–42.

103. Zema MJ. Colesevelam hydrochloride: evidence for its use in the treatment of hypercholesterolemia and type 2 diabetes mellitus with insights into mechanism of action. Core Evid. 2012;7:61–75.
104. Scheen AJ, Paquot N. Use of cannabinoid CB1 receptor antagonists for the treatment of metabolic disorders. Best Pract Res Clin Endocrinol Metab. 2009;23(1):103–16.
105. Silvestri C, Di Marzo V. Second generation CB1 receptor blockers and other inhibitors of peripheral endocannabinoid overactivity and the rationale of their use against metabolic disorders. Expert Opin Investig Drugs. 2012;21(9):1309–22.
106. Koffarnus RL, Wargo KA, Phillippe HM. Rivoglitazone: a new thiazolidinedione for the treatment of type 2 diabetes mellitus. Ann Pharmacother. 2013;47(6):877–85.
107. Van Cauter E, Polonsky KS, Scheen AJ. Roles of circadian rhythmicity and sleep in human glucose regulation. Endocr Rev. 1997;18(5):716–38.
108. Yki-Jarvinen H. Thiazolidinediones. N Engl J Med. 2004;351(11):1106–18.
109. Meier JJ. GLP-1 receptor agonists for individualized treatment of type 2 diabetes mellitus. Nat Rev Endocrinol. 2012;8(12):728–42.
110. Matthews DR, Hosker JP, Rudenski AS, Naylor BA, Treacher DF, Turner RC. Homeostasis model assessment: insulin resistance and beta-cell function from fasting plasma glucose and insulin concentrations in man. Diabetologia. 1985;28(7):412–9.
111. Levy JC, Matthews DR, Hermans MP. Correct homeostasis model assessment (HOMA) evaluation uses the computer program. Diabetes Care. 1998;21(12):2191–2.
112. Wallace TM, Levy JC, Matthews DR. Use and abuse of HOMA modeling. Diabetes Care. 2004; 27(6):1487–95.
113. Katz A, Nambi SS, Mather K, Baron AD, Follmann DA, Sullivan G, et al. Quantitative insulin sensitivity check index: a simple, accurate method for assessing insulin sensitivity in humans. J Clin Endocrinol Metab. 2000;85(7):2402–10.
114. Pacini G, Mari A. Methods for clinical assessment of insulin sensitivity and beta-cell function. Best Pract Res Clin Endocrinol Metab. 2003;17(3):305–22.
115. Manley SE, Luzio SD, Stratton IM, Wallace TM, Clark PM. Preanalytical, analytical, and computational factors affect homeostasis model assessment estimates. Diabetes Care. 2008;31(9):1877–83.
116. Reaven G. Wanted!: a standardized measurement of plasma insulin concentration. Arterioscler Thromb Vasc Biol. 2011;31(5):954–5.
117. Kim SH, Abbasi F, Reaven GM. Impact of degree of obesity on surrogate estimates of insulin resistance. Diabetes Care. 2004;27(8):1998–2002.
118. Wallace TM, Matthews DR. The assessment of insulin resistance in man. Diabet Med. 2002;19(7):527–34.
119. Jayagopal V, Kilpatrick ES, Jennings PE, Hepburn DA, Atkin SL. Biological variation of homeostasis model assessment-derived insulin resistance in type 2 diabetes. Diabetes Care. 2002;25(11):2022–5.
120. Aye MM, Kilpatrick ES, Afolabi P, Wootton SA, Rigby AS, Coady AM, et al. Postprandial effects of long-term niacin/laropiprant use on glucose and lipid metabolism and on cardiovascular risk in patients with polycystic ovary syndrome. Diabetes Obes Metab. 2014;16:545–52.
121. Yang Y, Wei RB, Xing Y, Tang L, Zheng XY, Wang ZC, et al. A meta-analysis of the effect of angiotensin receptor blockers and calcium channel blockers on blood pressure, glycemia and the HOMA-IR index in non-diabetic patients. Metabolism. 2013;62(12):1858–66.
122. Elliott WJ, Meyer PM. Incident diabetes in clinical trials of antihypertensive drugs: a network meta-analysis. Lancet. 2007;369(9557):201–7.
123. Asmar M, Holst JJ. Glucagon-like peptide 1 and glucose-dependent insulinotropic polypeptide: new advances. Curr Opin Endocrinol Diabetes Obes. 2010;17(1):57–62.
124. Schernthaner G, Grimaldi A, Di Mario U, Drzewoski J, Kempler P, Kvapil M, et al. GUIDE study: double-blind comparison of once-daily gliclazide MR and glimepiride in type 2 diabetic patients. Eur J Clin Invest. 2004;34(8):535–42.
125. Drucker DJ, Nauck MA. The incretin system: glucagon-like peptide-1 receptor agonists and dipeptidyl peptidase-4 inhibitors in type 2 diabetes. Lancet. 2006;368(9548):1696–705.
126. Bergman RN, Phillips LS, Cobelli C. Physiologic evaluation of factors controlling glucose tolerance in man: measurement of insulin sensitivity and beta-cell glucose sensitivity from the response to intravenous glucose. J Clin Invest. 1981;68(6):1456–67.
127. Beard JC, Bergman RN, Ward WK, Porte Jr D. The insulin sensitivity index in nondiabetic man. Correlation between clamp-derived and IVGTT-derived values. Diabetes. 1986;35(3):362–9.
128. Bergman RN, Ider YZ, Bowden CR, Cobelli C. Quantitative estimation of insulin sensitivity. Am J Physiol. 1979;236(6):E667–77.
129. Bergman RN, Finegood DT, Ader M. Assessment of insulin sensitivity in vivo. Endocr Rev. 1985;6(1):45–86.
130. Saad MF, Anderson RL, Laws A, Watanabe RM, Kades WW, Chen YD, et al. A comparison between the minimal model and the glucose clamp in the assessment of insulin sensitivity across the spectrum of glucose tolerance. Insulin resistance atherosclerosis study. Diabetes. 1994;43(9):1114–21.
131. Best JD, Kahn SE, Ader M, Watanabe RM, Ni TC, Bergman RN. Role of glucose effectiveness in the determination of glucose tolerance. Diabetes Care. 1996;19(9):1018–30.
132. Rayner CK, Horowitz M. Gastrointestinal motility and glycemic control in diabetes: the chicken and the egg revisited? J Clin Invest. 2006;116(2):299–302.

133. Holst JJ, Vilsboll T, Deacon CF. The incretin system and its role in type 2 diabetes mellitus. Mol Cell Endocrinol. 2009;297(1–2):127–36.
134. Ferrannini E, Mari A. How to measure insulin sensitivity. J Hypertens. 1998;16(7):895–906.
135. Muniyappa R, Lee S, Chen H, Quon MJ. Current approaches for assessing insulin sensitivity and resistance in vivo: advantages, limitations, and appropriate usage. Am J Physiol Endocrinol Metab. 2008;294(1):E15–26.
136. Kim SH. Measurement of insulin action: a tribute to Sir Harold Himsworth. Diabet Med. 2011;28(12):1487–93.
137. Schwartz MW, Seeley RJ, Tschop MH, Woods SC, Morton GJ, Myers MG, et al. Cooperation between brain and islet in glucose homeostasis and diabetes. Nature. 2013;503(7474):59–66.
138. Ko GT, Chan JC, Woo J, Lau E, Yeung VT, Chow CC, et al. The reproducibility and usefulness of the oral glucose tolerance test in screening for diabetes and other cardiovascular risk factors. Ann Clin Biochem. 1998;35(Pt 1):62–7.
139. Vinik AI, Maser RE, Mitchell BD, Freeman R. Diabetic autonomic neuropathy. Diabetes Care. 2003;26(5):1553–79.
140. Due A, Larsen TM, Hermansen K, Stender S, Holst JJ, Toubro S, et al. Comparison of the effects on insulin resistance and glucose tolerance of 6-mo high-monounsaturated-fat, low-fat, and control diets. Am J Clin Nutr. 2008;87(4):855–62.
141. Heer M, Egert S. Nutrients other than carbohydrates: their effects on glucose homeostasis in humans. Diabetes Metab Res Rev. 2014. doi: 10.1002/dmrr.2533. [Epub ahead of print].
142. Karlsson F, Tremaroli V, Nielsen J, Backhed F. Assessing the human gut microbiota in metabolic diseases. Diabetes. 2013;62(10):3341–9.
143. Alberti KG, Zimmet PZ. Definition, diagnosis and classification of diabetes mellitus and its complications. Part 1: diagnosis and classification of diabetes mellitus provisional report of a WHO consultation. Diabet Med. 1998;15(7):539–53.
144. Bilku DK, Dennison AR, Hall TC, Metcalfe MS, Garcea G. Role of preoperative carbohydrate loading: a systematic review. Ann R Coll Surg Engl. 2014;96(1):15–22.
145. Matsuda M, DeFronzo RA. Insulin sensitivity indices obtained from oral glucose tolerance testing: comparison with the euglycemic insulin clamp. Diabetes Care. 1999;22(9):1462–70.
146. Stumvoll M, Mitrakou A, Pimenta W, Jenssen T, Yki-Järvinen H, Van Haeften T, et al. Use of the oral glucose tolerance test to assess insulin release and insulin sensitivity. Diabetes Care. 2000;23(3):295–301.
147. Mari A, Pacini G, Murphy E, Ludvik B, Nolan JJ. A model-based method for assessing insulin sensitivity from the oral glucose tolerance test. Diabetes Care. 2001;24(3):539–48.
148. Dalla Man C, Campioni M, Polonsky KS, Basu R, Rizza RA, Toffolo G, et al. Two-hour seven-sample oral glucose tolerance test and meal protocol: minimal model assessment of beta-cell responsivity and insulin sensitivity in nondiabetic individuals. Diabetes. 2005;54(11):3265–73.
149. Beysen C, Murphy EJ, McLaughlin T, Riiff T, Lamendola C, Turner HC, et al. Whole-body glycolysis measured by the deuterated-glucose disposal test correlates highly with insulin resistance in vivo. Diabetes Care. 2007;30(5):1143–9.
150. Meyer C, Dostou JM, Welle SL, Gerich JE. Role of human liver, kidney, and skeletal muscle in postprandial glucose homeostasis. Am J Physiol Endocrinol Metab. 2002;282(2):E419–27.
151. Dube S, Errazuriz I, Cobelli C, Basu R, Basu A. Assessment of insulin action on carbohydrate metabolism: physiological and non-physiological methods. Diabet Med. 2013;30(6):664–70.
152. Polidori D, Sha S, Mudaliar S, Ciaraldi TP, Ghosh A, Vaccaro N, et al. Canagliflozin lowers postprandial glucose and insulin by delaying intestinal glucose absorption in addition to increasing urinary glucose excretion: results of a randomized, placebo-controlled study. Diabetes Care. 2013;36(8):2154–61.
153. Hucking K, Watanabe RM, Stefanovski D, Bergman RN. OGTT-derived measures of insulin sensitivity are confounded by factors other than insulin sensitivity itself. Obesity (Silver Spring). 2008;16(8):1938–45.
154. Chen CC, Wang TY, Hsu SY, Chen RH, Chang CT, Chen SJ. Is the short insulin tolerance test safe and reproducible? Diabet Med. 1998;15(11):924–7.
155. Gelding SV, Robinson S, Lowe S, Niththyananthan R, Johnston DG. Validation of the low dose short insulin tolerance test for evaluation of insulin sensitivity. Clin Endocrinol (Oxf). 1994;40(5):611–5.
156. Shen SW, Reaven GM, Farquhar JW. Comparison of impedance to insulin-mediated glucose uptake in normal subjects and in subjects with latent diabetes. J Clin Invest. 1970;49(12):2151–60.
157. Harano Y, Hidaka H, Takatsuki K, Ohgaku S, Haneda M, Motoi S, et al. Glucose, insulin, and somatostatin infusion for the determination of insulin sensitivity in vivo. Metabolism. 1978;27(9 Suppl 1):1449–52.
158. Pei D, Jones CN, Bhargava R, Chen YD, Reaven GM. Evaluation of octreotide to assess insulin-mediated glucose disposal by the insulin suppression test. Diabetologia. 1994;37(8):843–5.
159. Elahi D, Meneilly GS, Minaker KL, Andersen DK, Rowe JW. Escape of hepatic glucose production during hyperglycemic clamp. Am J Physiol. 1989;257(5 Pt 1):E704–11.
160. Kruzynska Y. In: Pickup JC, Williams G, editors. Textbook of diabetes. Oxford: Blackwell Science; 1997.
161. Rizza RA, Mandarino LJ, Gerich JE. Dose-response characteristics for effects of insulin on production and utilization of glucose in man. Am J Physiol. 1981;240(6):E630–9.

162. Stumvoll M, Meyer C, Mitrakou A, Gerich JE. Important role of the kidney in human carbohydrate metabolism. Med Hypotheses. 1999;52(5):363–6.
163. Gerich JE, Meyer C, Woerle HJ, Stumvoll M. Renal gluconeogenesis: its importance in human glucose homeostasis. Diabetes Care. 2001;24(2):382–91.
164. Krentz AJ, Nattrass M. Insulin resistance: a multifaceted metabolic syndrome. Insights gained using a low-dose insulin infusion technique. Diabet Med. 1996;13(1):30–9.
165. Conte C, Fabbrini E, Kars M, Mittendorfer B, Patterson BW, Klein S. Multiorgan insulin sensitivity in lean and obese subjects. Diabetes Care. 2012;35(6):1316–21.
166. Pratipanawatr T, Pratipanawatr W, Rosen C, Berria R, Bajaj M, Cusi K, et al. Effect of IGF-I on FFA and glucose metabolism in control and type 2 diabetic subjects. Am J Physiol Endocrinol Metab. 2002;282(6):E1360–8.
167. Van Pelt RE, Gozansky WS, Kohrt WM. A novel index of whole body antilipolytic insulin action. Obesity (Silver Spring). 2013;21(1):E162–5.
168. Glintborg D, Frystyk J, Hojlund K, Andersen KK, Henriksen JE, Hermann AP, et al. Total and high molecular weight (HMW) adiponectin levels and measures of glucose and lipid metabolism following pioglitazone treatment in a randomized placebo-controlled study in polycystic ovary syndrome. Clin Endocrinol (Oxf). 2008;68(2):165–74.
169. Morrow L, Hompesch M, Tideman AM, Matson J, Dunne N, Pardo S, et al. Evaluation of a novel continuous glucose measurement device in patients with diabetes mellitus across the glycemic range. J Diabetes Sci Technol. 2011;5(4):853–9.
170. Norjavaara E, Ericsson H, Sjoberg F, Leonsson-Zachrisson M, Sjöstrand M, Morrow LA, et al. Glucokinase activators AZD6370 and AZD1656 do not affect the central counterregulatory response to hypoglycemia in healthy males. J Clin Endocrinol Metab. 2012;97(9):3319–25.
171. Krentz AJ, Boyle PJ, Macdonald LM, Schade DS. Octreotide: a long-acting inhibitor of endogenous hormone secretion for human metabolic investigations. Metabolism. 1994;43(1):24–31.
172. DeFronzo RA, Hompesch M, Kasichayanula S, Liu X, Hong Y, Pfister M, et al. Characterization of renal glucose reabsorption in response to dapagliflozin in healthy subjects and subjects with type 2 diabetes. Diabetes Care. 2013;36(10):3169–76.
173. Tonelli J, Li W, Kishore P, Pajvani UB, Kwon E, Waever C, et al. Mechanisms of early insulin-sensitizing effects of thiazolidinediones in type 2 diabetes. Diabetes 2004;53:1621–9.
174. Del Prato S, Matsuda M, Simonson DC, Groop LC, Sheehan P, Leonetti F, et al. Studies on the mass action effect of glucose in NIDDM and IDDM: evidence for glucose resistance. Diabetologia. 1997;40(6):687–97.
175. Morris AD, Ueda S, Petrie JR, Connell JM, Elliott HL, Donnelly R. The euglycaemic hyperinsulinaemic clamp: an evaluation of current methodology. Clin Exp Pharmacol Physiol. 1997;24(7):513–8.
176. Sherwin RS, Kramer KJ, Tobin JD, Insel PA, Liljenquist JE, Berman M, et al. A model of the kinetics of insulin in man. J Clin Invest. 1974;53(5):1481–92.
177. Kampmann U, Hoeyem P, Mengel A, Schmitz O, Rungby J, Orskov L, et al. Insulin dose-response studies in severely insulin-resistant type 2 diabetes – evidence for effectiveness of very high insulin doses. Diabetes Obes Metab. 2011;13(6):511–6.
178. Hompesch M, Rave K. An analysis of how to measure glucose during glucose clamps: are glucose meters ready for research? J Diabetes Sci Technol. 2008;2(5):896–8.
179. Staehr P, Hother-Nielsen O, Levin K, Holst JJ, Beck-Nielsen H. Assessment of hepatic insulin action in obese type 2 diabetic patients. Diabetes. 2001;50(6):1363–70.
180. Nattrass M, Alberti KG, Dennis KJ, Gillibrand PN, Letchworth AT, Buckle AL. A glucose-controlled insulin infusion system for diabetic women during labour. Br Med J. 1978;2(6137):599–601.
181. Schock A, Schultz M, Kerner W, Maier V, Pfeiffer EF. The effect of three days of blood glucose normalization by means of an "artificial endocrine pancreas" on the concentrations of growth hormone, glucagon, and cortisol in juvenile diabetics. Horm Metab Res Suppl. 1979;8:93–6.
182. Brennan JR, Gebhart SS, Blackard WG. Pump-induced insulin aggregation. A problem with the Biostator. Diabetes. 1985;34(4):353–9.
183. Verdonk CA, Rizza RA, Westland RE, Nelson RL, Gerich JE, Service FJ. Glucose clamping using the Biostator GCIIS. Horm Metab Res. 1980;12(4):133–5.
184. Ponchner M, Heine RJ, Pernet A, Hanning I, Francis AJ, Cook D, et al. A comparison of the artificial pancreas (glucose controlled insulin infusion system) and a manual technique for assessing insulin sensitivity during euglycaemic clamping. Diabetologia. 1984;26(6):420–5.
185. Clemens AH, Hough DL, D'Orazio PA. Development of the Biostator glucose clamping algorithm. Clin Chem. 1982;28(9):1899–904.
186. Heinemann L, Ampudia-Blasco FJ. Glucose clamps with the Biostator: a critical reappraisal. Horm Metab Res. 1994;26(12):579–83.
187. Picchini U, De Gaetano A, Panunzi S, Ditlevsen S, Mingrone G. A mathematical model of the euglycemic hyperinsulinemic clamp. Theor Biol Med Model. 2005;2:44.
188. Doberne L, Greenfield MS, Schulz B, Reaven GM. Enhanced glucose utilization during prolonged glucose clamp studies. Diabetes. 1981;30(10):829–35.
189. Roden M, Price TB, Perseghin G, Petersen KF, Rothman DL, Cline GW, et al. Mechanism of free fatty acid-induced insulin resistance in humans. J Clin Invest. 1996;97(12):2859–65.
190. Revers RR, Kolterman OG, Olefsky JM. Relationship between serum glucose level and the metabolic

clearance rate of glucose in non-insulin-dependent diabetes mellitus. Diabetes. 1983;32(7):627–32.
191. Heise T, Rave K, Weyer C, Heinemann L. Measurement of insulin sensitivity with the euglycaemic clamp technique: methodological pitfalls. Int J Diabetes. 1998;6:70–5.
192. Kauh EA, Mixson LA, Shankar S, McCarthy J, Maridakis V, Morrow L, et al. Short-term metabolic effects of prednisone administration in healthy subjects. Diabetes Obes Metab. 2011;13(11):1001–7.
193. Merovci A, Solis-Herrera C, Daniele G, Eldor R, Fiorentino TV, Tripathy D, et al. Dapagliflozin improves muscle insulin sensitivity but enhances endogenous glucose production. J Clin Invest. 2014;124(2):509–14.
194. Ferrannini E, Muscelli E, Frascerra S, Baldi S, Mari A, Heise T, et al. Metabolic response to sodium-glucose cotransporter 2 inhibition in type 2 diabetic patients. J Clin Invest. 2014;124(2):499–508.
195. Soop M, Nygren J, Brismar K, Thorell A, Ljungqvist O. The hyperinsulinaemic-euglycaemic glucose clamp: reproducibility and metabolic effects of prolonged insulin infusion in healthy subjects. Clin Sci (Lond). 2000;98(4):367–74.
196. Dokcrmark L, Froden A, Attvall S, Wikstrand J, Fagerberg B. The euglycemic hyperinsulinemic clamp examination: variability and reproducibility. Scand J Clin Lab Invest. 2000;60(1):27–36.
197. Mak RH, DeFronzo RA. Glucose and insulin metabolism in uremia. Nephron. 1992;61(4):377–82.
198. Rave K, Heise T, Weyer C, Sawicki P, Heinemann L. Measurement of insulin sensitivity: influence of potassium supply during euglycaemic glucose clamps in healthy volunteers. Exp Clin Endocrinol Diabetes. 1999;107(5):313–7.
199. Nathan DM, Buse JB, Davidson MB, Ferrannini E, Holman RR, Sherwin R, et al. Medical management of hyperglycaemia in type 2 diabetes mellitus: a consensus algorithm for the initiation and adjustment of therapy: a consensus statement from the American Diabetes Association and the European Association for the Study of Diabetes. Diabetologia. 2009;52(1):17–30.
200. Inzucchi SE, Maggs DG, Spollett GR, Page SL, Rife FS, Walton V, et al. Efficacy and metabolic effects of metformin and troglitazone in type II diabetes mellitus. N Engl J Med. 1998;338(13):867–72.
201. Mayerson AB, Hundal RS, Dufour S, Lebon V, Befroy D, Cline GW, et al. The effects of rosiglitazone on insulin sensitivity, lipolysis, and hepatic and skeletal muscle triglyceride content in patients with type 2 diabetes. Diabetes. 2002;51(3):797–802.
202. Miyazaki Y, Matsuda M, DeFronzo RA. Dose-response effect of pioglitazone on insulin sensitivity and insulin secretion in type 2 diabetes. Diabetes Care. 2002;25(3):517–23.
203. Stern SE, Williams K, Ferrannini E, DeFronzo RA, Bogardus C, Stern MP. Identification of individuals with insulin resistance using routine clinical measurements. Diabetes. 2005;54(2):333–9.
204. Krentz AJ, Morrow L, Hompesch M. Developing new drugs for diabetes and cardiometabolic disorders: a changing paradigm. Drugs. 2012;72(13):1709–11.
205. Deanfield JE, Halcox JP, Rabelink TJ. Endothelial function and dysfunction: testing and clinical relevance. Circulation. 2007;115(10):1285–95.
206. Sidhu JS, Kaposzta Z, Markus HS, Kaski JC. Effect of rosiglitazone on common carotid intima-media thickness progression in coronary artery disease patients without diabetes mellitus. Arterioscler Thromb Vasc Biol. 2004;24(5):930–4.
207. Kang S, Brange J, Burch A, Volund A, Owens DR. Absorption kinetics and action profiles of subcutaneously administered insulin analogues (AspB9GluB27, AspB10, AspB28) in healthy subjects. Diabetes Care. 1991;14(11):1057–65.
208. Weinges K, Ehrhardt M, Enzmann F. Comparison of biosynthetic human insulin and pork insulin in the Gerritzen test. Diabetes Care. 1981;4(2):180–2.
209. Davidson MB, Navar MD, Echeverry D, Duran P. U-500 regular insulin: clinical experience and pharmacokinetics in obese, severely insulin-resistant type 2 diabetic patients. Diabetes Care. 2010;33(2):281–3.
210. Ampudia Blasco FJ, Heinemann L, Bender R, Schmidt A, Heise T, Berger M, et al. Comparative dose-related time-action profiles of glibenclamide and a new non-sulphonylurea drug, AG-EE 623 ZW, during euglycaemic clamp in healthy subjects. Diabetologia. 1994;37(7):703–7.
211. Wolzt M, de la Pena A, Berclaz PY, Tibaldi FS, Gates JR, Muchmore DB. AIR inhaled insulin versus subcutaneous insulin: pharmacokinetics, glucodynamics, and pulmonary function in asthma. Diabetes Care. 2008;31(4):735–40.
212. Committee for Proprietary Medicinal Products. Note on guidance on clinical investigation of medicinal products in the treatment of diabetes mellitus. 2002; London: European Agency for the Evaluation of Medicinal Products. http://www.ema.europa.eu/docs/en_GB/document_library/Scientific_guideline/2009/09/WC500003262.pdf.
213. Food and Drug Administration. Guidance for industry. Diabetes mellitus: developing drugs and therapeutic biologics for treatment and prevention. 2008. http://www.fda.gov/downloads/Drugs/Guidances/ucm071624.pdf.
214. Owen WE, Roberts WL. Cross-reactivity of three recombinant insulin analogs with five commercial insulin immunoassays. Clin Chem. 2004;50(1):257–9.
215. Hilgenfeld R, Seipke G, Berchtold H, Owens DR. The evolution of insulin glargine and its continuing contribution to diabetes care. Drugs. 2014;74:911–27.
216. Swinnen SG, Holleman F, DeVries JH. The interpretation of glucose clamp studies of long-acting insulin analogues: from physiology to marketing and back. Diabetologia. 2008;51(10):1790–5.
217. Wang L, Lovejoy NF, Faustman DL. Persistence of prolonged C-peptide production in type 1 diabetes

as measured with an ultrasensitive C-peptide assay. Diabetes Care. 2012;35(3):465–70.
218. Oram RA, Jones AG, Besser RE, Knight BA, Shields BM, Brown RJ, et al. The majority of patients with long-duration type 1 diabetes are insulin microsecretors and have functioning beta cells. Diabetologia. 2014;57(1):187–91.
219. Greenbaum CJ, Mandrup-Poulsen T, McGee PF, Battelino T, Haastert B, Ludvigsson J, et al. Mixed-meal tolerance test versus glucagon stimulation test for the assessment of beta-cell function in therapeutic trials in type 1 diabetes. Diabetes Care. 2008;31(10):1966–71.
220. Zangeneh F, Arora PS, Dyck PJ, Bekris L, Lernmark A, Achenbach SJ, et al. Effects of duration of type 2 diabetes mellitus on insulin secretion. Endocr Pract. 2006;12(4):388–93.
221. Ocheltree SM, Hompesch M, Wondmagegnehu ET, Morrow L, Win K, Jacober SJ. Comparison of pharmacodynamic intrasubject variability of insulin lispro protamine suspension and insulin glargine in subjects with type 1 diabetes. Eur J Endocrinol. 2010;163(2):217–23.
222. Hompesch M, Kang J, Morrow L, Yun N, Kwon S, Lim CG, Trautmanm M, Krentz AJ, Win K, Chapel S, Son J. The ultra-long-acting insulin HM12460A demonstrates safety and efficacy in patients with type 1 diabetes: a phase 1 single dose explorative glucose clamp study. Diabetes. 2014;63 Suppl 1:A229.
223. Morrow L, Muchmore DB, Hompesch M, Ludington EA, Vaughn DE. Comparative pharmacokinetics and insulin action for three rapid-acting insulin analogs injected subcutaneously with and without hyaluronidase. Diabetes Care. 2013;36(2):273–5.
224. Lepore M, Pampanelli S, Fanelli C, Porcellati F, Bartocci L, Di Vincenzo A, et al. Pharmacokinetics and pharmacodynamics of subcutaneous injection of long-acting human insulin analog glargine, NPH insulin, and ultralente human insulin and continuous subcutaneous infusion of insulin lispro. Diabetes. 2000;49(12):2142–8.
225. Zinman B. Newer insulin analogs: advances in basal insulin replacement. Diabetes Obes Metab. 2013;15 Suppl 1:6–10.
226. Meneghini L, Atkin SL, Gough SC, Raz I, Blonde L, Shestakova M, et al. The efficacy and safety of insulin degludec given in variable once-daily dosing intervals compared with insulin glargine and insulin degludec dosed at the same time daily: a 26-week, randomized, open-label, parallel-group, treat-to-target trial in individuals with type 2 diabetes. Diabetes Care. 2013;36(4):858–64.
227. Gough SC, Harris S, Woo V, Davies M. Insulin degludec: overview of a novel ultra long-acting basal insulin. Diabetes Obes Metab. 2013;15(4):301–9.
228. Bergenstal RM, Rosenstock J, Arakaki RF, Prince MJ, Qu Y, Sinha VP, et al. A randomized, controlled study of once-daily LY2605541, a novel long-acting basal insulin, versus insulin glargine in basal insulin-treated patients with type 2 diabetes. Diabetes Care. 2012;35(11):2140–7.
229. Heinemann L, Linkeschova R, Rave K, Hompesch B, Sedlak M, Heise T. Time-action profile of the long-acting insulin analog insulin glargine (HOE901) in comparison with those of NPH insulin and placebo. Diabetes Care. 2000;23(5):644–9.
230. Scholtz HE, Pretorius SG, Wessels DH, Becker RH. Pharmacokinetic and glucodynamic variability: assessment of insulin glargine, NPH insulin and insulin ultralente in healthy volunteers using a euglycaemic clamp technique. Diabetologia. 2005;48(10):1988–95.
231. Riddle MC, Rosenstock J, Gerich J. The treat-to-target trial: randomized addition of glargine or human NPH insulin to oral therapy of type 2 diabetic patients. Diabetes Care. 2003;26(11):3080–6.
232. Ratner RE, Hirsch IB, Neifing JL, Garg SK, Mecca TE, Wilson CA. Less hypoglycemia with insulin glargine in intensive insulin therapy for type 1 diabetes. U.S. study group of insulin glargine in type 1 diabetes. Diabetes Care. 2000;23(5):639–43.
233. Morrow L, Muchmore DB, Ludington EA, Vaughn DE, Hompesch M. Reduction in intrasubject variability in the pharmacokinetic response to insulin after subcutaneous co-administration with recombinant human hyaluronidase in healthy volunteers. Diabetes Technol Ther. 2011;13(10):1039–45.
234. Heise T, Nosek L, Ronn BB, Endahl L, Heinemann L, Kapitza C, et al. Lower within-subject variability of insulin detemir in comparison to NPH insulin and insulin glargine in people with type 1 diabetes. Diabetes. 2004;53(6):1614–20.
235. Madsbad S. LY2605541 – a preferential hepato-specific insulin analogue. Diabetes. 2014;63(2):390–2.
236. Sciacca L, Cassarino MF, Genua M, Pandini G, Le Moli R, Squatrito S, et al. Insulin analogues differently activate insulin receptor isoforms and post-receptor signalling. Diabetologia. 2010;53(8):1743–53.
237. Karlstad O, Starup-Linde J, Vestergaard P, Hjellvik V, Bazelier MT, Schmidt MK, et al. Use of insulin and insulin analogs and risk of cancer – systematic review and meta-analysis of observational studies. Curr Drug Saf. 2013;8(5):333–48.
238. ORIGIN Trial Investigators, Gerstein HC, Bosch J, Dagenais GR, Díaz R, Jung H, et al. Basal insulin and cardiovascular and other outcomes in dysglycemia. N Engl J Med. 2012;367(4):319–28.
239. Bordeleau L, Yakubovich N, Dagenais GR, Rosenstock J, Probstfield J, Chang Yu P, et al. The association of basal insulin glargine and/or n-3 fatty acids with incident cancers in patients with dysglycemia. Diabetes Care. 2014;37(5):1360–6.
240. Krentz AJ, Hompesch M. Cardiovascular safety of new drugs for diabetes: getting the balance right? Pharm Med. 2014;28:109–17.
241. Heinemann L, Hompesch M. Biosimilar insulins: basic considerations. J Diabetes Sci Technol. 2014;8(1):6–13.
242. Kramer I, Sauer T. The new world of biosimilars: what diabetologists need to know about biosimilar insulins. Br J Diabetes Vasc Dis. 2010;10:163–71.

243. Heinemann L, Hompesch M. Biosimilar insulins: how similar is similar? J Diabetes Sci Technol. 2011;5(3):741–54.
244. Kuhlmann M, Marre M. Lessons learned from biosimilar epoetins and insulins. Br J Diabetes Vasc Dis. 2010;10:90–7.
245. Wang J, Chow SC. On the regulatory approval pathway of biosimilar products. Pharmaceuticals (Basel). 2012;5(4):353–68.
246. European Medicines Agency. Guideline on non-clinical and clinical development of similar biological medicinal products containing recombinant human insulin and insulin analogues. Draft. Available from: http://www.ema.europa.eu/docs/en_GB/document_library/Scientific_guideline/2014/04/WC500165988.pdf.
247. Owens DR, Landgraf W, Schmidt A, Bretzel RG, Kuhlmann MK. The emergence of biosimilar insulin preparations – a cause for concern? Diabetes Technol Ther. 2012;14(11):989–96.
248. Anonymous. Approval of biosimilars in the USA – dead ringers? Lancet. 2012;379(9817):686.
249. Food and Drug Administration. Guidance for industry. Scientific considerations in demonstrating biosimilarity to a reference product. 2012. Available from: http://www.fda.gov/downloads/Drugs/GuidanceComplianceRegulatoryInformation/Guidances/UCM291128.pdf.
250. Heise T, Hermanski L, Nosek L, Feldman A, Rasmussen S, Haahr H. Insulin degludec: four times lower pharmacodynamic variability than insulin glargine under steady-state conditions in type 1 diabetes. Diabetes Obes Metab. 2012;14(9):859–64.

Assessment of β-Cell Function

Andrew J. Krentz, Lutz Heinemann, and Marcus Hompesch

Keywords
β-cell • Insulin • Insulin secretion • Diabetes

Summary

Background

Defective insulin secretion is a fundamental defect in the pathogenesis of diabetes. In patients with type 1 diabetes, absolute insulin deficiency resulting from autoimmune destruction of islet β-cells necessitates lifelong replacement therapy with exogenous insulin or insulin analogues. Strategies to prevent type 1 diabetes or to preserve β-cell function have been tested in clinical trials, albeit with limited success to date. In patients with type 2 diabetes, insulin deficiency is relative rather than absolute but insufficient to compensate for insulin resistance which is usually present, leading to an increase in blood glucose by insufficient handling of a glucose load. Sulphonylureas (which directly stimulate insulin release), dipeptidyl peptidase (DPP)-4 inhibitors (which enhance levels of incretin hormones), and glucagon-like peptide-1 analogues (which enhance glucose-stimulated insulin secretion via activation of the incretin system) are widely used in the treatment of patients with type 2 diabetes. Progressive loss of β-cell mass and/or function usually requires escalating polypharmacy and ultimately insulin replacement therapy also in many patients with type 2 diabetes. Novel classes of insulin secretagogues, e.g. GPR40 and GPR119 agonists, have recently entered clinical trials.

Key Methods

Tests of basal insulin secretion measure circulating β-cell products after an overnight fast. Dynamic tests assess the response of the β-cells to oral or intravenous glucose ± non-glucose secretagogues.

A.J. Krentz, MD, FRCP (✉) • L. Heinemann, PhD
M. Hompesch, MD
Profil Institute for Clinical Research,
Chula Vista, CA, USA
e-mail: andrew.krentz@profilinstitute.com;
lutz.heinemann@profilinstitute.com;
marcus.hompesch@profilinstitute.com

Tests of Basal Insulin Secretion

	Method	Measurement	Advantages	Disadvantages	Value in drug development decisions
Fasting serum insulin and/or C-peptide[a]	Serum insulin and/or C-peptide measured after an overnight fast	Fasting insulin; homeostasis model assessment (HOMA-B) is a mathematical index calculated from insulin and glucose concentrations	Simple; relatively inexpensive	Provides no information about stimulated insulin secretion; relatively high day-to-day variability	Relatively limited; of value as an exploratory endpoint requiring confirmation with a dynamic test of β-cell function

[a]Measurement of proinsulin and partially processed proinsulin products released from the β-cell may provide additional evidence of compromised β-cell function

Tests of Stimulated Insulin Secretion

	Method	Measurement	Advantages	Disadvantages	Value in drug development decisions
75 g oral glucose tolerance test	Insulin and/or C-peptide responses to 75 g oral glucose	Area under the curve for insulin; insulinogenic index (Δinsulin/Δglucose at $t=30$ min)	Assesses β-cell response to the principal dietary secretagogue under well-standardized and internationally accepted conditions; extensive scientific literature against which to reference data; assesses integrated response that includes the effect of incretin hormones	Relatively high intra-individual and between-individual variability; β-cell response to secretagogues other than glucose not assessed; may be affected by gastric emptying rate	Similar to mixed meal tolerance test but less comprehensive assessment since restricted to glucose-stimulated insulin secretion; provides additional categorical data on glucose tolerance, i.e. progression/regression of diabetes
Mixed meal tolerance test	Serum insulin and/or C-peptide to a meal of defined composition	Area under the curve for insulin; insulinogenic index (Δinsulin/Δglucose at $t=30$ min)	Provides data relevant to normal physiology; flexible, i.e. nutrient components can be adjusted; assesses integrity of incretin axis	Relatively high intra-individual and between-individual variability; affected by gastric emptying rate	Provides dynamic data of physiological relevance; sensitive techniques for preliminary assessment of drug effects on insulin secretion; incretin axis is integral to responses

	Method	Measurement	Advantages	Disadvantages	Value in drug development decisions
Intravenous glucose tolerance test	Insulin and C-peptide responses to an intravenous bolus of glucose	Acute insulin response (AIR)	Provides dynamic data; widely used in clinical metabolic research	Relevance to normal physiology uncertain; does not generate dose–response data; incretin axis not assessed	May be a useful indicator of drug-induced effects on insulin secretion
Hyperglycaemic clamp	Serum insulin and C-peptide responses to sustained hyperglycaemia generated by constant infusion of hypertonic glucose	First- and second-phase insulin responses to hyperglycaemia	Provides standardized assessment of insulin secretion	Insulin secretion is assessed in an unphysiological state of sustained hyperglycaemia; does not provide dose–response data; incretin axis not assessed	Moderately useful technique for assessing drug effects on insulin secretion
Arginine potentiation test	Intravenous infusion of arginine superimposed on hyperglycaemic clamp	Acute insulin response to arginine (AIR_{max}) usually in the setting of controlled hyperglycaemia	Provides an assessment of near-maximal insulin secretion	Of limited physiological relevance; incretin axis not assessed	Of limited application in the context of drug development
Graded glucose infusion	Serum insulin and C-peptide responses to a stepped incremental intravenous glucose infusion	Insulin secretion dose–response vs. glucose concentration; displacement of curve to left indicative of improved β-cell function	Provides detailed insulin-glucose dose–response data over range of glycaemia relevant to normal physiology as well as the pathophysiology of glucose intolerance and type 2 diabetes	Incretin axis not assessed; lengthy and labour intensive	Sensitive and reproducible technique that can provide robust data about drug-induced changes in insulin secretion, albeit without information about the incretin axis

Conclusions

The range of different techniques for the assessment of insulin secretion and response to therapeutic interventions reflects the absence of a true reference method for drug development. No single method adequately captures all potentially relevant aspects of β-cell function. Selection of the most appropriate tests should be guided by the putative mechanism of action, e.g. direct secretagogue and activation of the incretin axis. A plurality of methods may be required to provide a comprehensive picture sufficient for making drug development decisions. Assessing the integrity of the incretin axis has come to prominence in recent years.

Introduction

Insulin is the principal anabolic hormone of the body and is essential for life [1]. The hormone exerts wide-ranging effects on carbohydrate, lipid and protein metabolism and regulates aspects of cell growth and differentiation [2]. Human insulin is composed of 51 amino acids and has a molecular weight of 5.8 kDa. The insulin molecule is a dimer comprised of an A-chain and a B-chain. The insulin gene is located on the short arm of chromosome 11 [3]. Insulin is synthesized within the β-cells of the pancreatic islets as a 110-amino-acid precursor. Preproinsulin is cleaved to proinsulin, and the latter is processed to insulin and C-peptide by specific endopeptidases and processed in the endoplasmic reticulum [4]. After passage through the Golgi apparatus, insulin is stored as hexamers in secretory granules awaiting release [5]. Insulin has a compact three-dimensional structure consisting of three helices and three conserved disulphide bridges [6]. This conformation is important for binding to and activating the insulin receptor. In the presence of zinc, the flux of which is regulated by zinc transporter proteins [7], and at a pH of approximately 6.0, insulin monomers assemble into higher order hexameric conformations [8]. The concentration of insulin within the storage granules of the β-cells is approximately 40 mmol/L [9]. The synthesis of insulin is regulated at both the transcriptional and translational level. Glucose metabolism within the β-cells stimulates the secretion of preformed insulin. Glucose is also the major physiological stimulator of the insulin gene [10].

Islet Physiology

The human pancreas contains approximately one million islets that comprise 1–2 % of the total mass of the gland. Islets contain four different endocrine cell types:
- β-cells that produce insulin and constitute ~60–80 % of the endocrine cell mass
- α-cells (~10–20 %) that produce glucagon
- δ-cells (~5 %) that produce somatostatin
- PP cells (<1 %) that produce pancreatic polypeptide

In order that β-cells can respond rapidly to prevailing blood glucose concentrations, islets receive approximately tenfold the blood flow of the surrounding exocrine cells of the pancreas. The capillaries surrounding islets have numerous fenestrations that facilitate nutrient exchange [11]. Heterogeneity in β-cell numbers between islets may be relevant to insulin secretion [12]. The activity of β-cells is synchronized both within and across islets. Endogenous insulin secretion is characterized by a pulsatile secretion with a periodicity of approximately 5 min and higher order swings [13, 14]. Alterations in the pulsatile secretion of insulin have been reported in patients with type 2 diabetes [15, 16] and also in glucose-intolerant first-degree relatives [17]. The increase in β-cell insulin secretion following ingestion of a meal normally signals a decrease or maintenance of glucagon secretion [18]. In the setting of deficient insulin secretion, relative hyperglucagonaemia contributes to hyperglycaemia in diabetes [18]. The higher proportion of α-cells to β-cell in the islets of some patients with type 2 diabetes has been attributed to a decrease in β-cell number rather than an increase in α-cell number [19]. Somatostatin, the pulsatility of which is aligned with insulin [20], inhibits the secretion of both insulin and glucagon [21].

Glucose-Stimulated Insulin Secretion

In health, insulin is secreted to precisely meet metabolic demand and maintain circulating glucose concentration within strict limits. The rates of hepatic glucose production and glucose utilization are regulated by circulating insulin levels, remaining closely matched and relatively constant from day to day. Endogenous insulin secretion is stimulated primarily by increases in blood glucose levels. Non-glucose initiators of insulin secretion include certain monosaccharides, amino acids and fatty acids [11, 22]. It has been suggested that insulin secretion may also be influenced by other factors acting directly via cell surface receptors [23]. The discovery of G-protein fatty acid receptors that are either directly (GPR40) or indirectly (e.g. GPR120) involved in insulin secretion has generated new targets for diabetes drug development (see below) [24].

Glucose is transported from the blood into the β-cell via the high-capacity glucose transporter (GLUT2) system. Inside the cells, it is metabolized by glucokinase to generate glucose-6-phosphate [25]. Glycolytic and oxidative metabolism of glucose elevates the cytosolic adenosine triphosphate/adenosine diphosphate (ATP/ADP) ratio. This closes ATP-sensitive potassium channels in the cell membrane. The resulting depolarization triggers opening of voltage-gated calcium channels. Increased intracellular calcium concentration allows the fusion of insulin-containing granules with plasma membrane and the subsequent release of stored insulin through interactions with Ca^{2+}-sensitive proteins (Fig. 2.1).

- *Initiators of insulin secretion* – These induce insulin secretion both by triggering, i.e. involving closure of the K_{ATP} channels, and amplifying effects.
- *Potentiators of insulin secretion* – The incretin hormone glucagon-like peptide (GLP)-1 (see below) and arginine do not initiate insulin secretion by themselves, but enhance insulin secretion in the presence of an initiator, e.g. glucose.

Even in the unstimulated (basal) state, insulin secretion is continually tuned by numerous stimulatory and inhibitory signals [26]. Insulin secretion is influenced by central neural activity [27] and paracrine factors [28, 29]. Autocrine regulation of insulin secretion has been proposed [30, 31], although the physiological relevance of such a mechanism in humans has been questioned [32].

Glucose-stimulated insulin secretion to a rapid and sustained increment in plasma glucose is characteristically biphasic (Fig. 2.2) [33]. A transient first phase of insulin secretion with an early peak is followed by a gradually developing and more prolonged second phase. It has been suggested that the first phase may represent release of insulin from rapidly mobilized storage granules, triggered by the influx of Ca^{2+}; the second phase of insulin secretion may reflect ATP-dependent recruitment and release of granules

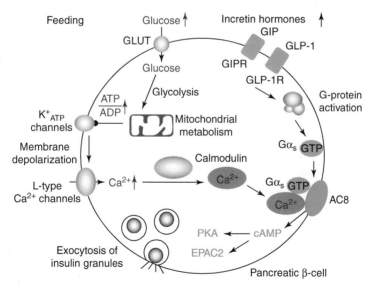

Fig. 2.1 Insulin secretion after a meal is typically initiated by a rise in extracellular glucose, which is detected by a metabolic signalling pathway. Aerobic glycolysis and mitochondrial oxidation produce metabolic signals, such as a rise in the ATP to ADP concentration ratio. This closes K+ATP-channels, depolarizes the plasma membrane and causes calcium influx that stimulates exocytosis. At the same time, the incretin hormones GLP-1 and GIP bind to their receptors, which are highly expressed on human pancreatic β-cells. This causes the activation of G proteins. The glucose and GLP1 signalling pathways converge on AC8, an isoform of adenylate cyclase that is abundant in pancreatic β-cells and fully activated when both Gαs–GTP and calcium–calmodulin are bound. The subsequent rise in cellular cAMP triggers exocytosis by protein kinase A (PKA) and EPAC2 (also known as RAPGEF4) (Reprinted by permission from β-cells Macmillan Publishers Ltd: Nature Cell Biology, Integrating insulin secretion and ER stress in pancreatic β-cells, K Lemaire and F Schuit, copyright 2012)

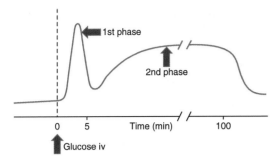

Fig. 2.2 Glucose-induced insulin secretion. A rapid first phase is followed by a slower and more sustained second phase of insulin release. *iv* intravenous. The biphasic response is observed in response to acute sustained experimental hyperglycaemia as induced by the hyperglycaemic clamp technique. See DeFronzo et al. [33] for methodological details

from a reserve pool [5, 34]. The relevance of first-phase insulin secretion to glucose homeostasis in human physiology remains uncertain [35].

Role of the Incretin System in Insulin Secretion

At matched plasma glucose concentrations, orally ingested glucose elicits a substantially greater insulin secretory response than intravenous glucose; this is the so-called incretin effect [36]. The main incretin hormones, GLP-1 and glucose-dependent insulinotropic polypeptide (GIP), are released from intestinal endocrine cells (L cells and K cells, respectively) within minutes of nutrient ingestion. The potentiation of glucose-stimulated insulin secretion by the incretin hormones may account for approximately 50–70 % of postprandial insulin secretion [37, 38]. GLP-1 and GIP circulating in the blood are rapidly inactivated via enzymatic cleavage by dipeptidyl peptidase 4 (DPP-4) [39, 40]. GLP-1 and GIP act via specific G-protein-coupled cellular receptors to raise intracellular levels of cyclic adenosine monophosphate (AMP) and inhibit ATP-sensitive K^+ channels, actions which induce β-cell exocytosis of insulin (see Fig. 2.1) [41]. Incretin-mediated augmentation of insulin secretion and inhibition of glucagon secretion are dependent on ambient glucose concentrations [42]. In addition, GLP-1 reduces gastric emptying, increases satiety and reduces food intake [43] as well as stimulating the transcription of glucokinase and the GLUT 2 transporter gene [44].

Defects in incretin axis physiology are implicated in the pathogenesis of type 2 diabetes. Delineation of these defects has led to the development of important new classes of glucose-lowering drugs, i.e. the DPP-4 inhibitors and GLP-1 analogues [40]. Reported reductions in GLP-1 responses in patients with type 2 diabetes provided the theoretical basis for these incretin-based glucose-lowering drugs [45]. The impact of hyperglycaemia and incretin effect on insulin secretion and β-cell function continues to be unravelled [46, 47]. In a placebo-controlled study of subjects ($n=22$) with impaired fasting glucose, sitagliptin increased intact circulating GLP-1 concentrations but had no effect on postprandial plasma glucose, insulin or C-peptide concentrations [48]. While the secretion of GIP is near normal in patients with type 2 diabetes, the effect of this incretin on insulin secretion, particularly the late phase, is impaired [38].

Hepatic Clearance of Insulin

Insulin and C-peptide are co-secreted into blood that is directed to the portal vein, and insulin directly regulates hepatic glucose metabolism [16]. Hepatic first-pass clearance of insulin removes >50 % of insulin ensuring that the portal:systemic insulin gradient is 2:1 or higher. Insulin clearance, of which hepatic extraction is the main determinant, may be altered in common metabolic diseases [49] and possibly by certain glucose-lowering drugs [50]. Since it is not cleared by the liver, the serum concentration of C-peptide in the peripheral circulation provides a more reliable indicator of endogenous insulin secretion. The most robust assessment of dynamic β-cell insulin secretion would require blood samples drawn directly from the hepatic portal vein. Such a highly invasive approach is not feasible in clinical research, although the technique has been applied in nonhuman primate studies [51]. Prehepatic insulin secretion may be estimated by mathematical deconvolution of serum C-peptide in peripheral blood (see below) [52]. The half-life of serum C-peptide is longer than that of insulin (~20–30 vs. ~3–5 min). During dynamic tests of insulin secretion, the longer half-life in the circulation of serum C-peptide requires that blood sampling time points for measurement of C-peptide be adjusted relative to those for insulin. Impaired renal function reduces C-peptide clearance [53].

β-Cell Dysfunction in the Pathogenesis of Diabetes

Glucose metabolism is regulated via a feedback loop between islet β-cells and insulin-sensitive target tissues [54]. Within this physiological regulatory system, the sensitivity of the liver and muscle cells to insulin modulates the β-cell response [55]. When insulin resistance develops, usually due to combinations of genetic and lifestyle factors, β-cells maintain normal glucose tolerance via an appropriate increase in endogenous insulin secretion [56]. According to a widely accepted model of the pathogenesis of type 2 diabetes, hyperglycaemia results when sufficient amounts of insulin cannot be secreted to fully compensate for insulin resistance (see below) [55, 57]. In this scenario, the relative contributions of decreased β-cell mass versus decreased β-cell function remain uncertain [58]. In humans, β-cell mass increases through cellular proliferation during the first decade of life before stabilizing during adolescence [59]. In adulthood, hyperplasia and hypertrophy permit a degree of plasticity in compensation for insulin resistance [60]. If issues of sensitivity and precision can be resolved [61], quantitative imaging techniques, e.g. fluorescent exendin-4 derivatives [61, 62], may eventually complement conventional metabolic approaches for estimating β-cell mass [63]. Type 1 diabetes and type 2 diabetes are both characterized by progressive β-cell destruction (see below) in which apoptosis (programmed cell death) predominates. Since a low rate of β-cell turnover may continue throughout the human lifespan, β-cell number will fall if the rate of apoptosis or dedifferentiation is increased relative to neogenesis [64, 65].

Type 1 Diabetes

Selective immune destruction of β-cells is the principal pathogenic defect of type 1 diabetes [66]. The resulting insulin deficiency necessitates lifelong replacement therapy with subcutaneous administration of insulin or insulin analogues (or a successful pancreas or islet transplant). However, recent data suggest that even patients with type 1 diabetes of long duration may have low levels of residual insulin secretion [67, 68].

In clinical trials of patients with type 1 diabetes, β-cell function is commonly assessed by the serum C-peptide response to intravenous glucagon [69] or a mixed meal [70]. Glucagon is injected as an intravenous bolus with timed measurements of serum C-peptide [69]. The glucagon stimulation test may also be of value in clinical practice when therapeutic decisions may be are informed by assessment of endogenous insulin secretion [71].

Type 2 Diabetes

Islet β-cell insufficiency is central to the development and progression of type 2 diabetes. A decline in β-cell function antedates and predicts the onset of clinical diabetes [61]. Genetic and environmental factors are strongly implicated [55]. Characterization of defective insulin secretion in the precursor states of impaired fasting glucose (IFG) and impaired glucose tolerance (IGT) has provided valuable insights into the pathogenesis of type 2 diabetes [72]. In the United Kingdom Prospective Diabetes Study (UKPDS), β-cell function, determined using a modelling method (HOMA-B, see below), was reduced by approximately 50 % in middle-aged subjects at the time of diagnosis [73]. This is in line with estimates based on autopsies place the reduction of β-cell mass at approximately 40–65 % at the time of clinical presentation of type 2 diabetes [74]. A reduction in functional β-cell mass is evident during the long preclinical phase of type 2 diabetes. In parallel, the regulation of blood glucose both postprandially and in the fasting state deteriorates through stages of glucose intolerance before rising to levels diagnostic of diabetes. Insulin secretion rates rise through the range between normal glucose tolerance to IGT and decline thereafter [75]. Longitudinal studies have demonstrated progressive and variable, but not inevitable, loss of β-cell function in patients with type 2 diabetes [76, 77]. As the number of β-cells per islet falls, plaques of amyloid fibrils, which may contribute to β-cell loss, are deposited [78, 79]. Hyperglycaemia (glucotoxicity), both acute [80] and chronic [81], and prolonged elevations of plasma concentration of nonesterified ('free') fatty acid concentrations (lipotoxicity) [82] are detrimental to β-cell function and viability [10, 83]. Oxidative and endoplasmic reticulum stress together with inflammation have been identified as pathways to β-cell loss that are potentially amenable to targeted therapeutic interventions [84]. As hyperglycaemia develops, insulin pulses are attenuated [85] and circulating levels of proinsulin and partially processed proinsulin products become are elevated, albeit remaining at low concentrations relative to insulin [86]. Loss of acute glucose-stimulated insulin secretion is accompanied by alterations in β-cell phenotype and in gene and protein expression.

Uncommon monogenic forms of diabetes in which β-cell defects have been well delineated, e.g. forms of maturity-onset diabetes of the young (MODY) [87, 88], contrast with the complexity of type 2 diabetes in which the relative contributions of genetic, epigenetic and nongenetic factors to β-cell failure remain uncertain [61, 89]. To date, the utility of molecular genetics in identifying personalized therapeutic approaches for diabetes has been confined to relatively small subgroups of patients. Diabetes due to hepatic nuclear factor-1α mutations is especially sensitive to sulphonylureas [90]. Neonatal diabetes due to rare activating mutations in genes encoding the ATP-sensitive potassium channel subunits Kir6.2 or SUR1 can be successfully treated with high-dose sulphonylureas [90].

Strategies to Improve β-Cell Function for the Treatment and Prevention of Diabetes

Type 1 Diabetes

The causes of type 1 are complex and multifactorial, involving genetic and environmental factors [91]. The natural history of type 1 diabetes involves a prolonged and variable latent preclinical period that culminates in the destruction of pancreatic β-cells [92]. When autoimmune-mediated β-cell loss reaches a critical point, hyperglycaemia develops. A temporary partial recovery of β-cell function may occur after initiation of insulin therapy – the so-called honeymoon period – before waning again thereafter. A diverse range of strategies for averting type 1 diabetes (primary prevention) or preserving β-cell function in subjects with recently diagnosed type 1 diabetes (secondary prevention) have been explored in clinical trials [93]. Examples of interventions directed at arresting the immune process include nicotinamide, insulin injections, oral insulin, nasal insulin, glutamic acid decarboxylase, cyclosporine, teplizumab and abatacept [93]. These challenging intervention studies have been aided by the development of biomarkers of autoimmunity [94] and serial tests of β-cell function [95]. The latter include the mixed meal tolerance test (see below) and glucagon-stimulated serum C-peptide response; these methods should not be assumed to provide equivalent results [96]. Recent research has shown that endogenous glucagon dynamics are also altered early in the course of type 1 diabetes with elevated levels in response to a mixed meal challenge [97]. The plurality of aforementioned therapeutic targets attests to the complex pathophysiology of β-cell attrition in type 1 diabetes. Novel non-immunomodulatory strategies are being explored. For example, preclinical evidence suggests that verapamil, a calcium channel blocker used for the treatment of hypertension and cardiac arrhythmias, may enhance β-cell survival and function [98]. In a recent study of patients with newly diagnosed type 1 diabetes the lipid-modifying agent atorvastatin appeared to slow the decline of β-cell function (stimulated C-peptide secretion), in a subgroup defined by higher levels of inflammation-associated immune mediators [99].

Type 2 Diabetes

In obese subjects with glucose intolerance behavioural interventions that indirectly improve insulin secretion reduce the risk of progression to diabetes [100]. Many drugs have been shown to increase insulin secretion in vitro, but few have therapeutic potential [101]. Thiazolidinediones, which do not directly stimulate insulin secretion, have also been shown to improve β-cell function and reduce the risk of new-onset diabetes in insulin-resistant women with a history of gestational diabetes [102]. The latter observation illustrates the pathophysiological relevance of the feedback loop between insulin secretion and insulin action [103]. Lifestyle modification is the cornerstone of controlling hyperglycaemia in established type 2 diabetes [104]. Bariatric surgery procedures [105] or voluntary dietary calorie restriction of a sufficient degree can rapidly lower blood glucose concentrations and improve β-cell function [106]. A doubling of β-cell function in obese patients with type 2 diabetes 1 year after gastric bypass surgery has been reported [107]. When standard behavioural changes prove insufficient, pharmacotherapy is required to control hyperglycaemia. Sulphonylureas have the mainstay of pharmacological strategies to enhance insulin secretion for decades [108]. Agents in this class act primarily by blocking ATP-sensitive potassium channels in the β-cells thereby stimulating insulin release [109]. Dipeptidyl peptidase (DPP)-4 inhibitors, which potentiate insulin secretion in a glucose-dependent fashion by reducing the breakdown of GLP-1, have superior safety and tolerability profiles to sulphonylureas [110]. Unlike sulphonylureas, which continue to stimulate insulin secretion even during hypoglycaemia [111], DPP-4 inhibitors and GLP-1 analogues promote insulin exocytosis only when blood glucose levels are elevated.

This property reduces the risk of hypoglycaemia when these drugs are used as monotherapy or in combination with other agents that have a low propensity to cause hypoglycaemia [112, 113]. Preclinical data suggesting effects of DPP-4 inhibitors on functional β-cell mass and pancreatic insulin content in rodent models raised hopes that the natural history of type 2 diabetes might be modified [114]. The UKPDS demonstrated an inexorable loss of β-cell function with sulphonylureas and insulin [73]. As yet, however, there is no firm evidence from clinical studies that GLP-1 agonists [115] or DPP-4 inhibitors [114] have durable effects on β-cell function. Progressive loss of β-cell function is regarded as the main reason that many patients with type 2 diabetes ultimately require insulin replacement therapy [73]. The hypothesis that β-cell function may be preserved by using specific combinations of glucose-lowering drugs is being tested in clinical trials [116]. New drugs designed to improve β-cell function that have entered clinical trials in recent years include:

- DDP-4 inhibitors (including agents requiring only once-weekly dosing) [117]
- Novel GLP-1 agonists [118] (including new delivery routes) [119]
- Bile acid sequestrants with indirect effects on incretin secretion [120]
- GPR40 agonists [121]
- GPR119 agonists [122]
- Unimolecular dual agonists of GLP-1 and GIP [118, 123]
- Glucokinase activators [124]
- Interleukin-1 β antagonists [125] (Table 2.1)

In parallel, potential cardioprotective actions of GLP-1, highly attractive in the context of the enhanced risk of cardiovascular disease in type 2 diabetes, have also been explored [126]. A novel hypothesis that extends to the broader cardiometabolic risk profile of patients with type 2 diabetes is that strategies to raise high-density lipoprotein (HDL) levels may improve β-cell function [127]. The cholesteryl ester transfer protein inhibitor torcetrapib improved glycaemic control in atorvastatin-treated patients with

Table 2.1 Current and future pharmaceutical agents with direct or indirect actions on islet β-cells for the treatment of diabetes

Primary pharmacological effect on β-cells[a]	
Insulinotropic agents	
Sulphonylureas[b]	Direct: closure of K_{ATP} channels; stimulation of insulin secretion
Meglitinides	Direct: closure of K_{ATP} channels; stimulation of insulin secretion
DPP-4 inhibitors	Indirect: elevation of GLP-1 levels; potentiation of insulin secretion
Incretin mimetics[c]	Direct: stimulation of GLP-1 receptors; potentiation of insulin secretion
Insulin sensitizers	
Metformin	Indirect: reduction in insulin resistance; elevation of GLP-1 levels
Thiazolidinediones	Indirect: reduction in insulin resistance; reduction in lipotoxicity
Glucose-lowering drugs with non-insulin-dependent actions	
α-glucosidase inhibitors	Indirect: reduction in glucotoxicity
SGLT-2 inhibitors	Indirect: reduction in glucotoxicity
Insulin; insulin analogues	Indirect: reduction in glucotoxicity
Potential agents and/or targets for future treatment of type 2 diabetes	
Bile acid sequestrants	Indirect: stimulation of intestinal GLP-1 secretion
GPR40 agonists	Direct: activation of FFA1 receptor
GPR119 agonists	Direct and indirect: activation of GPR119 receptor; activation of incretin axis
Dual GLP-1/GIP agonists	Direct: stimulation of GLP-1 and GIP receptors
Glucokinase activators	Direct: activation of glucose-sensing enzyme glucokinase
IL-1β antagonist	Direct: reduced intracellular cytokine signalling
HDL lipoproteins[d]	Direct: calcium-dependent insulin secretion

DPP-4 dipeptidyl peptidase, *FFA* free fatty acid, *GIP* glucose-dependent insulinotropic peptide, *IL* interleukin
[a]Multiple mechanisms may contribute to effects on insulin secretion for some drugs. Furthermore, not all putative mechanisms have been demonstrated in humans to date
[b]High-dose sulphonylureas are also used in the treatment of neonatal diabetes due to activating mutations in genes encoding the ATP-sensitive potassium channel subunits Kir6.2 or SUR1
[c]Glucagon-like peptide (GLP)-1 receptor agonists
[d]HDL (high-density lipoprotein), apolipoprotein-A-I, apolipoprotein-A-II

type 2 diabetes. However, it remains to be determined whether this effect was a direct consequence of raising HDL levels [128]. Further elucidation of the molecular regulation of β-cell mass and function offers the prospect of additional therapeutic agents to preserve insulin secretion [129].

Other Drugs with Effects on β-Cell Function

In the design of studies of novel therapies for diabetes, the potential for confounding by drugs that have effects on β-cell function should be carefully considered (Tables 2.1 and 2.2). In studies of new pharmacological entities for type 2 diabetes, individuals who are treatment naïve or on stable metformin monotherapy are preferred (see Chap. 9). Washing off sulphonylureas and DPP-4 inhibitors is a routine practice in early-phase studies of diabetes drugs although careful monitoring of glycaemic control is required according to regulatory guidelines [130]. When thiazolidinediones [131] or GLP-1 analogues [132] are temporarily withdrawn, a sufficient length of time is required to ensure that the any metabolic effects of these drugs have fully dissipated [130].

Aside from glucose-lowering medications, many patients with diabetes are treated with antihypertensive and lipid-modifying drugs that may have class-specific effects to either increase or decrease endogenous insulin secretion [133, 134]. Recent reports of adverse effects of statins on glucose metabolism are pertinent in this context [135]. Certain statins may affect insulin secretion through direct and/or indirect effects on β-cell calcium channels [136].

Table 2.2 Selected drugs commonly used in the treatment of disorders other than diabetes with reported direct effects on β-cell function

Effect on insulin secretion	
Anti-hypertensive drugs	
β-adrenergic blockers[a]	Decreased
Angiotensin-converting enzyme inhibitors	Increased
Angiotensin receptor	Increased
Calcium channel blockers[b,c]	Decreased
Imidazoline agonists	Increased
Diazoxide[b]	Decreased
Lipid-modifying drugs	
Statins[d]	Decreased
Antipsychotic drugs	
Second-generation antipsychotic agents[d]	Decreased
Calcineurin inhibitors	
Cyclosporine, tacrolimus	Decreased
Somatostatin receptor agonists[b]	
Octreotide, lanreotide	Decreased

[a]Nonselective β-adrenergic blockers impair β-cell function, whereas β-blockers with vasodilator activity may improve insulin secretion
[b]These drugs or individual members of the class have been used in the treatment of endogenous and/or iatrogenic hyperinsulinaemia
[c]Nifedipine has been used in the treatment of hyperinsulinaemia. Other calcium channels blockers, e.g. amlodipine, reportedly have neutral effects on insulin secretion
[d]Differences may be evident between drugs within the class. Current evidence incomplete and of uncertain significance in the context of drug-induced diabetes. Other iatrogenic metabolic defects, e.g. impaired insulin sensitivity, may coexist with effects on insulin secretion

Clinical Research Methods for Quantifying β-Cell Function

No consensus exists on a reference method for assessing endogenous insulin secretion in humans [103]. It has been argued that conclusions concerning insulin secretion and the impact of therapeutic interventions may vary according to the use of different methodologies [137]. Each of the commonly used methods focuses on a defined facet of β-cell function [138]. Assessment of β-cell function may be undertaken either in the basal, i.e. non-stimulated state, or following challenge with various secretagogues, either in isolation or combination [139]. The administered stimuli may be either physiological, i.e. a test meal of known macronutrient composition, or pharmacological, e.g. intravenous injection of glucose or arginine.

The advent of the therapeutic era of incretin mimetics has focused attention on the incretin axis and broader aspects of islet function. The effect of DPP-4 inhibitors on insulin secretion is indirect, mediated through improvements in incretin axis signalling [140]. Comprehensive evaluation of a novel incretin mimetic requires assessment of both the incretin axis and the resulting effect on insulin secretion [37]. Approximately 30–50 % of circulating GLP-1 in the postprandial state consists of active GLP-1, the rest being the inactive truncated fragment [141]. During treatment with DPP-4 inhibitors, the relative proportion of the active form of the hormone, i.e. GLP-1_{7-36}, is increased [142]. DPP-4 inhibitors preferentially lower postprandial glucose, with less marked effects on fasting hyperglycaemia [110]. Metformin [143] and α-glucosidase inhibitors [144] have also been shown to increase circulating GLP-1 levels. Part of the glucose-lowering effect of incretin mimetics is mediated via reductions in glucagon secretion [145–147]. Clinical methods for the assessment of α-cell function are not as sophisticated as those directed towards β-cell function [72]. The glucagon receptor has been identified as a therapeutic target for type 2 diabetes [148]. However, toxicity issues including elevations in hepatic transaminases direc and plasma lipids have been reported with glucagon receptor antagonists [148].

Non-stimulated (Basal) Assessments

Fasting Insulin and/or C-Peptide

The feedback loop between the β-cells and insulin-responsive tissues requires that circulating insulin concentrations be interpreted in the context of the prevailing blood glucose level. Changes in both insulin sensitivity and β-cell function are evident as glucose tolerance deteriorates [149]. When fasting hyperglycaemia is present, the predicted level of hyperinsulinaemia would be higher if β-cells were able to fully overcome any defect in insulin action through compensatory increased insulin secretion [150].

Demonstration of an effect on residual β-cell function is an important consideration in studies of new drug therapies for type 2 diabetes. This is most readily accomplished by measurement of serum or plasma C-peptide after an overnight fast. Several classes of diabetes drugs either stimulate insulin secretion (e.g. sulphonylureas, DPP-4 inhibitors) or require the presence of sufficient insulin to exert their glucose-lowering effects (e.g. metformin, thiazolidinediones) [108]. Exceptions include α-glucosidase inhibitors [151] and sodium glucose cotransporter 2 (SGLT2) inhibitors [152].

Proinsulin

The use of insulin-specific immunoradiometric assays eliminates cross-reactivity with proinsulin and partially processed proinsulin molecules [153]. Loss of the normal pulsatile oscillations in insulin secretion [85] and increased ratios of circulating proinsulin to insulin [153, 154] are regarded as markers of compromised β-cell function in prediabetic states of glucose intolerance. In patients with type 2 diabetes, the ratio of proinsulin to insulin is inversely related to β-cell function [155]. In studies of an insulin secretagogue and an insulin sensitizer in patients with type 2 diabetes, a differential effect of the two classes of glucose-lowering drugs was observed on plasma proinsulin and the proinsulin to immunoreactive insulin ratio [155]. Glibenclamide (glyburide) increased, whereas rosiglitazone decreased, the concentration of proinsulin and the proinsulin-to-insulin ratio [155]. In a 12-month head-to-head study of these two drugs, rosiglitazone reduced the concentrations of insulin, proinsulin and split proinsulin compared to glibenclamide [156]. As expected, rosiglitazone improved insulin sensitivity, whereas glibenclamide therapy was associated with worsening insulin resistance [156]. These results were replicated in ADOPT (A Diabetes Outcome Progression Trial) [157]. Over the 4-year course of ADOPT, rosiglitazone had more favourable effects on β-cell function than glibenclamide [158]. The improvements in β-cell function with rosiglitazone, which were accompanied by a decrease in insulin resistance, were associated with a more durable effect on glycaemic control [157, 158]. Whether the beneficial effects of rosiglitazone on β-cell function were indirect via improved insulin sensitivity or resulted from a direct β-cell action [159] could not be determined from this study (see below). Metformin, which was also studied in ADOPT, had effects on β-cell function and glycaemic control that were intermediate to those observed with rosiglitazone and glibenclamide [157, 158].

HOMA-B

Homeostasis model assessment is a method for assessing insulin secretory capacity from fasting plasma insulin and glucose concentrations. HOMA-B has been widely applied in clinical metabolic research, including diabetes drug development.

$$\text{HOMA } \beta\text{-cell function} = \frac{20 \times \text{insulin}\,(\text{mU}/\text{L})}{\text{glucose}\,(\text{mmol}/\text{L}) - 3.5}$$

An early study of diabetic and nondiabetic subjects reported a coefficient of variation (CV) for HOMA-B measured on two occasions of approximately 30–40 % [160]. Subsequent studies using specific insulin assays in larger samples have yielded CVs closer to 10 % [138]. The use of triplicate samples may improve the CV with smaller sample sizes [138]. In comparative studies, HOMA-B has been shown to correlate with measures of insulin secretion obtained using the hyperglycaemic clamp (see below) in diabetic ($r=0.59$) and nondiabetic subjects ($r=0.71$) [160]. Since HOMA values are rarely normally distributed, the data should be logarithmically transformed and presented as geometric means with appropriate measures of dispersion.

The HOMA model apportions the basal state of insulin and glucose in terms of insulin resistance and β-cell function [138]. Insulin sensitivity and insulin secretion are mutually related as a hyperbolic function in which insulin resistance is compensated by increased insulin secretion [54, 103]. Reporting HOMA-B data in isolation, i.e. without considering the prevailing level of insulin sensitivity for the individual, could lead to erroneous conclusions about β-cell function [103, 138]. The validity of assumptions inherent in HOMA-B has been challenged [161]. It has been argued that measures of β-cell function and insulin sensitivity should be as independent as possible; clearly, HOMA does not satisfy this requirement [103]. HOMA-B is a measure of β-cell activity rather than health; accordingly, the temporary improvement observed in response to a classic secretagogue, i.e. a sulphonylurea, should be regarded as reflecting the mechanism of action of the drug rather than any intrinsic change in functional capacity [73].

HOMA-B provides an index of insulin secretory capacity in the non-stimulated state at serum insulin levels primarily of relevance to hepatic glucose regulation [162]. This focus may detract from the ability of HOMA-B to quantify defective β-cell function relative to dynamic tests. In the Insulin Resistance Atherosclerosis Study (IRAS), HOMA-B underestimated the magnitude of the β-cell defect in subjects with IGT and newly diagnosed diabetes compared with the acute insulin response assessed using an intravenous glucose challenge (see below) [163]. In a study in which insulin secretion was compared with pancreatic histology, the glucose-stimulated C-peptide-to-glucose ratio appeared to predict β-cell area better than HOMA [164]. With these caveats in mind, HOMA-B offers a simple and useful approach for assessing β-cell function that can be of value in evaluating the actions of new diabetes drugs. For example, the insulin sensitizer pioglitazone lowers blood glucose in patients with type 2 diabetes primarily by improving insulin action [131]. Thiazolidinediones also improve β-cell function through indirect mechanisms, an effect demonstrable as an increase in HOMA-B [165]. For DDP-4 inhibitors, which primarily enhance postprandial insulin secretion, an oral glucose challenge would be more logical than an assessment of fasting β-cell function. However, in a recent meta-analysis of placebo-controlled clinical trials of sitagliptin, improved β-cell function was evident as an increased HOMA-B index [166]. Note that HOMA-B cannot be used in patients treated with exogenous insulin.

Dynamic Tests of β-Cell Function

Oral Glucose Tolerance Test

The 75 g oral glucose tolerance test (OGTT) is the reference method for diagnosing diabetes and other categories of glucose dysregulation [167]. Thus, regression from one diagnostic category to another, e.g. IGT to normal glucose tolerance, in response to therapy can be determined. For example, in the DREAM (Diabetes Reduction Assessment with Ramipril and Rosiglitazone Medication) study in adults with IFG and/or IGT, rosiglitazone significantly reduced the incidence of type 2 diabetes and increased the likelihood of regression to normoglycaemia compared to placebo [168].

The OGTT can also provide an integrated assessment to the β-cell response to an intestinal glucose stimulus that includes activation of the incretin axis. As discussed above, the incretin effect on the islets includes enhancement of glucose-stimulated insulin secretion in concert with reduced glucagon release [169]. When assessing the response to therapeutic agents whose primary mode of action is mediated via the incretin axis, e.g. DDP-4 inhibitors, the response of the major incretin hormones (GLP-1, GIP) can be quantified and related to the stimulation of insulin secretion and suppression of glucagon secretion. For example, in a placebo-controlled crossover study performed in patients with type 2 diabetes, a single oral dose of sitagliptin (25 mg or 200 mg) dose-dependently inhibited plasma DPP-4 activity over 24 h [170]. Sitagliptin increased active levels of GLP-1 and GIP, increased serum insulin and C-peptide levels, decreased plasma glucagon levels and reduced the rise in blood glucose during a 75 g OGTT [170].

For paired comparisons, the area under the curve (AUC) for serum insulin (or C-peptide) offers a simple exploratory assessment of the change in endogenous insulin secretion in response to a therapeutic intervention that incorporates early and later phases of insulin release. Consideration should be given to the methods used for data analysis in this scenario [171]. Since the OGTT is not standardized in terms of attained blood glucose concentrations, methods for normalizing insulin secretion to the glucose stimulus have been developed. A number of empirical indexes of modelling approaches have been proposed which relate insulin responses to increments in blood glucose. For example, the *insulinogenic index*, which reportedly correlates with first-phase insulin release assessed using an intravenous glucose bolus, is calculated as the ratio of the increment of insulin to glucose above baseline 30 min (Δinsulin/Δglucose) after an oral glucose challenge [172]. In ADOPT [157] (see above), the insulinogenic index was used to study the β-cell responses to rosiglitazone, glibenclamide and metformin. A higher acute change in the insulinogenic index was observed over the first 6 months with glibenclamide than with rosiglitazone or metformin [158]. Thereafter, glibenclamide was associated with a significantly faster rate of decline in insulinogenic index versus rosiglitazone (11.1 vs. 6.0 % per year), the decline with metformin being intermediate. Despite the fact that glibenclamide is a classic insulin secretagogue, the mean insulinogenic index with glibenclamide was lower than those in the other treatment groups beyond 2 years [158]. Patients who failed monotherapy (with any agent) had a lower median insulinogenic index at baseline compared to those who completed the 4-year trial [158]. High within-subject variability for the insulinogenic index has been reported [173] which should be considered in the design of studies with smaller sample sizes.

Mixed Meal Tolerance Test

The mixed meal tolerance test (MMTT) has the advantage over the OGTT of providing a more physiological assessment of β-cell function. The β-cell response to a meal of varied macronutrient composition is complex and includes activation of the incretin system and direct contributions of glucose and other stimuli the phases of insulin secretion to the overall β-cell response cannot be readily identified. The MMTT is a relatively straightforward procedure requiring only an overnight fast. This, like the OGTT, makes it suitable for use in an outpatient research setting. However, admission to a clinical research facility 1–2 days in advance is recommended in order that preceding meals and physical activity levels can be standardized. This precaution helps to reduce the impact of these sources of variability, a principle that pertains to any quantitative test of β-cell function.

Test meals of specified macronutrient composition can be prepared in a metabolic kitchen. Alternatively, proprietary liquid nutritional products may be used, e.g. Sustacal (Mead Johnson Nutritionals, Greenville, IL, USA). The MMTT has been widely applied in drug development studies. For example, Cosma et al. used a 500 kcal test meal to assess the insulinogenic index (Δinsulin30/Δglucose30) and AUC for insulin in response to the meglitinide derivative repaglinide in doses of 0.5, 1, 2 and 4 mg versus placebo in patients with diet-treated type 2 diabetes [174]. Dose-dependent increases in insulin secretion were noted. On subgroup analysis, incremental insulin responses were apparent only in patients who had a fasting plasma glucose <9 mmol/L (162 mg/dL) [174]. In a 24-week placebo-controlled study conducted in metformin-treated patients with type 2 diabetes, sitagliptin 100 mg daily led to a reduction in glycated haemoglobin (haemoglobin A_{1c}, HbA_{1c}) which was associated with improved post-meal serum insulin and C-peptide AUCs and in post-meal insulin AUC-to-glucose AUC ratio ($p<0.001$ for all) [175]. Fasting serum insulin, fasting serum C-peptide, fasting proinsulin-to-insulin ratio and HOMA-B were also significantly improved by sitagliptin [175]. Ahren et al. performed a mechanistic study in patients with type 2 diabetes in which placebo or vildagliptin (50 mg daily) was added to metformin (1.5–3.0 mg/day) [176]. In patients who completed 52 weeks ($n=57$), HbA_{1c} decreased in the vildagliptin/metformin group ($n=31$) but increased in the placebo/metformin group. In response to a standardized 465 kcal breakfast, insulin secretion (post-meal suprabasal area under the 0–30 min C-peptide curve divided by the 30 min increase in plasma glucose) increased in the vildagliptin-treated group but was reduced in the patients who received placebo (Fig. 2.3). Insulin sensitivity during meal ingestion (assessed using a modelling method) [177] increased in the vildagliptin treatment group but

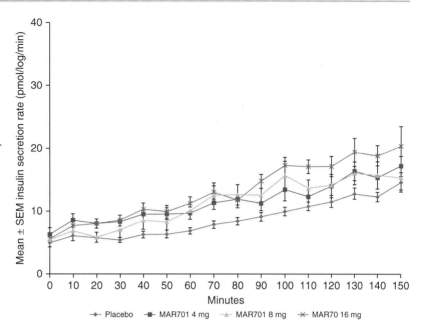

Fig. 2.3 Effect of exenatide (Byetta®; 5A) and MAR701 (a dual agonist of glucagon-like peptide-1/glucose-dependent insulinotropic peptide; 5B) on insulin secretion rate in healthy volunteers ($n=6$ for each). $p<0.0001$ for exenatide vs. placebo and $p<0.0001$ for MAR701 vs. placebo at each step (From Hompesch et al. [205] with permission)

was not altered with placebo. Insulin secretion related to insulin sensitivity (i.e. adaptation index) increased in the patients in the vildagliptin group but decreased in those in the placebo group. The change in adaptation index correlated to the change in HbA$_{1C}$ ($r=-0.39$, $p=0.004$) which was interpreted as supporting improved β-cell function in the improvement observed in glucose metabolism [176].

An *oral minimal model method* has been proposed for the estimation of β-cell responses along with insulin sensitivity and hepatic insulin extraction from an MMTT (or an OGTT) [178]. Proponents argue that the oral minimal model is both more physiological and simpler to administer than the intravenous alternatives, e.g. the intravenous glucose tolerance test and the glucose clamp technique (see below).

Intravenous Glucose Tolerance Test

The intravenous glucose tolerance test (IVGTT) measures direct β-cell responses to glucose in the absence of the modulating effect of the incretin axis. Thus, the IVGTT provides at best a partial assessment of β-cell physiology. During an IVGTT, the subject lies supine or semi-supine. After an overnight fast, basal blood samples for measurement of glucose, insulin and C-peptide are drawn at t −10 and −5 min. At 0 min, a bolus of glucose (0.3 g/kg body weight given as a 50 % solution in sterile water) is administered via an intravenous line and completed within 2 min. The cannula is then flushed with 20–30 mL 0.9 % sterile saline to reduce the risk of venous irritation and thrombosis. Blood samples are withdrawn at 2, 4, 6, 8 and 10 min. As discussed above, the early phase – or acute – insulin response, during the first 5–10 min, is held to reflect the rapid release of insulin from storage granules into the circulation [34]. The acute insulin response (AIR) is defined as the increment of insulin above the baseline, i.e. fasting level. Several aspects of the IVGTT have been standardized to reduce variability between tests, including glucose load and the timing of sample collection [179].

The AIR is dependent on the stimulus, i.e. the glucose load and the increase in blood glucose concentration. The latter will vary as a function of the insulin sensitivity of the individual, even if the glucose bolus is standardized. For this reason, comparisons of AIR between groups of subjects with different degrees of insulin sensitivity should be made with caution [103]. The pathophysiological significance of a reduced AIR, as derived using the IVGTT, has been the subject of debate. Individuals may still show a response to oral glucose in the absence of a discernable acute phase insulin response during an IVGTT [180, 181]. If the caveat is accepted that an impaired AIR may have limited relevance to broader aspects of β-cell function, then the AIR may nevertheless be a useful marker of response to a therapeutic intervention. For example, Fehse et al. demonstrated restoration of impaired first-phase insulin secretion with intravenous exenatide during an IVGTT in patients with type 2 diabetes [182]. Second-phase insulin secretion was also improved in this study [182]. A mechanistic study of the DPP-4 inhibitor vildagliptin for 6 weeks in subjects with impaired fasting glucose showed an improved AIR ($p<0.05$) during an IVGTT together with a decrease in glucose AUC in response to a MMTT ($p=0.002$) [183]. The improvement in first-phase insulin secretion using a method that excludes acute activation of the incretin axis, i.e. the IVGTT, suggests a therapeutic effect of vildagliptin indepedent of acute elevation of incretin hormones. While the mechanism remains uncertain, a concomitant improvement in insulin sensitivity (S_I) suggests that multiple aspects of metabolism may be influenced by DPP-4 inhibition. A reduction in glucose toxicity has been hypothesized [183].

The IVGTT has also been used extensively in prevention studies of type 1 diabetes. Using data from the Diabetes Prevention Trial Type 1 (DPT-1) which involved serial IVGTT data, Sosenko et al. observed a distinct pattern of first-phase insulin response among subjects identified as being at elevated risk who progressed to type 1 diabetes [184]. While prophylactic parenteral and oral insulin failed to slowed the progression of type 1 diabetes the identification of an optimal point during the natural history of declining β-cell function may help to guide the design of future early intervention studies [185].

The *insulin-modified frequently sampled IVGTT* permits calculation of endogenous insulin secretion that follows the AIR [186]. However, the administration of exogenous insulin may confound the results by partially suppressing insulin secretion. As originally described by Philip Eaton and colleagues at the University of New Mexico, USA deconvolution analysis requires knowledge of C-peptide kinetics [187]. The necessity to collect data on serum C-peptide kinetics in individual study subjects was superseded by a method in which approximate kinetics are derived from anthropometric measurements [188, 189]. Deconvolution analysis has been applied in the evaluation of the effects of GLP-1 [190] and GLP-1 analogues on endogenous insulin secretion [191]. Where serum C-peptide levels are not available, an alternative method for determining pre-hepatic insulin secretion based on plasma insulin concentrations after an oral glucose tolerance test has been described [192]. Deconvolution analysis of C-peptide can also be applied to meal-derived data [193].

Continuous Infusion of Glucose with Model Assessment (CIGMA)

In this method, increases in circulating insulin levels are measured in response to a low-dose intravenous infusion of glucose. This provides a simple and non-labour-intensive test in which β-cell function is expressed as a percentage of that expected in healthy subjects [194]. However, CIGMA has not found wide application in the development of metabolically active drugs [195].

Hyperglycaemic Clamp

This technique permits the biphasic insulin response to glucose to be quantified. Both the first and second phases of insulin secretion can be assessed, albeit in the setting of the non-physiological construct of a sustained increment of blood glucose [33]. In the fasting state, an intravenous bolus of glucose is followed by a continuous glucose infusion delivered at a variable rate in order to achieve and maintain a target level of hyperglycaemia, e.g. 10 mmol/L (180 mg/dL) or higher [196]. Frequent measurements of blood glucose at the bedside guide a variable rate intravenous infusion of glucose. Samples for measurement of blood glucose and endogenous insulin responses are taken at frequent intervals during the first 10 min or so in order to assess first-phase insulin secretion. Thereafter, during the plateau hyperglycaemic phase, less frequent sampling is required. An intravenous bolus of 5 g arginine may then be given as an additional non-glucose stimulus (see below) [191]. Indices of glucose-stimulated insulin secretion that may be calculated from the hyperglycaemic clamp include the amplitude of the first phase, the final attained plasma insulin concentration and the rise above fasting levels. The hyperglycaemic clamp provides a robust and reproducible stimulus to the β-cells. In a proof-of-concept study, Krentz et al. used the hyperglycaemic clamp to assess the completeness of pharmacological inhibition of endogenous insulin secretion achieved using an intravenous infusion of the somatostatin analogue octreotide in healthy volunteers [197]. Insulin, glucagon and growth hormone were infused to provide basal replacement levels of the hormones. This study supported the use of octreotide in place of the native hormone somatostatin in the *pancreatic* or *islet cell clamp technique* [197].

While the hyperglycaemic clamp provides a robust stimulus to both phases of insulin secretion, the technique is labour intensive and requires technical expertise [196]. The enhancement of endogenous insulin secretion attributable to the entero-insular axis is not assessed using this method. Henry et al. addressed this limitation by performing randomized, parallel-group, placebo-controlled study of 12 weeks of treatment with saxagliptin in a dose of 5 mg daily. The investigators used the hyperglycaemic glucose clamp to assess insulin secretion in the fasting state and then tested integrated incretin-enhanced insulin secretion by following the clamp with a 75 g oral glucose challenge. Using this combined approach, it was confirmed that treatment with saxagliptin improved pancreatic β-cell responsiveness to glucose in the fasting ($p<0.02$) and postprandial states ($p<0.04$) [198]. The effect on fasting glucose-stimulated insulin secretion is congruent with the lowering of fasting plasma glucose that is usually observed during DPP-4 therapy [199].

Arginine Stimulation Test

While glucose is the chief physiological regulator of β-cells, arginine, which is the direct precursor of nitric oxide, may also be used to provoke an acute insulin response. An intravenous injection of arginine elicits insulin release that may exceed the response observed during an IVGTT. In the 1960s, it was demonstrated that intravenous arginine increased circulating insulin concentrations and was the most potent among several essential amino acids [200]. In a method originally described by Daniel Porte's group at the University of Washington, USA injections of arginine are superimposed upon multiple levels of hyperglycaemia achieved by intravenous glucose infusion [201]. This approach, which has been widely applied by investigators, aims to generate a near-maximal insulin secretory response. The greater insulin response from the combination of arginine and hyperglycaemia is thought to result from release of a larger intracellular pool of insulin within storage granules. Arginine is injected in the basal (fasting) state and then after raising and maintaining blood glucose using a stepped hyperglycaemic clamp up to levels of approximately 35 mmol/L (630 mg/dL). Thus, the β-cell response to arginine is modulated by short-term hyperglycaemia to provide a synergistic stimulus to insulin secretion. It should be noted that arginine also stimulates glucagon secretion from islet α-cells, and so glucagon release occurs in addition to insulin secretion [202].

Using this approach, Ward et al. in early studies documented a decreased maximal insulin responsiveness to the potentiating effects of glucose on arginine-stimulated insulin secretion in patients with type 2 diabetes [201]. In addition to quantifying the absolute response of insulin (AIR_{max}), the so-called glucose potentiation slope may be calculated by plotting the AIR to arginine during the basal and first level of hyperglycaemia. The arginine potentiation test has been used in the assessment of new therapies for type 2 diabetes. For example, Bunck et al. studied metformin-treated patients with type 2 diabetes randomly assigned to the GLP-1 analogue exenatide or insulin glargine titrated to target according to a prespecified algorithm [115]. Arginine-stimulated hyperglycaemic clamps were performed at baseline, at week 52 and after a 4-week off-drug period. An intravenous bolus of arginine was administered at steady-state hyperglycaemia of 15 mmol/L (270 mg/dL). Exenatide significantly improved arginine-stimulated C-peptide levels ($p<0.0001$) during 1 year of treatment compared with titrated insulin glargine. After cessation of both exenatide and insulin glargine therapy, β-cell function returned to pretreatment values [115].

Graded Glucose Infusion

In 1995, Ken Polonsky and colleagues at the University of Chicago, USA described a low-dose graded glucose infusion protocol designed to explore the dose–response relationship between glucose and insulin secretion [203]. After an overnight fast, a basal (control) period is followed by sequential incremental intravenous infusions of glucose calculated to raise the blood glucose concentration from fasting to approximately 12 mmol/L (216 mg/dL). Venous blood samples for measurement of glucose and serum C-peptide are drawn, and the pre-hepatic insulin secretion rate for each step of hyperglycaemia is calculated by deconvolution of peripheral serum C-peptide levels. The mean insulin secretion rate at the end of each step may be plotted against mean blood glucose to generate a dose–response curve for β-cell function. Changes in the relationship between glucose and insulin secretion rate, e.g. as a result of an intervention that improves β-cell function, can be identified as shifts in the mean dose–response curve. In their original report, Byrne et al. observed an increased insulin secretion rate with a shift of the dose–response curve to the left indicative of improved β-cell responsiveness following a 42-h glucose infusion in healthy volunteers [203]. The graded glucose infusion provides reproducible data over blood glucose concentrations spanning the physiological and pathological range. In our view, this places the graded glucose infusion at the forefront of techniques available for quantifying β-cell function in clinical diabetes drug development studies. An important limitation of the technique is the inability to directly assess the contribution of the incretin response to insulin secretion.

The graded glucose infusion provides a standardized method for examining the effect of novel pharmacotherapies for patients with type 2 diabetes. For example, Kjems and colleagues assessed the effect of intravenous infusions of GLP-1 on insulin secretion in patients with type 2 diabetes and a group of matched healthy controls [204]. Small doses of intravenous insulin were used to bring fasting plasma glucose concentrations in the patients with diabetes down to a level similar to the healthy controls. A graded infusion of 20 % glucose was then administered at 2, 4, 6, 8 and 12 mg/kg/min each for 30 min. Blood samples were drawn at 10, 20 and 30 min during each 30 min period for measurement of glucose, insulin and plasma C-peptide. Pre-hepatic insulin secretion rates for each individual were derived by deconvolution of peripheral C-peptide concentrations. Infusion of GLP-1 increased pre-hepatic insulin secretion in both groups in a dose-dependent manner. GLP-1 restored insulin secretion and β-cell responsiveness to glucose in the patients with diabetes to levels observed in the normal subjects in the absence of GLP-1 infusion [204]. However, the dose–response relation between β-cell responsiveness to glucose and GLP-1 was severely impaired in the patients with type 2 diabetes when compared with the healthy controls. Using a similar experimental approach, Hompesch et al. in a proof-of-concept study. Compared the effect of a dual agonist of GLP-1 and GIP (MAR701) with exenatide and placebo on endogenous insulin secretion rate in healthy volunteers [205]. Dose-dependent increases in insulin secretion rate were observed at each glucose infusion rate with exenatide (and MAR701 compared to placebo ($p<0.001$ for each) (Fig. 2.3).

Choosing Between Different Tests of β-Cell Function

As the centennial of the naming of insulin approaches [206], the evaluation of β-cell function continues to present challenges to clinical researchers. No clear best choice exists for the assessment of β-cell function. The absence of a reference method reflects the complexity of β-cell function which cannot be completely captured using a single test. The most informative standardized assessments require a specialist clinical investigation unit with experienced research staff and strict observance of the experimental protocol. The choice of a test – or combination of tests – may be influenced by considerations that not only include the required (minimum vs. optimal) information about β-cell function but also the study budget, available clinical facilities and subject acceptability of the time, complexity and invasiveness of specific methods.

References

1. Ashcroft F, Ashcroft SH. Insulin: molecular biology to pathology. Oxford: IRL Press; 1992.
2. Pessin JE, Saltiel AR. Signaling pathways in insulin action: molecular targets of insulin resistance. J Clin Invest. 2000;106(2):165–9.
3. Owerbach D, Bell GI, Rutter WJ, Shows TB. The insulin gene is located on chromosome 11 in humans. Nature. 1980;286(5768):82–4.
4. Liu M, Wright J, Guo H, Xiong Y, Arvan P. Proinsulin entry and transit through the endoplasmic reticulum in pancreatic beta cells. Vitam Horm. 2014;95:35–62.
5. Hou JC, Min L, Pessin JE. Insulin granule biogenesis, trafficking and exocytosis. Vitam Horm. 2009;80:473–506.
6. Chang SG, Choi KD, Jang SH, Shin HC. Role of disulfide bonds in the structure and activity of human insulin. Mol Cells. 2003;16(3):323–30.
7. Lemaire K, Chimienti F, Schuit F. Zinc transporters and their role in the pancreatic beta-cell. J Diabetes Investig. 2012;3(3):202–11.
8. Smith GD, Pangborn WA, Blessing RH. The structure of T6 human insulin at 1.0 A resolution. Acta Crystallogr D Biol Crystallogr. 2003;59(Pt 3):474–82.
9. De Meyts P. Insulin and its receptor: structure, function and evolution. Bioessays. 2004;26(12):1351–62.
10. Poitout V, Hagman D, Stein R, et al. Regulation of the insulin gene by glucose and fatty acids. J Nutr. 2006;136(4):873–6.
11. Fu Z, Gilbert ER, Liu D. Regulation of insulin synthesis and secretion and pancreatic beta-cell dysfunction in diabetes. Curr Diabetes Rev. 2013;9(1):25–53.
12. Farhat B, Almelkar A, Ramachandran K, Williams SJ, Huang HH, Zamierowksi D, et al. Small human islets comprised of more beta-cells with higher insulin content than large islets. Islets. 2013;5(2):87–94.
13. Menge BA, Gruber L, Jorgensen SM, Deacon CF, Schmidt WE, Veldhuis JD, et al. Loss of inverse relationship between pulsatile insulin and glucagon secretion in patients with type 2 diabetes. Diabetes. 2011;60(8):2160–8.
14. Song SH, McIntyre SS, Shah H, Veldhuis JD, Hayes PC, Butler PC. Direct measurement of pulsatile insulin secretion from the portal vein in human subjects. J Clin Endocrinol Metab. 2000;85(12):4491–9.
15. Matthews DR, Lang DA, Burnett MA, Turner RC. Control of pulsatile insulin secretion in man. Diabetologia. 1983;24(4):231–7.
16. Wahren J, Kallas A. Loss of pulsatile insulin secretion: a factor in the pathogenesis of type 2 diabetes? Diabetes. 2012;61(9):2228–9.
17. O'Rahilly S, Turner RC, Matthews DR. Impaired pulsatile secretion of insulin in relatives of patients with non-insulin-dependent diabetes. N Engl J Med. 1988;318(19):1225–30.
18. Cryer PE. Minireview: glucagon in the pathogenesis of hypoglycemia and hyperglycemia in diabetes. Endocrinology. 2012;153(3):1039–48.
19. Henquin JC, Rahier J. Pancreatic alpha cell mass in European subjects with type 2 diabetes. Diabetologia. 2011;54(7):1720–5.
20. Hellman B, Salehi A, Gylfe E, Dansk H, Grapengiesser E. Glucose generates coincident insulin and somatostatin pulses and antisynchronous glucagon pulses from human pancreatic islets. Endocrinology. 2009;150(12):5334–40.
21. Pfeifer MA, Halter JB, Porte Jr D. Insulin secretion in diabetes mellitus. Am J Med. 1981;70(3):579–88.
22. Salinari S, Bertuzzi A, Manco M, Mingrone G. NEFA-glucose comodulation model of beta-cell insulin secretion in 24-h multiple-meal test. Am J Physiol Endocrinol Metab. 2007;292(6):E1890–8.
23. Malaisse WJ. Insulin release: the receptor hypothesis. Diabetologia. 2014;57(7):1287–90.
24. Hirasawa A, Hara T, Katsuma S, Adachi T, Tsujimoto G. Free fatty acid receptors and drug discovery. Biol Pharm Bull. 2008;31(10):1847–51.
25. Matschinsky FM. Glucokinase as glucose sensor and metabolic signal generator in pancreatic beta-cells and hepatocytes. Diabetes. 1990;39(6):647–52.
26. Komatsu M, Takei M, Ishii H, Sato Y. Glucose-stimulated insulin secretion: a newer perspective. J Diabetes Investig. 2013;4(6):511–6.
27. Thorens B. Brain glucose sensing and neural regulation of insulin and glucagon secretion. Diabetes Obes Metab. 2011;13 Suppl 1:82–8.
28. Rodriguez-Diaz R, Menegaz D, Caicedo A. Neurotransmitters act as paracrine signals to regulate insulin secretion from the human pancreatic islet. J Physiol. 2014;592:3413–7.
29. Molina J, Rodriguez-Diaz R, Fachado A, Jacques-Silva MC, Berggren PO, Caicedo A. Control of insulin secretion by cholinergic signaling in the human pancreatic islet. Diabetes. 2014;63:2714–26.
30. Braun M, Ramracheya R, Rorsman P. Autocrine regulation of insulin secretion. Diabetes Obes Metab. 2012;14 Suppl 3:143–51.

31. McKillop AM, Ng MT, Abdel-Wahab YH, Flatt PR. Evidence for inhibitory autocrine effects of proinsulin C-peptide on pancreatic beta cell function and insulin secretion. Diabetes Obes Metab. 2014;16:937–46.
32. Rhodes CJ, White MF, Leahy JL, Kahn SE. Direct autocrine action of insulin on beta-cells: does it make physiological sense? Diabetes. 2013;62(7): 2157–63.
33. DeFronzo RA, Tobin JD, Andres R. Glucose clamp technique: a method for quantifying insulin secretion and resistance. Am J Physiol. 1979;237(3):E214–23.
34. Rorsman P, Eliasson L, Renstrom E, Gromada J, Barg S, Göpel S. The cell physiology of biphasic insulin secretion. News Physiol Sci. 2000;15:72–7.
35. Caumo A, Luzi L. First-phase insulin secretion: does it exist in real life? Considerations on shape and function. Am J Physiol Endocrinol Metab. 2004;287(3):E371–85.
36. Creutzfeldt W. The incretin concept today. Diabetologia. 1979;16(2):75–85.
37. Kim W, Egan JM. The role of incretins in glucose homeostasis and diabetes treatment. Pharmacol Rev. 2008;60(4):470–512.
38. Holst JJ, Vilsboll T, Deacon CF. The incretin system and its role in type 2 diabetes mellitus. Mol Cell Endocrinol. 2009;297(1–2):127–36.
39. Holst JJ. The physiology of glucagon-like peptide 1. Physiol Rev. 2007;87(4):1409–39.
40. Drucker DJ, Nauck MA. The incretin system: glucagon-like peptide-1 receptor agonists and dipeptidyl peptidase-4 inhibitors in type 2 diabetes. Lancet. 2006;368(9548):1696–705.
41. Drucker DJ. The role of gut hormones in glucose homeostasis. J Clin Invest. 2007;117(1):24–32.
42. Drucker DJ. Incretin action in the pancreas: potential promise, possible perils, and pathological pitfalls. Diabetes. 2013;62(10):3316–23.
43. Baggio LL, Drucker DJ. Biology of incretins: GLP-1 and GIP. Gastroenterology. 2007;132(6):2131–57.
44. Buteau J, Roduit R, Susini S, Prentki M. Glucagon-like peptide-1 promotes DNA synthesis, activates phosphatidylinositol 3-kinase and increases transcription factor pancreatic and duodenal homeobox gene 1 (PDX-1) DNA binding activity in beta (INS-1)-cells. Diabetologia. 1999;42(7):856–64.
45. Vilsboll T. On the role of the incretin hormones GIP and GLP-1 in the pathogenesis of Type 2 diabetes mellitus. Dan Med Bull. 2004;51(4):364–70.
46. Tura A, Muscelli E, Gastaldelli A, Ferrannini E, Mari A. Altered pattern of the incretin effect as assessed by modelling in individuals with glucose tolerance ranging from normal to diabetic. Diabetologia. 2014;57(6):1199–203.
47. Calanna S, Christensen M, Holst JJ, Laferrère B, Gluud LL, Vilsbøll T, et al. Secretion of glucagon-like peptide-1 in patients with type 2 diabetes mellitus: systematic review and meta-analyses of clinical studies. Diabetologia. 2013;56(5):965–72.
48. Bock G, Dalla Man C, Micheletto F, Basu R, Giesler PD, Laugen J, et al. The effect of DPP-4 inhibition with sitagliptin on incretin secretion and on fasting and postprandial glucose turnover in subjects with impaired fasting glucose. Clin Endocrinol (Oxf). 2010;73(2):189–96.
49. Duckworth WC, Bennett RG, Hamel FG. Insulin degradation: progress and potential. Endocr Rev. 1998;19(5):608–24.
50. Barzilai N, Groop PH, Groop L, DeFronzo RA. A novel mechanism of glipizide sulfonylurea action: decreased metabolic clearance rate of insulin. Acta Diabetol. 1995;32(4):273–8.
51. Hansen BC, Striffler JS, Bodkin NL. Decreased hepatic insulin extraction precedes overt noninsulin dependent (Type II) diabetes in obese monkeys. Obes Res. 1993;1(4):252–60.
52. Polonsky KS. Lilly lecture 1994. The beta-cell in diabetes: from molecular genetics to clinical research. Diabetes. 1995;44(6):705–17.
53. Henriksen JH, Tronier B, Bulow JB. Kinetics of circulating endogenous insulin, C-peptide, and proinsulin in fasting nondiabetic man. Metabolism. 1987;36(5):463–8.
54. Kahn SE. The relative contributions of insulin resistance and beta-cell dysfunction to the pathophysiology of type 2 diabetes. Diabetologia. 2003;46(1):3–19.
55. Kahn SE, Cooper ME, Del Prato S. Pathophysiology and treatment of type 2 diabetes: perspectives on the past, present, and future. Lancet. 2014;383(9922): 1068–83.
56. Reaven GM. Role of insulin resistance in the pathophysiology of non-insulin dependent diabetes mellitus. Diabetes Metab Rev. 1993;9 Suppl 1:5S–12S.
57. DeFronzo RA. Pathogenesis of type 2 diabetes mellitus. Med Clin North Am. 2004;88(4):787–835, ix.
58. Meier JJ, Bonadonna RC. Role of reduced beta-cell mass versus impaired beta-cell function in the pathogenesis of type 2 diabetes. Diabetes Care. 2013;36 Suppl 2:S113–9.
59. Gregg BE, Moore PC, Demozay D, Hall BA, Li M, Husain A, et al. Formation of a human beta-cell population within pancreatic islets is set early in life. J Clin Endocrinol Metab. 2012;97(9):3197–206.
60. Rhodes CJ. Type 2 diabetes-a matter of beta-cell life and death? Science. 2005;307(5708):380–4.
61. Halban PA, Polonsky KS, Bowden DW, Hawkins MA, Ling C, Mather KJ, et al. Beta-cell failure in type 2 diabetes: postulated mechanisms and prospects for prevention and treatment. Diabetes Care. 2014;37(6):1751–8.
62. Ichise M, Harris PE. Imaging of beta-cell mass and function. J Nucl Med. 2010;51(7):1001–4.
63. Robertson RP. Estimation of beta-cell mass by metabolic tests: necessary, but how sufficient? Diabetes. 2007;56(10):2420–4.
64. Bonner-Weir S. Beta-cell turnover: its assessment and implications. Diabetes. 2001;50 Suppl 1:S20–4.
65. Dor Y, Glaser B. Beta-cell dedifferentiation and type 2 diabetes. N Engl J Med. 2013;368(6):572–3.
66. Bluestone JA, Herold K, Eisenbarth G. Genetics, pathogenesis and clinical interventions in type 1 diabetes. Nature. 2010;464(7293):1293–300.

67. McGee P, Steffes M, Nowicki M, Bayless M, Gubitosi-Klug R, Cleary P, et al. Insulin secretion measured by stimulated C-peptide in long-established type 1 diabetes in the Diabetes Control and Complications Trial (DCCT)/Epidemiology of Diabetes Interventions and Complications (EDIC) cohort: a pilot study. Diabet Med. 2014;31:1264–8.
68. Oram RA, Jones AG, Besser RE, Knight BA, Shields BM, Brown RJ, et al. The majority of patients with long-duration type 1 diabetes are insulin microsecretors and have functioning beta cells. Diabetologia. 2014;57(1):187–91.
69. Greenbaum CJ, Mandrup-Poulsen T, McGee PF, Battelino T, Haastert B, Ludvigsson J, et al. Mixed-meal tolerance test versus glucagon stimulation test for the assessment of beta-cell function in therapeutic trials in type 1 diabetes. Diabetes Care. 2008;31(10):1966–71.
70. Besser RE, Jones AG, McDonald TJ, Shields BM, Knight BA, Hattersley AT. The impact of insulin administration during the mixed meal tolerance test. Diabet Med. 2012;29(10):1279–84.
71. Vague P, Nguyen L. Rationale and methods for the estimation of insulin secretion in a given patient: from research to clinical practice. Diabetes. 2002;51 Suppl 1:S240–4.
72. Ahren B, Pratley RE, Soubt M, Dunning BE, Foley JE. Clinical measures of islet function: usefulness to characterize defects in diabetes. Curr Diabetes Rev. 2008;4(2):129–45.
73. U.K. prospective diabetes study 16. Overview of 6 years' therapy of type II diabetes: a progressive disease. U.K. Prospective Diabetes Study Group. Diabetes. 1995;44(11):1249–58.
74. Butler AE, Janson J, Bonner-Weir S, Ritzel R, Rizza RA, Butler PC. Beta-cell deficit and increased beta-cell apoptosis in humans with type 2 diabetes. Diabetes. 2003;52(1):102–10.
75. Ferrannini E, Gastaldelli A, Miyazaki Y, Matsuda M, Mari A, DeFronzo RA. Beta-cell function in subjects spanning the range from normal glucose tolerance to overt diabetes: a new analysis. J Clin Endocrinol Metab. 2005;90(1):493–500.
76. Turner RC. The U.K. prospective diabetes study. A review. Diabetes Care. 1998;21 Suppl 3:C35–8.
77. Zangeneh F, Arora PS, Dyck PJ, Bekris L, Lernmark A, Achenbach SJ, et al. Effects of duration of type 2 diabetes mellitus on insulin secretion. Endocr Pract. 2006;12(4):388–93.
78. Jaikaran ET, Clark A. Islet amyloid and type 2 diabetes: from molecular misfolding to islet pathophysiology. Biochim Biophys Acta. 2001;1537(3):179–203.
79. Westermark GT, Westermark P. Islet amyloid polypeptide and diabetes. Curr Protein Pept Sci. 2013;14(4):330–7.
80. Toschi E, Camastra S, Sironi AM, Masoni A, Gastaldelli A, Mari A, et al. Effect of acute hyperglycemia on insulin secretion in humans. Diabetes. 2002;51 Suppl 1:S130–3.
81. Weir GC, Marselli L, Marchetti P, Katsuta H, Jung MH, Bonner-Weir S. Towards better understanding of the contributions of overwork and glucotoxicity to the beta-cell inadequacy of type 2 diabetes. Diabetes Obes Metab. 2009;11 Suppl 4:82–90.
82. Cusi K. The role of adipose tissue and lipotoxicity in the pathogenesis of type 2 diabetes. Curr Diab Rep. 2010;10(4):306–15.
83. Marchetti P, Del Prato S, Lupi R, Del Guerra S. The pancreatic beta-cell in human type 2 diabetes. Nutr Metab Cardiovasc Dis. 2006;16 Suppl 1:S3–6.
84. Montane J, Cadavez L, Novials A. Stress and the inflammatory process: a major cause of pancreatic cell death in type 2 diabetes. Diabetes Metab Syndr Obes. 2014;7:25–34.
85. Porksen N, Munn S, Steers J, Vore S, Veldhuis J, Butler P. Pulsatile insulin secretion accounts for 70 % of total insulin secretion during fasting. Am J Physiol. 1995;269(3 Pt 1):E478–88.
86. Temple RC, Carrington CA, Luzio SD, Owens DR, Schneider AE, Sobey WJ, et al. Insulin deficiency in non-insulin-dependent diabetes. Lancet. 1989;1(8633):293–5.
87. Owen K, Hattersley AT. Maturity-onset diabetes of the young: from clinical description to molecular genetic characterization. Best Pract Res Clin Endocrinol Metab. 2001;15(3):309–23.
88. Schwitzgebel VM. Many faces of monogenic diabetes. J Diabetes Investig. 2014;5(2):121–33.
89. Pal A, McCarthy MI. The genetics of type 2 diabetes and its clinical relevance. Clin Genet. 2013;83(4):297–306.
90. Hattersley AT, Pearson ER. Minireview: pharmacogenetics and beyond: the interaction of therapeutic response, beta-cell physiology, and genetics in diabetes. Endocrinology. 2006;147(6):2657–63.
91. Thrower SL, Bingley PJ. Prevention of type 1 diabetes. Br Med Bull. 2011;99:73–88.
92. Atkinson MA, Eisenbarth GS, Michels AW. Type 1 diabetes. Lancet. 2014;383(9911):69–82.
93. Skyler JS. Primary and secondary prevention of type 1 diabetes. Diabet Med. 2013;30(2):161–9.
94. Sherry NA, Tsai EB, Herold KC. Natural history of beta-cell function in type 1 diabetes. Diabetes. 2005;54 Suppl 2:S32–9.
95. Watkins RA, Evans-Molina C, Blum JS, Dimeglio LA. Established and emerging biomarkers for the prediction of type 1 diabetes: a systematic review. Transl Res. 2014;164:110–21.
96. Skyler JS. Struggles with clinical translation of immune intervention trials. Diabetes Care. 2014;37(5):1173–5.
97. Sherr J, Tsalikian E, Fox L, Buckingham B, Weinzimer S, Tamborlane WV, et al. Evolution of abnormal plasma glucagon responses to mixed meal feedings in youth with type 1 diabetes during the first two years after diagnosis. Diabetes Care. 2014;37:1741–4.
98. Xu G, Chen J, Jing G, Shalev A. Preventing beta-cell loss and diabetes with calcium channel blockers. Diabetes. 2012;61(4):848–56.

99. Strom A, Kolb H, Martin S, Herder C, Simon MC, Koenig W, et al. Improved preservation of residual beta cell function by atorvastatin in patients with recent onset type 1 diabetes and high CRP levels (DIATOR trial). PLoS One. 2012;7(3):e33108.
100. Kitabchi AE, Temprosa M, Knowler WC, Kahn SE, Fowler SE, Haffner SM, et al. Role of insulin secretion and sensitivity in the evolution of type 2 diabetes in the diabetes prevention program: effects of lifestyle intervention and metformin. Diabetes. 2005;54(8):2404–14.
101. Doyle ME, Egan JM. Pharmacological agents that directly modulate insulin secretion. Pharmacol Rev. 2003;55(1):105–31.
102. Buchanan TA, Xiang AH, Peters RK, Kjos SL, Marroquin A, Goico J, et al. Preservation of pancreatic beta-cell function and prevention of type 2 diabetes by pharmacological treatment of insulin resistance in high-risk hispanic women. Diabetes. 2002;51(9):2796–803.
103. Ahren B, Pacini G. Importance of quantifying insulin secretion in relation to insulin sensitivity to accurately assess beta cell function in clinical studies. Eur J Endocrinol. 2004;150(2):97–104.
104. Gumbiner B, Polonsky KS, Beltz WF, Griver K, Wallace P, Brechtel G, et al. Effects of weight loss and reduced hyperglycemia on the kinetics of insulin secretion in obese non-insulin dependent diabetes mellitus. J Clin Endocrinol Metab. 1990;70(6): 1594–602.
105. Thaler JP, Cummings DE. Minireview: hormonal and metabolic mechanisms of diabetes remission after gastrointestinal surgery. Endocrinology. 2009;150(6):2518–25.
106. Taylor R. Type 2 diabetes: etiology and reversibility. Diabetes Care. 2013;36(4):1047–55.
107. Camastra S, Muscelli E, Gastaldelli A, et al. Long-term effects of bariatric surgery on meal disposal and beta-cell function in diabetic and nondiabetic patients. Diabetes. 2013;62(11):3709–17.
108. Krentz AJ, Bailey CJ. Oral antidiabetic agents: current role in type 2 diabetes mellitus. Drugs. 2005;65(3):385–411.
109. Ashcroft FM. Mechanisms of the glycaemic effects of sulfonylureas. Horm Metab Res. 1996;28(9):456–63.
110. Deacon CF. Dipeptidyl peptidase-4 inhibitors in the treatment of type 2 diabetes: a comparative review. Diabetes Obes Metab. 2011;13(1):7–18.
111. Proks P, Reimann F, Green N, Gribble F, Ashcroft F. Sulfonylurea stimulation of insulin secretion. Diabetes. 2002;51 Suppl 3:S368–76.
112. Stein SA, Lamos EM, Davis SN. A review of the efficacy and safety of oral antidiabetic drugs. Expert Opin Drug Saf. 2013;12(2):153–75.
113. Drucker DJ. Enhancing incretin action for the treatment of type 2 diabetes. Diabetes Care. 2003;26(10):2929–40.
114. van Genugten RE, van Raalte DH, Diamant M. Dipeptidyl peptidase-4 inhibitors and preservation of pancreatic islet-cell function: a critical appraisal of the evidence. Diabetes Obes Metab. 2012;14(2):101–11.
115. Bunck MC, Diamant M, Corner A, Eliasson B, Malloy JL, Shaginian RM, et al. One-year treatment with exenatide improves beta-cell function, compared with insulin glargine, in metformin-treated type 2 diabetic patients: a randomized, controlled trial. Diabetes Care. 2009;32(5):762–8.
116. DeFronzo RA, Eldor R, Abdul-Ghani M. Pathophysiologic approach to therapy in patients with newly diagnosed type 2 diabetes. Diabetes Care. 2013;36 Suppl 2:S127–38.
117. Cahn A, Raz I. Emerging gliptins for type 2 diabetes. Expert Opin Emerg Drugs. 2013;18(2):245–58.
118. Lee YS, Jun HS. Anti-diabetic actions of glucagon-like peptide-1 on pancreatic beta-cells. Metabolism. 2014;63(1):9–19.
119. Ueno H, Mizuta M, Shiiya T, Tsuchimochi W, Noma K, Nakashima N, et al. Exploratory trial of intranasal administration of glucagon-like peptide-1 in Japanese patients with type 2 diabetes. Diabetes Care. 2014;37:2024–7.
120. Sonne DP, Hansen M, Knop FK. Mechanisms in endocrinology: bile acid sequestrants in type 2 diabetes: potential effects on GLP1 secretion. Eur J Endocrinol. 2014;171(2):R47–65.
121. Burant CF. Activation of GPR40 as a therapeutic target for the treatment of type 2 diabetes. Diabetes Care. 2013;36 Suppl 2:S175–9.
122. Ohishi T, Yoshida S. The therapeutic potential of GPR119 agonists for type 2 diabetes. Expert Opin Investig Drugs. 2012;21(3):321–8.
123. Finan B, Ma T, Ottaway N, Müller TD, Habegger KM, Heppner KM, et al. Unimolecular dual incretins maximize metabolic benefits in rodents, monkeys, and humans. Sci Transl Med. 2013;5(209): 209ra151.
124. Matschinsky FM, Porte D. Glucokinase activators (GKAs) promise a new pharmacotherapy for diabetics. F1000 Med Rep. 2010;2:43.
125. Larsen CM, Faulenbach M, Vaag A, Vølund A, Ehses JA, Seifert B, et al. Interleukin-1-receptor antagonist in type 2 diabetes mellitus. N Engl J Med. 2007;356(15):1517–26.
126. Angeli FS, Shannon RP. Incretin-based therapies: can we achieve glycemic control and cardioprotection? J Endocrinol. 2014;221(1):T17–30.
127. Barter PJ. High density lipoprotein: a therapeutic target in type 2 diabetes. Endocrinol Metab (Seoul). 2013;28(3):169–77.
128. Barter PJ, Rye KA, Tardif JC, Waters DD, Boekholdt SM, Breazna A, et al. Effect of torcetrapib on glucose, insulin, and hemoglobin A1c in subjects in the Investigation of Lipid Level Management to Understand its Impact in Atherosclerotic Events (ILLUMINATE) trial. Circulation. 2011;124(5): 555–62.
129. Puddu A, Sanguineti R, Mach F, Dallegri F, Viviani GL, Montecucco F. Update on the protective molec-

ular pathways improving pancreatic beta-cell dysfunction. Mediat Inflamm. 2013;2013:750540.
130. Food and Drug Administration, Guidance for industry. Diabetes mellitus: developing drugs and therapeutic biologics for treatment and prevention. 2008. http://www.fda.gov/downloads/Drugs/Guidances/ucm071624.pdf
131. Yki-Jarvinen H. Thiazolidinediones. N Engl J Med. 2004;351(11):1106–18.
132. Samson SL, Garber A. GLP-1R agonist therapy for diabetes: benefits and potential risks. Curr Opin Endocrinol Diabetes Obes. 2013;20(2):87–97.
133. Elliott WJ, Meyer PM. Incident diabetes in clinical trials of antihypertensive drugs: a network meta-analysis. Lancet. 2007;369(9557):201–7.
134. Ong KL, Barter PJ, Waters DD. Cardiovascular drugs that increase the risk of new-onset diabetes. Am Heart J. 2014;167(4):421–8.
135. Axsom K, Berger JS, Schwartzbard AZ. Statins and diabetes: the good, the bad, and the unknown. Curr Atheroscler Rep. 2013;15(2):299.
136. Brault M, Ray J, Gomez YH, Mantzoros CS, Daskalopoulou SS. Statin treatment and new-onset diabetes: a review of proposed mechanisms. Metabolism. 2014;63(6):735–45.
137. Reaven GM. Insulin secretory function in type 2 diabetes: does it matter how you measure it? J Diabetes. 2009;1(3):142–50.
138. Wallace TM, Levy JC, Matthews DR. Use and abuse of HOMA modeling. Diabetes Care. 2004;27(6):1487–95.
139. Wallace TM, Matthews DR. The assessment of insulin resistance in man. Diabet Med. 2002;19(7): 527–34.
140. Holst JJ. Glucagon-like peptide-1: from extract to agent. The Claude Bernard lecture, 2005. Diabetologia. 2006;49(2):253–60.
141. Vilsboll T, Krarup T, Deacon CF, Madsbad S, Holst JJ. Reduced postprandial concentrations of intact biologically active glucagon-like peptide 1 in type 2 diabetic patients. Diabetes. 2001;50(3):609–13.
142. Kieffer TJ, McIntosh CH, Pederson RA. Degradation of glucose-dependent insulinotropic polypeptide and truncated glucagon-like peptide 1 in vitro and in vivo by dipeptidyl peptidase IV. Endocrinology. 1995;136(8):3585–96.
143. Mannucci E, Tesi F, Bardini G, Ognibene A, Petracca MG, Ciani S, et al. Effects of metformin on glucagon-like peptide-1 levels in obese patients with and without Type 2 diabetes. Diabetes Nutr Metab. 2004;17(6):336–42.
144. Arakawa M, Ebato C, Mita T, Fujitani Y, Shimizu T, Watada H, et al. Miglitol suppresses the postprandial increase in interleukin 6 and enhances active glucagon-like peptide 1 secretion in viscerally obese subjects. Metabolism. 2008;57(9):1299–306.
145. D'Alessio D. The role of dysregulated glucagon secretion in type 2 diabetes. Diabetes Obes Metab. 2011;13 Suppl 1:126–32.
146. Holst JJ, Christensen M, Lund A, de Heer J, Svendsen B, Kielgast U, et al. Regulation of glucagon secretion by incretins. Diabetes Obes Metab. 2011;13 Suppl 1:89–94.
147. Cho YM, Merchant CE, Kieffer TJ. Targeting the glucagon receptor family for diabetes and obesity therapy. Pharmacol Ther. 2012;135(3):247–78.
148. Christensen M, Bagger JI, Vilsboll T, Knop FK. The alpha-cell as target for type 2 diabetes therapy. Rev Diabet Stud. 2011;8(3):369–81.
149. Ferrannini E, Natali A, Muscelli E, Nilsson PM, Golay A, Laakso M, et al. Natural history and physiological determinants of changes in glucose tolerance in a non-diabetic population: the RISC study. Diabetologia. 2011;54(6):1507–16.
150. Krentz AJ. Insulin resistance: a clinical handbook. Oxford: Blackwell Science; 2002.
151. Godbout A, Chiasson JL. Who should benefit from the use of alpha-glucosidase inhibitors? Curr Diab Rep. 2007;7(5):333–9.
152. Hasan FM, Alsahli M, Gerich JE. SGLT2 inhibitors in the treatment of type 2 diabetes. Diabetes Res Clin Pract. 2014;104:297–322.
153. Temple R, Clark PM, Hales CN. Measurement of insulin secretion in type 2 diabetes: problems and pitfalls. Diabet Med. 1992;9(6):503–12.
154. Krentz AJ, Clark PM, Cox L, Nattrass M. Hyperproinsulinaemia in impaired glucose tolerance. Clin Sci (Lond). 1993;85(1):97–100.
155. Smith SA, Porter LE, Biswas N, Freed MI. Rosiglitazone, but not glyburide, reduces circulating proinsulin and the proinsulin: insulin ratio in type 2 diabetes. J Clin Endocrinol Metab. 2004;89(12):6048–53.
156. Hanefeld M, Patwardhan R, Jones NP, Rosiglitazone Clinical Trials Study Group. A one-year study comparing the efficacy and safety of rosiglitazone and glibenclamide in the treatment of type 2 diabetes. Nutr Metab Cardiovasc Dis. 2007;17(1):13–23.
157. Kahn SE, Haffner SM, Heise MA, Herman WH, Holman RR, Jones NP, et al. Glycemic durability of rosiglitazone, metformin, or glyburide monotherapy. N Engl J Med. 2006;355(23):2427–43.
158. Kahn SE, Lachin JM, Zinman B, Haffner SM, Aftring RP, Paul G, et al. Effects of rosiglitazone, glyburide, and metformin on beta-cell function and insulin sensitivity in ADOPT. Diabetes. 2011;60(5):1552–60.
159. Vandewalle B, Moerman E, Lefebvre B, Defrance F, Gmyr V, Lukowiak B, et al. PPARgamma-dependent and -independent effects of rosiglitazone on lipotoxic human pancreatic islets. Biochem Biophys Res Commun. 2008;366(4):1096–101.
160. Matthews DR, Hosker JP, Rudenski AS, Naylor BA, Treacher DF, Turner RC. Homeostasis model assessment: insulin resistance and beta-cell function from fasting plasma glucose and insulin concentrations in man. Diabetologia. 1985;28(7):412–9.
161. Reaven GM. HOMA-beta in the UKPDS and ADOPT. Is the natural history of type 2 diabetes characterised by a progressive and inexorable loss of

insulin secretory function? Maybe? Maybe not? Diab Vasc Dis Res. 2009;6(2):133–8.
162. Rizza RA, Mandarino LJ, Gerich JE. Dose-response characteristics for effects of insulin on production and utilization of glucose in man. Am J Physiol. 1981;240(6):E630–9.
163. Festa A, Williams K, Hanley AJ, Haffner SM. Beta-cell dysfunction in subjects with impaired glucose tolerance and early type 2 diabetes: comparison of surrogate markers with first-phase insulin secretion from an intravenous glucose tolerance test. Diabetes. 2008;57(6):1638–44.
164. Meier JJ, Menge BA, Breuer TG, Müller CA, Tannapfel A, Uhl W, et al. Functional assessment of pancreatic beta-cell area in humans. Diabetes. 2009;58(7):1595–603.
165. Rosenblatt S, Miskin B, Glazer NB, Prince MJ, Robertson KE, Pioglitazone 026 Study Group. The impact of pioglitazone on glycemic control and atherogenic dyslipidemia in patients with type 2 diabetes mellitus. Coron Artery Dis. 2001;12(5):413–23.
166. Zhan M, Xu T, Wu F, Tang Y. Sitagliptin in the treatment of type 2 diabetes: a meta-analysis. J Evid Based Med. 2012;5(3):154–65.
167. Nathan DM, Davidson MB, DeFronzo RA, Heine RJ, Henry RR, Pratley R, et al. Impaired fasting glucose and impaired glucose tolerance: implications for care. Diabetes Care. 2007;30(3):753–9.
168. Gerstein HC, Yusuf S, Bosch J, Pogue J, Sheridan P, Dinccag N, et al. Effect of rosiglitazone on the frequency of diabetes in patients with impaired glucose tolerance or impaired fasting glucose: a randomised controlled trial. Lancet. 2006;368(9541):1096–105.
169. Vilsboll T, Holst JJ. Incretins, insulin secretion and type 2 diabetes mellitus. Diabetologia. 2004;47(3):357–66.
170. Herman GA, Bergman A, Stevens C, Kotey P, Yi B, Zhao P, et al. Effect of single oral doses of sitagliptin, a dipeptidyl peptidase-4 inhibitor, on incretin and plasma glucose levels after an oral glucose tolerance test in patients with type 2 diabetes. J Clin Endocrinol Metab. 2006;91(11):4612–9.
171. Potteiger JA, Jacobsen DJ, Donnelly JE. A comparison of methods for analyzing glucose and insulin areas under the curve following nine months of exercise in overweight adults. Int J Obes Relat Metab Disord. 2002;26(1):87–9.
172. Phillips DI, Clark PM, Hales CN, Osmond C. Understanding oral glucose tolerance: comparison of glucose or insulin measurements during the oral glucose tolerance test with specific measurements of insulin resistance and insulin secretion. Diabet Med. 1994;11(3):286–92.
173. Utzschneider KM, Prigeon RL, Tong J, Gerchman F, Carr DB, Zraika S, et al. Within-subject variability of measures of beta cell function derived from a 2 h OGTT: implications for research studies. Diabetologia. 2007;50(12):2516–25.
174. Cozma LS, Luzio SD, Dunseath GJ, Underwood PM, Owens DR. Beta-cell response during a meal test: a comparative study of incremental doses of repaglinide in type 2 diabetic patients. Diabetes Care. 2005;28(5):1001–7.
175. Charbonnel B, Karasik A, Liu J, Wu M, Meininger G, Sitagliptin Study 020 Group. Efficacy and safety of the dipeptidyl peptidase-4 inhibitor sitagliptin added to ongoing metformin therapy in patients with type 2 diabetes inadequately controlled with metformin alone. Diabetes Care. 2006;29(12):2638–43.
176. Ahren B, Pacini G, Foley JE, Schweizer A. Improved meal-related beta-cell function and insulin sensitivity by the dipeptidyl peptidase-IV inhibitor vildagliptin in metformin-treated patients with type 2 diabetes over 1 year. Diabetes Care. 2005;28(8):1936–40.
177. Mari A, Pacini G, Murphy E, Ludvik B, Nolan JJ. A model-based method for assessing insulin sensitivity from the oral glucose tolerance test. Diabetes Care. 2001;24(3):539–48.
178. Cobelli C, Dalla Man C, Toffolo G, Basu R, Vella A, Rizza R. The oral minimal model method. Diabetes. 2014;63(4):1203–13.
179. Bingley PJ, Colman P, Eisenbarth GS, Jackson RA, McCulloch DK, Riley WJ, et al. Standardization of IVGTT to predict IDDM. Diabetes Care. 1992;15(10):1313–6.
180. Ferrannini E, Mari A. Beta cell function and its relation to insulin action in humans: a critical appraisal. Diabetologia. 2004;47(5):943–56.
181. Mari A, Tura A, Pacini G, Kautzky-Willer A, Ferrannini E. Relationships between insulin secretion after intravenous and oral glucose administration in subjects with glucose tolerance ranging from normal to overt diabetes. Diabet Med. 2008;25(6):671–7.
182. Fehse F, Trautmann M, Holst JJ, Halseth AE, Nanayakkara N, Nielsen LL, et al. Exenatide augments first- and second-phase insulin secretion in response to intravenous glucose in subjects with type 2 diabetes. J Clin Endocrinol Metab. 2005;90(11):5991–7.
183. Utzschneider KM, Tong J, Montgomery B, Udayasankar J, Gerchman F, Marcovina SM, et al. The dipeptidyl peptidase-4 inhibitor vildagliptin improves beta-cell function and insulin sensitivity in subjects with impaired fasting glucose. Diabetes Care. 2008;31(1):108–13.
184. Sosenko JM, Skyler JS, Beam CA, Krischer JP, Greenbaum CJ, Mahon J, et al. Acceleration of the loss of the first-phase insulin response during the progression to type 1 diabetes in diabetes prevention trial-type 1 participants. Diabetes. 2013;62(12):4179–83.
185. Williams AJ, Long AE. Following the fate of the failing beta-cell: new insights from first-phase insulin responses. Diabetes. 2013;62(12):3990–2.
186. Toffolo G, Cefalu WT, Cobelli C. Beta-cell function during insulin-modified intravenous glucose tolerance test successfully assessed by the C-peptide minimal model. Metabolism. 1999;48(9):1162–6.
187. Eaton RP, Allen RC, Schade DS, Erickson KM, Standefer J. Prehepatic insulin production in man: kinetic analysis using peripheral connecting peptide

behavior. J Clin Endocrinol Metab. 1980;51(3):520–8.
188. Van Cauter E, Mestrez F, Sturis J, Polonsky KS. Estimation of insulin secretion rates from C-peptide levels. Comparison of individual and standard kinetic parameters for C-peptide clearance. Diabetes. 1992;41(3):368–77.
189. Hovorka R, Jones RH. How to measure insulin secretion. Diabetes Metab Rev. 1994;10(2):91–117.
190. Ahren B, Holst JJ, Mari A. Characterization of GLP-1 effects on beta-cell function after meal ingestion in humans. Diabetes Care. 2003;26(10):2860–4.
191. Degn KB, Juhl CB, Sturis J, Jakobsen G, Brock B, Chandramouli V, et al. One week's treatment with the long-acting glucagon-like peptide 1 derivative liraglutide (NN2211) markedly improves 24-h glycemia and alpha- and beta-cell function and reduces endogenous glucose release in patients with type 2 diabetes. Diabetes. 2004;53(5):1187–94.
192. Tura A, Pacini G, Kautzky-Willer A, Gastaldelli A, DeFronzo RA, Ferrannini E, et al. Estimation of prehepatic insulin secretion: comparison between standardized C-peptide and insulin kinetic models. Metabolism. 2012;61(3):434–43.
193. Kahleova H, Belinova L, Malinska H, Oliyarnyk O, Trnovska J, Skop V, et al. Eating two larger meals a day (breakfast and lunch) is more effective than six smaller meals in a reduced-energy regimen for patients with type 2 diabetes: a randomised crossover study. Diabetologia. 2014;57:1552–60.
194. Hosker JP, Matthews DR, Rudenski AS, Burnett MA, Darling P, Bown EG, et al. Continuous infusion of glucose with model assessment: measurement of insulin resistance and beta-cell function in man. Diabetologia. 1985;28(7):401–11.
195. Zandbergen AA, Lamberts SW, Janssen JA, Bootsma AH. Short-term administration of an angiotensin-receptor antagonist in patients with impaired fasting glucose improves insulin sensitivity and increases free IGF-I. Eur J Endocrinol. 2006;155(2):293–6.
196. Elahi D. In praise of the hyperglycemic clamp. A method for assessment of beta-cell sensitivity and insulin resistance. Diabetes Care. 1996;19(3):278–86.
197. Krentz AJ, Boyle PJ, Macdonald LM, Schade DS. Octreotide: a long-acting inhibitor of endogenous hormone secretion for human metabolic investigations. Metabolism. 1994;43(1):24–31.
198. Henry RR, Smith SR, Schwartz SL, Mudaliar SR, Deacon CF, Holst JJ, et al. Effects of saxagliptin on beta-cell stimulation and insulin secretion in patients with type 2 diabetes. Diabetes Obes Metab. 2011;13(9):850–8.
199. Krentz AJ, Patel MB, Bailey CJ. New drugs for type 2 diabetes mellitus : what is their place in therapy? Drugs. 2008;68(15):2131–62.
200. Floyd Jr JC, Fajans SS, Conn JW, Knopf RF, Rull J. Stimulation of insulin secretion by amino acids. J Clin Invest. 1966;45(9):1487–502.
201. Ward WK, Bolgiano DC, McKnight B, Halter JB, Porte Jr D. Diminished B cell secretory capacity in patients with noninsulin-dependent diabetes mellitus. J Clin Invest. 1984;74(4):1318–28.
202. Palmer JP, Benson JW, Walter RM, Ensinck JW. Arginine-stimulated acute phase of insulin and glucagon secretion in diabetic subjects. J Clin Invest. 1976;58(3):565–70.
203. Byrne MM, Sturis J, Polonsky KS. Insulin secretion and clearance during low-dose graded glucose infusion. Am J Physiol. 1995;268(1 Pt 1):E21–7.
204. Kjems LL, Holst JJ, Volund A, Madsbad S. The influence of GLP-1 on glucose-stimulated insulin secretion: effects on beta-cell sensitivity in type 2 and nondiabetic subjects. Diabetes. 2003;52(2):380–6.
205. Hompesch M, ML, Win K, Vignati L, Hautpmann J, Hompesch M, et al. Oral presentation #148. European Association for the Study of Diabetes, Barcelona, 2013.
206. Schafer E. The endocrine organs. London: Longman, Green & Company; 1916.

Isotopic Tracers for the Measurement of Metabolic Flux Rates

3

Carine Beysen, Marc K. Hellerstein, and Scott M. Turner

> **Keywords**
>
> Glucose metabolism • Lipid metabolism • Lipoprotein metabolism • Metabolic flux • Isotope tracer • De novo lipogenesis • Liver • Adipose • Translational • Endogenous glucose production • Gluconeogenesis • Glycogenolysis • Dual tracer test • Glucose absorption • Glycolysis • Deuterated water • GC/MS • LC-MS/MS • Protein synthesis • In vivo

Summary

Background

Stable isotopes have been used for more than 75 years to assess the rates of synthesis and degradation, or turnover, of proteins, lipids, and carbohydrates in animals and humans. Advances in the sensitivity and sophistication of mass spectrometry and modelling and interpretation of tracer data have made possible the development of numerous useful tools for determining the turnover or many pathways that are important targets in disease development and treatment with pharmacological agents for cardio-metabolic disease. Stable isotope tracers are safe and simple to administer in a clinical research setting and allow – using minimally invasive techniques – the activity of synthetic and catabolic pathways to be quantified. The activity of agents that target the synthesis or degradation of fatty acids, triglycerides, glucose, or proteins can be directly assessed in individual subjects before and after treatment. The sensitive and quantitative nature of these measurements generally provides clear significant results with fewer than 20 subjects, allowing early assessment of pharmacologic activity in clinical studies. Because these measurements are quantitative, they can be very useful for defining dose response and pharmacokinetic/pharmacodynamic (PK/PD) relationships.

C. Beysen, PhD • M.K. Hellerstein, MD, PhD
S.M. Turner, PhD (✉)
KineMed, Inc., Emeryville, CA, USA
e-mail: sturner@kinemed.com

Key Methods

There are numerous publications describing isotope tracer methods. Our aim here is to provide methods and approaches that have worked well in our hands and with collaborators for investigations of pathophysiology and treatment interventions in early clinical trials. In many instances these isotope methods can be performed in tandem providing a "multiplexed" approach to metabolic flux analysis. Several examples of multiplexed study designs will be provided. Methods are divided in the table below according to the metabolic pathway assessed.

Lipid Metabolism

	Method	Measurement	Advantages	Disadvantages	Value in drug development decisions
Fasting hepatic DNL	2–3 days of oral administration of deuterated water (^2H_2O)	The fraction of palmitate that is newly synthesized in the liver	Outpatient, single blood sample, real world measurement	Repeat measurement variable depending on recent diet	Can be used to assess diet/drug interactions in response to chronic treatment; useful for evaluating nonalcoholic fatty liver disease
Fasting hepatic DNL	^{13}C-acetate infusion	The fraction of palmitate that is newly synthesized in the liver	Single blood measurement, known precursor pool enrichment	Requires overnight intravenous infusion. Repeat measurement variable depending on recent diet	Accurately assesses metabolic status and response to chronic treatment
Fructose-stimulated hepatic DNL	^{13}C-acetate infusion and continuous oral fructose feeding	The fraction of palmitate that is newly synthesized in the liver in response to fructose feeding	Very reproducible; less between subject variability compared to fasting hepatic DNL; known precursor pool enrichment	Requires 24-h inpatient intravenous infusion and repeated fructose dosing	Accurate assessment of acute or chronic inhibition of DNL; particularly useful for evaluation of lipogenesis inhibitors
Adipose DNL and triglyceride synthesis	14–21 days of oral administration of deuterated water (^2H_2O)	The fraction of palmitate and triglyceride that are newly synthesized in adipose tissue	In vivo assessment of fatty acid and triglyceride synthesis rates in adipose tissue; can be combined with adipocyte cell proliferation measurement	Requires adipose tissue sample	Can evaluate chronic effects on adipose growth/metabolism; particularly valuable for weight loss and insulin-sensitizing agents

DNL de novo lipogenesis, *TG* triglyceride, ^2H_2O deuterated water

Glucose Metabolism

	Method	Measurement	Advantages	Disadvantages	Value in drug development decisions
Fasting endogenous glucose production (infusion)	Infusion of a stable isotope-labeled glucose	Rate of endogenous glucose production into plasma	Gold standard, quantifies hepatic and renal contribution to fasting glucose	5–7-h IV required	Demonstrate effects on regulation of fasting glucose
Suppression of endogenous glucose production (clamp)	Infusion of a stable isotope-labeled glucose during a hyperinsulinaemic euglycaemic clamp	Rate of endogenous glucose production into plasma	Gold standard for the measurement of hepatic insulin sensitivity, simultaneous measurement of peripheral insulin sensitivity	IV and glucose clamp required, prior knowledge of endogenous glucose production rates needed for optimal infusion protocol design	Evaluation of PK/PD effects on hepatic and peripheral insulin sensitivity

	Method	Measurement	Advantages	Disadvantages	Value in drug development decisions
Fasting endogenous glucose production (bolus)	Intravenous bolus of a stable isotope-labeled glucose with frequent blood sampling	Rate of endogenous glucose production into plasma	Easy to perform, shorter duration than intravenous method	Less validated, data modelling required, frequent blood sampling	Demonstrate effects on regulation of fasting glucose
Glycolysis	Oral administration of [6,6-^{2}H$_2$] glucose as part of a mixed meal of an oral glucose tolerance test (OGTT)	Disposal of oral glucose through glycolytic pathway (vs. glycogen storage)	Simple oral test to assess glycolysis	Accurate insulin measurements required to properly interpret	Adds additional information about the metabolic fate of glucose in an OGTT or mixed meal
Postprandial glucose fluxes	Dual tracer approach	Glucose absorption, glucose disposal an endogenous glucose production during a mixed meal	Simplified version of the triple tracer; can be combined with glycolysis measurement	IV and frequent blood sampling required, calculation of parameters based on some assumptions	Useful for evaluating PK/PD effects of glucose absorption inhibitors
Gluconeogenesis/ glycogenolysis	Infusion of ^{13}C-glycerol in combination with mass isotopomer distribution analysis (MIDA)	Contribution of gluconeogenesis vs. glycogenolysis to endogenous glucose production	Can be simultaneously assessed with endogenous glucose production	Glycogenolysis is calculated and not directly measured, MIDA requires highly accurate measurements	Can determine hepatic pathways contributing to hepatic glucose output

Lipoprotein and Protein Metabolism

	Method	Measurement	Advantages	Disadvantages	Value in drug development decisions
Intravenous bolus	Intravenous bolus of ^{13}C- leucine, multi-compartment modelling	Lipoproteins and protein synthesis rates	Gold standard, Simple administration of tracer, many model parameters accessible	Frequent blood sampling and multi-compartment modelling required	Can determine numerous mechanisms of altering lipoprotein concentrations
Primed constant infusion	Constant infusion of ^{2}H or ^{13}C labeled leucine and simple precursor/ product model	Lipoproteins and protein synthesis rates	Fewer samples required, straightforward modelling	Simple model, ignores some parameters	Can determine mechanisms of altering lipoprotein concentrations and turnover of regulatory proteins
Deuterated water	Oral administration of ^{2}H$_2$O	Tissue and whole-body protein synthesis rates	Simple oral tracer administration; simple lipoprotein and protein kinetics can be determined from a single blood draw or finger prick	Less useful for careful assessment of rapidly turning over proteins	Suitable for large trials, can concurrently assess lipid and carbohydrate metabolism with same tracer

Conclusions

Stable isotope tracer methods offer the early clinical investigator unique quantitative tools to evaluate pharmacodynamics in small clinical studies. These methods can also be performed in preclinical studies and provide early proof of mechanism and dose response in humans by demonstrating direct modulation of pathways in cardio-metabolic disease.

Introduction

Metabolic flux refers to transformations of chemicals in living systems in the dimension of time. These transformations may be biochemical in nature and involve synthesis, degradation, intermediary metabolism, storage, or other processes, or they may be spatial in nature and involve processes such as transport, uptake, or secretion. A central element to the definition of metabolic flux is that it is best described quantitatively in terms of the rate (mass/per unit time) at which the processes occur. Careful regulation of the flux through metabolic pathways may be seen as the unifying theme governing all cellular regulatory machinery, the central defining feature of a cell type, and the basis of phenotypic variability among cells and organisms.

There are few fields where measurements of metabolic fluxes have been more effectively utilized than in the study of cardio-metabolic disease. From the elucidation of carbon fluxes in the Krebs cycle [1] to the effect of diet on protein and lipid synthesis [2, 3], isotopes, both radioactive and stable, have been essential in understanding the source and fate of metabolites in cell biology and physiology. With the development of modern mass spectrometric methods, there has been an explosion in the number of pathways which can be accurately measured in vivo using stable isotope labeling techniques. Dozens of analytical methods and clinical protocols can be found in the literature dating back more than 70 years [4].

Regardless of the specific methodology used, the in vivo measurement of fluxes is a unique and powerful approach to assess disease physiology and clinical responses. The measurement of flux rates provides information about what is new within a biological system and how rapidly molecules are being synthesized and degraded. It is useful to see the flux of molecules as consisting of the production (rate of entry) and removal (rate of exit) of a molecule into a compartment in the body, such as the cytosol of a tissue or the bloodstream. Static measurements, in contrast to flux measurements, may provide information on the concentration, content, or structure of components of a system in a compartment in the body, which in turn reflects the balance between the input and output rates. When the input and output rates are the same, the system is at steady state, i.e., there are no changes in concentrations of molecules in the system over the time period studied. However, a system at steady state can have either high flux rates (large numbers of new molecules entering and replacing old molecules) or low flux rates (a small number of new molecules entering and replacing old molecules). Static measurements cannot reveal the turnover within the dynamic system that is at steady state and differentiate between these very different states. Understanding the dynamic state within a biological system and the effect of interventions on that state is especially important in early clinical trials where the duration of intervention is often not sufficient to reach a new steady-state condition as, for example, when a treatment targets a slow turnover molecular process, such as tissue fibrosis and brain myelin content. It is axiomatic that changes in flux necessarily precede changes in concentration and is often of a greater magnitude as counter regulatory pathways will typically feedback and "defend" steady-state concentrations [5, 6].

For the evaluation of early clinical responses to novel therapies, it is important that methods be relatively simple in order to be minimally burdensome on the subjects as well as the clinical research team. Here we present selected applications for the in vivo assessment of lipid, glucose, and protein metabolic flux using stable isotope tracers. The focus will be on methods that have been used effectively in early clinical research studies to study disease pathology and drug efficacy. This is by no means intended to be a review of all the available methods for measuring metabolic fluxes in vivo. Many of the methods described here may be performed with single quadrupole gas chromatography/mass spectroscopy (GC/MS) analysis methods, such as the Agilent 6890's series instruments which are inexpensive, widely available, and provide excellent quantitative isotope enrichment measurements when carried out properly. In principle, however, any instrument that can accurately measure the relative isotopomer abundance for a specific analyte can be used. Methods such as GC/MS, isotope ratio mass spectrometry (IR/MS), liquid chromatography-tandem mass spectrometry (LC-MS/MS), and nuclear magnetic resonance (NMR) can be combined with stable isotope tracers to measure metabolic fluxes in vivo very accurately, provided appropriate analytical expertise is applied. The tracers presented herein reflect what we feel to be the most practical choices in terms of cost and utility. Although in certain cases substitutions are possible, care must be taken and careful consideration given to the fate of specific labeled carbon or hydrogen atoms.

The well-established safety and straightforward regulatory status of stable isotope tracers are worth mentioning. Stable isotopes have been safely administered in human research for decades. The long-standing policy of the US Food and Drug Administration is that "if a substance does not otherwise require submission of an IND (i.e., investigational new drug application), then that substance enriched with a stable isotope does not require an IND either. Thus, INDs are not required for metabolic tracer studies using stable isotope-enriched substances such as water, glucose and individual amino acids." This policy is based on extensive biological evidence that the introduction of tracer levels of stable isotope-perturbed molecules carries no additional risks compared to their natural abundance congeners [7–9]. This is certainly well established for stable isotope-tagged glucose, glycerol, acetate, fatty acids, and amino acids which can be given safely orally or intravenously provided usual US Pharmacopeia (USP) precautions are taken [9].

Deuterated or heavy water is an increasingly common and highly versatile stable isotope-tagged precursor used in clinical and preclinical research [10, 11]. Deuterated water (^2H_2O) as a tracer for clinical studies is safe and well tolerated, as well as being simple to administer [7–9]. Deuterated water does have some biological effects at very high doses (>20 % enrichment in cellular water in an organism), but these levels are more than an order of magnitude greater than is required or achieved for flux rate measurements in people and would never be achieved in a clinical setting [12]; in general the body water enrichments (% ^2H_2O) used range from 1 to 2 % in clinical studies and <10 % in animal studies. The only notable side effect of giving deuterated water to humans is a transient feeling of dizziness or vertigo if the tracer is initially administered too quickly. This is thought to be the result of slight changes in the fluid dynamics in the inner ear. This effect has been reported to occur in approximately 1 in 30 subjects but can be essentially completely eliminated if the dose of deuterated water for an adult is less than 40 mL every 3 h [12].

It is recognized in the field of enzymology that there are "isotope" effects on certain reactions, comparing the rate of a 100 % labeled site vs. natural abundance. In principle this could have a small but measurable effect on stable isotope tracer studies in vivo. These theoretical isotope effects are relevant to any reaction wherein a chemical bond containing the heavy atom is broken. In vivo, however, the observed isotope effect for ^{13}C or deuterium is minimal for almost all reactions, with the exception of certain carboxylation/decarboxylation reactions. This is confirmed by the observation that over the lifetime of a mammal, there is not a significant accumulation or depletion of heavy atom-containing molecules (as is seen in some plant metabolic processes, such as carbon dioxide fixation which may exhibit isotope effect and differential retention of ^{13}C). Moreover, studies comparing deuterated water labeling with ^{13}C labeling of the same pathways have repeatedly given the same results when directly compared [13] in spite of having significantly different theoretical isotope effects.

Stable isotope administration combined with mass spectrometry can reliably determine the flux rates through many metabolic pathways involved in cardio-metabolic diseases. Quantitative assessments of pathways of glucose metabolism [14, 15], fatty acid [16, 17], triglyceride [18, 19], and lipoprotein metabolism [20, 21] as well as muscle protein turnover [22, 23] including mitochondria biogenesis [24] can be studied using minimally invasive techniques applicable in early clinical as well as in preclinical studies.

De Novo Lipogenesis

Introduction

De novo lipogenesis (DNL) is the synthesis of fatty acids from their metabolic precursor, acetyl-CoA. This process can in principle occur in all cells but in humans is primarily performed, in quantitative terms, by adipose and liver tissues. Other tissues, however, such as skeletal muscle, pancreatic β-cells, skin, blood cells, and hypothalamus, have been shown to carry out DNL to some extent, with what may be critical regulatory functions in cellular metabolism. Indeed, where it was once believed to simply be an "overflow" pathway for excess carbohydrate intake, DNL is increasingly recognized to be a key regulatory pathway influencing lipid metabolism, fuel oxidation, plasma triglyceride production, tissue insulin resistance, and obesity [25, 26]. Abnormal regulation of DNL has been observed in numerous animal models of metabolic syndrome and diabetes, and recent clinical research has demonstrated increased hepatic DNL in nonalcoholic fatty liver disease (NAFLD) [27] and impaired adipose DNL in insulin resistance [28]. Finally, DNL may also play a significant role in the detrimental effects of certain dietary factors (e.g., fructose) which contribute to the etiology of cardio-metabolic diseases [29, 30]. Measurement of DNL and other lipid synthesis pathways may also be useful in the study of adipose metabolism and obesity. During the development of obesity, there is accumulation of lipid in adipose tissues. Accordingly, quantifying adipose tissue triglyceride and fatty acid synthesis is likely to be important in studying the development of obesity. The dynamic state of adipose lipid stores may play a role in the development and treatment of obesity [18].

DNL may be a viable pathway to target directly with pharmacological agents. Inhibition of DNL may increase fatty acid oxidation, relieve ectopic fat accumulation, and improve insulin sensitivity [25, 31]. Furthermore, the observation that DNL is increased in insulin resistance and NAFLD may make measurement of DNL useful for evaluating improved metabolic status in response to interventions which do not directly target lipid synthesis. It should be pointed out that simply measuring the concentrations of palmitate (the primary end product of DNL) is generally insufficient to evaluate DNL pathway activity, because DNL generally contributes a minority of circulating or stored palmitate, the majority of which is derived from diet.

There are numerous ways to approach measuring these pathways in vivo [18, 32, 33]. Here we will focus on describing a few examples of useful clinical stable isotope tracer approaches for evaluating hepatic and adipose lipid synthesis with an emphasis on the physiological and pharmacological questions they address. Specifically, two approaches to measuring lipid fluxes in vivo will be described; deuterated water labeling is useful for long-term and comprehensive analysis, and ^{13}C-acetate labeling is an attractive option when short-term quantitative sensitivity and minimum variability of the pathway is desired.

Background

The use of stable isotope tracers to measure lipid synthesis began in the Department of Biological Chemistry of the Columbia College of Physicians and Surgeons in New York in 1935. Rudolf Schoenheimer developed the first approaches using deuterated water to measure the "dynamic state of body constituents" [34]. Many talented researchers have since utilized stable and radioactive isotopes to provide our current body of knowledge on the regulation of lipid synthesis. Contemporary measurement of DNL is performed using either deuterated water or ^{13}C-acetate. Both of these labeling approaches have intrinsic advantages and limitations, which are highlighted below. In general, however, when utilized properly, the two methods deliver nearly identical results. While it is beyond the scope of this text to detail the analytical methods or derive calculation parameters, several excellent reviews and texts are available [3, 19, 32, 33].

Key Methods

De Novo Lipogenesis Measured Using Deuterated Water

Deuterated water can be used to assess the contribution of DNL to total palmitate in adipose samples and plasma very low-density lipoprotein (VLDL) triglycerides. Orally administered deuterated water is freely permeable across almost all biological membranes, is well mixed in the body, and its enrichment within the body water compartment is easily maintained for extended periods of time because of relatively slow turnover of body water (half-life 7–10 days). Labeled hydrogen atoms from deuterated water (^{2}H$_2$O) enter into biosynthetic pathways by exchange with cellular water or by specific incorporation of H from NAD(P)H. Deuterated water is a particularly useful tracer for assessment of lipid synthesis because it can be administered for long periods of time, and the label is incorporated into multiple lipid components so that, if desired, the synthesis rate of cholesterol, phospholipid, triglyceride, and fatty acids can be determined in a single experiment. Cell proliferation, i.e., deoxyribonucleic (DNA) synthesis [18, 35] as well as protein synthesis, can also be measured through deuterated water labeling [11, 22, 36] (see protein synthesis).

Deuterated water has been given to humans for more than 70 years without significant adverse effects, and animals have been raised for sequential generations on relatively high levels of deuterium water (e.g., up to 15–20 %), without phenotypic consequences or adverse effects. Additionally, no known risks have been observed in studies examining the effect of deuterated water on male or female reproductive tissues, including sperm function. As mentioned, the only minor adverse effect reported for deuterated water at these doses is transient dizziness when the initial rate of deuterated water intake is too rapid, occurring in approximately 1 in 30 individuals, which typically resolves completely within 3 h. Accordingly, care must be taken in the initial loading rate of deuterated water that is administered.

Method

Deuterated water labeling studies generally consist of several short outpatient visits for blood or tissue sampling, while the deuterated water is consumed daily at home. For proof of concept studies in healthy subjects, adult female and male volunteers are appropriate. Bulk deuterated water is available from several vendors and can be administered as 100 % or a more dilute solution, typically 70 %. Deuterated water is most conveniently prepared in single-use bottles which should be tested for sterility to ensure safe use and durable shelf life. Plasma, urine, or saliva samples are appropriate for measurement of body water enrichments provided they are collected in tubes with no additional liquid (e.g., spray-dried anticoagulants should be used). Often frequent ^{2}H$_2$O measurements are desired, and this can be easily done by the subject collecting saliva at home in salivette containers that are mailed to the laboratory or frozen and brought to the site during a scheduled visit. The dose of deuterated water given is dependent on the specific study design; however, a typical labeling paradigm that works well in most settings is as follows: Subjects receive loading doses of 70 % deuterated water for 2 days administered as oral doses of 50–60 mL four times daily to achieve approximately 1 % body water enrichment. Subjects then continue to take a single daily oral deuterated water dose (50–60 mL of 70 % deuterated water) until completion of the study. Subjects return to the site outpatient visits for blood collection. At all outpatient visits, plasma, urine, or saliva samples are collected to determine body deuterated water enrichments and to determine fractional

DNL in very low-density lipoprotein triglyceride or total plasma triglyceride. Adipose samples can be collected after 7 days for assessment of DNL. Subcutaneous adipose tissue biopsy samples are obtained under sterile conditions and local anesthesia with 1 % lidocaine. After a small incision, a biopsy needle (Bard Biopsy Systems, Crawley, UK) is used to obtain tissue samples. The portion of adipose tissue used for lipid synthesis should be rinsed in saline and immediately frozen. Alternatively subcutaneous adipose tissue can be collected though aspiration. Examples of typical values for body water enrichment, DNL, triglyceride, and cholesterol synthesis in the plasma compartment are shown in Fig. 3.1.

Advantages/Disadvantages

Using deuterated water labeling for assessing de novo lipid synthesis has several intrinsic advantages over other approaches. The flexibility in timing from hours to weeks allows for measurements in different metabolic compartments to be made in the same subject. The ubiquitous nature of deuterated water labeling also allows the turnover of multiple metabolites to be assessed simultaneously. The ability to assess lipogenesis at metabolic steady state integrates diurnal and dietary fluctuations into a single real world measurement. Finally, the simple route of administration (oral, once daily) unburdens the patient and research sites from requiring overnight intravenous infusions.

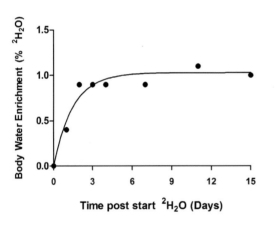
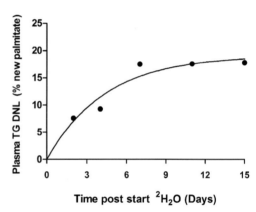
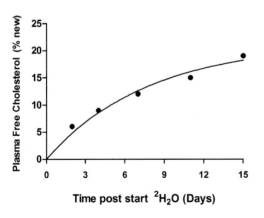
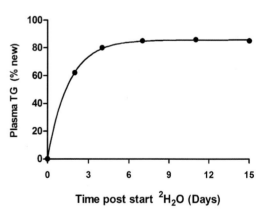

Fig. 3.1 An example of the use of oral deuterated water (^2H_2O) as a metabolic tracer for the simultaneous measurement of de novo lipogenesis (DNL), triglyceride (TG) and cholesterol turnover in the plasma compartment in a human volunteer. The subject received loading doses of 70 % ^2H_2O for 2 days (four aliquots of 60 ml of 70 % ^2H_2O given at least 3 h apart on day 1 and day 2) followed by a single dose of 60 ml of 70 % ^2H_2O once daily until the end of the experiment to achieve steady-state body deuterated water enrichments of approximately 1 %

There are some drawbacks to this labeling approach, principally around the interaction between behavior and metabolism. Because deuterated water labeling is generally used in the outpatient setting, potential variability or changes in diet or other behaviors need to be considered. Deuterated water labeling also requires some time to reach the optimal enrichment in the body water pool and thus is not ideal for very short-term kinetic studies that require high precursor pool enrichments. Deuterated water also has a long half-life in the body which prevents short-term (<3 weeks) restudy of subjects. For studies where very tight metabolic control over the short-term is desired, we recommend using ^{13}C-acetate infusion method.

De Novo Lipogenesis Measured Using ^{13}C-Acetate

Intravenous infusion of ^{13}C-acetate is another common method used to measure hepatic DNL. Oral or intravenous acetate is efficiently taken up by the liver and the intrahepatic acetyl-CoA pool is labeled. As lipids are synthesized, ^{13}C acetyl-CoA is incorporated into the new fatty acids and the fractional synthesis can in principle be calculated from a simple precursor/product ratio. The challenge historically has been the difficulty in accurately determining the isotope enrichment in the intrahepatic acetyl-CoA precursor pool. Additionally, other concerns regarding the lack of equilibrium of acetate across the liver have also been raised. Both of these methodological considerations have been largely resolved. The intracellular acetyl-CoA pool enrichment can be noninvasively determined using mass isotopomer distribution analysis (MIDA) [33, 37] or other similar combinatorial algorithms [38] which largely correct for any transhepatic disequilibrium [39] and have been shown to give results in line with deuterated water labeling methods where equilibration is not an issue. There are many possible ways to utilize this approach for assessing hepatic DNL. ^{13}C-acetate can be safely infused for several days, and diurnal changes in DNL can be monitored [40, 41]. For proof of concept studies focused on the regulation of hepatic DNL, we have found the use of a controlled dietary stimulation to deliver very reproducible results in cross-sectional and particularly longitudinal studies where subjects can serve as their own controls.

While obese and diabetic subjects are known to have higher than normal basal fasting levels of hepatic fractional DNL, on the order of 15–20 % contribution to VLDL palmitate, healthy lean individuals have fasting hepatic fractional DNL on the order of 3–5 % after a brief 8–12-h infusion of labeled acetate [40, 42]. Fasting DNL varies considerably within as well as among subjects, due to influences from changes in exercise, alcohol, diet (both caloric content and carbohydrate composition) [30, 43], energy balance, weight, etc. [26]. A high carbohydrate diet can increase DNL from 5 % or less to 20 % in the fasting state, for example. Accordingly, study cohorts should be carefully enrolled to match for these physiological factors, as well as body mass index (BMI), sex, age, etc. when fasting DNL is the measurement of interest. It is known that acute ingestion of ethanol and fructose can increase fractional DNL contribution to circulating fatty acids in VLDL triglyceride from baseline to approximately 35 %, and we have shown that fructose-stimulated DNL assessments are very reproducible compared to fasting DNL [44]. The improvement in variability in the DNL measurement with fructose feeding will require fewer subjects to find certain effects in clinical studies.

Method

Subjects receive a standardized eucaloric dinner on day 0 and abstain from all foods and drinks (except water), until the oral fructose intake begins the next morning. On day 0 (e.g., 10:00 PM) a continuous infusion of 1-^{13}C-acetic acid (sodium salt) is started and continuous until the last sample for DNL is drawn. An infusion rate of approximately 10 mg ^{13}C-acetate per minute is ideal. A fasting blood draw is taken in the morning of day 1 prior to fructose dosing, then oral fructose (approximately 10 mg/kg fat free mass/min) is given as a drink every 30 min (e.g., 20 drinks given over 9.5 h). Blood samples are obtained regularly until 10 h post. There should be a minimum of a 5-day washout interval between fructose/[1-^{13}C]acetate administration studies to allow labeled fatty acids to be cleared from hepatic lipid stores.

Fasting- and fructose-stimulated hepatic DNL is determined by measuring the incorporation of [1-^{13}C] acetate into palmitate in circulating VLDL triglyceride by use of mass isotopomer distribution analysis (MIDA) [33]. VLDL is isolated from frozen plasma samples (1 mL) by ultracentrifugation. Lipoprotein triglyceride should be prepared by thin-layer chromatography (TLC), and VLDL-triglyceride fatty acids are then trans-esterified to fatty acid methyl esters in preparation for GC/MS analysis. Fractional DNL should be calculated using MIDA as described. This method for determining hepatic precursor pool enrichment is important in this setting as the acetyl-CoA pool is significantly diluted by fructose in humans. An example of changes in plasma DNL and hepatic acetyl-CoA pool dilution with fructose feeding are shown in Fig. 3.2. In practice, fructose can be replaced with other dietary components. In our hands, fructose stimulation offers a very direct and predictable model for assessing hepatic lipogenesis [44]. Mixed meal stimulation have also been shown to work well.

Advantages/Disadvantages

Using ^{13}C-acetate combined with fructose administration to assess de novo lipid synthesis has several intrinsic advantages over other approaches. Because the fructose administration results in a reproducible individual response over time [44], the metabolic response to a treatment intervention such as a putative inhibitor of DNL (e.g., an acetyl-CoA carboxylase inhibitor or ATP-citrate lyase inhibitor) can be accurately quantified relative to dose and time of exposure in a small number of patients. This approach can be used for single and multiple dose studies as well as long-term interventions.

Drawbacks to this approach are largely operational; it requires overnight intravenous administration of acetate and repeated dosing of fructose during the day which can occasionally cause gastrointestinal discomfort.

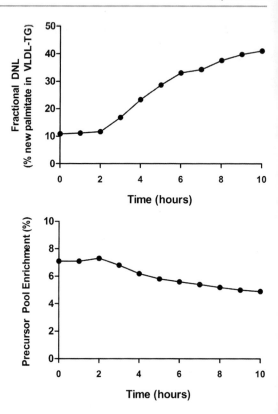

Fig. 3.2 Example of the response of hepatic de novo lipogenesis (DNL) and its precursor pool (hepatic acetyl-CoA) to acute fructose feeding in a healthy subject. The volunteer was confined to the Clinical Research Unit throughout the study under standardized conditions. At approximately 10:00 PM on day 0, an intravenous administration of [1-^{13}C] acetate (9–9.5 mg/min) was started and continued for approximately 19.5 h. Immediately following the fasting blood draw (8:00 AM on day 1 or 0 h), oral fructose (0.25 g per kg body weight) was started (8:30 AM on day 1 or 0.5 h) and given as a drink every 30 min (20 drinks given over 9.5 h). Blood samples were obtained hourly for 10 h post fructose for the assessment of hepatic DNL

Translating Results into Clinical Practice

Direct measurement of DNL can be extremely valuable in making early decisions in cardiometabolic drug development. Just as DNL sensitively responds to diet, it can be a very sensitive barometer of metabolic changes induced by a therapeutic intervention, making it an excellent pharmacodynamic marker and in some circumstances may predict treatment response or identify candidate populations for particular therapeutic targets. The role of DNL in the pathophysiology of fatty liver, obesity, and insulin resistance all point to this being an important pathway reflecting metabolic health which is also responsive to interventions. Assessment of DNL can be useful for evaluating diabetes, fatty liver, inflammation, obesity, and dyslipidemia and is particularly informative when combined with complementary assessments such as energy expenditure, food intake, triglyceride, or lipoprotein production, to name a few.

Because the role of DNL is varied and highly context-dependent, it is a challenge to tie alterations in DNL to a single clinical endpoint. Furthermore, direct inhibitors of DNL have not been studied for the clinical pharmacodynamics of DNL reduction in relation to specific disease components. On the other hand, several studies have examined the cross-sectional relationship between DNL and disease phenotype as well as examining dietary interventions which increase DNL specifically. Using the ^{13}C-acetate approach, Stanhope et al. [30] demonstrated that overfeeding of fructose beverages for 10 weeks increased meal-stimulated DNL by 50 % and resulted in a doubling of the postprandial triglyceride AUC (area under the curve). Interestingly, no increase was seen in fasting triglyceride or DNL in this study. Comparing insulin-resistant elderly subjects to young controls using deuterated water, Flannery et al. [45] observed a twofold higher rate of DNL in the insulin-resistant group, with corresponding increases in postprandial triglyceride concentrations, insulin level, and intrahepatic lipid content. Similarly in obese hypertriglyceridemic diabetic and nondiabetic subjects, a threefold increase in DNL was observed [40]. In a separate study, a 50 % reduction in DNL corresponded to 30 % drop in fasting plasma triglyceride. Finally, in fatty liver disease DNL has been consistently shown to be two to threefold elevated compared to controls [27]. Taking these results together it is evident that increased postprandial DNL is closely associated with clinically relevant aspects of cardiometabolic disease.

Conclusions

DNL is a relatively straightforward metabolic pathway to measure in vivo using a variety of stable isotope methodologies. Postprandial or stimulated DNL appears to have the most relevance when translating results into clinical practice and can be performed with either ^{13}C-acetate or deuterated water. The quantitative nature of these measurements make them well suited for early clinical trials and with the relative ease of administration of deuterated water for the study of DNL performing large clinical trials with quantitative flux measurements are now possible.

Glucose Metabolism

Introduction

Blood glucose concentrations are tightly controlled in healthy people through the regulation of both glucose disposal and glucose delivery by glucose, insulin, and other signals. In the fasting state, glucose circulating in the plasma is mainly produced by the liver whereas the brain is the major organ of glucose disposal. After a meal, glucose is absorbed from the intestine into the circulation, endogenous glucose production (EGP) is suppressed, and tissue glucose disposal is increased. Following a meal in a healthy person, glucose concentrations return to fasting levels within a few hours [46].

Type 2 diabetes is characterized by hyperglycaemia in both the fasting and the postprandial state. Even though type 2 diabetes is defined as a single disease, most clinicians recognize that type 2 diabetes is a complex, multifactorial disorder which may be the result of dysregulation of one or more pathways in glucose metabolism. Measurements of glucose concentrations are, of course, important but do not provide any mechanistic information of the metabolic events leading to type 2 diabetes. The metabolic flux of glucose through the different pathways can be measured using stable isotope tracer methodologies. These methods have been shown to be sensitive to detect changes in glucose pathways with disease and treatment, often before changes in glucose concentrations are detected. Because diabetes is such a multifactorial disease usually requiring polypharmacy for effective management, it is important to have the best possible understanding of the effect of new therapies on the metabolic pathways regulating glucose homeostasis.

Key Methods

Fasting Endogenous Glucose Production

Fasting EGP can be assessed using the isotope dilution technique [47]. Originally the method involved the use of radioactive tracers but the introduction of stable isotope-labeled glucose resulted in extensive research exploring the effect of disease and drug treatment on EGP in the postabsorptive state. Isotopic measurement of EGP represents glucose release from both the liver and the kidney, and although the quantitative contribution of renal glucose release (between 5 % and 28 % in healthy subjects) is small compared to that of the liver, one should not equate whole-body isotopically measured EGP with hepatic glucose production alone [48].

A variety of experimental protocols for the measurement of fasting endogenous glucose production have been described in the literature. Methodological differences are noted in the type of glucose tracer, administration of the tracer (continuous infusion vs. bolus), priming technique, tracer infusion time, timing, and number of sample collection and calculation models (steady-state vs. non-steady-state equations) used. It is generally accepted that the use of [U-^{13}C$_6$]-glucose and [6,6-^{2}H$_2$]-glucose provide the most relevant and easily interpretable measurement of total EGP in context of isotope loss or recycling during partial metabolism of glucose taken up by the liver [49]. Detailed description of the different tracers for the use of glucose production has been published by Wolfe [3]. Often, the tracer is administered as a primed-continuous infusion for 2–5 h, and plasma glucose enrichments are determined by GC/MS during the last 30–60 min of the steady-state period. The rate of EGP is then calculated using the steady-state equation:

$$\text{EGP} = \text{rate of tracer infusion} / \text{plasma glucose enrichment} - \text{rate of tracer infusion}.$$

In healthy subjects a fixed priming dose corresponding to a 100-min infusion is usually used. However, in insulin-resistant states, where the glucose pool size is increased, the priming dose should be adjusted for plasma glucose concentrations, and a prolonged infusion (4–6 h) is required for valid measurements when using steady-state equations, because of slower turnover rate of the larger extracellular glucose pool. An insufficient priming and infusion time when hyperglycaemia is present has been shown to overestimate EGP due to failure to reach true plateau glucose enrichments in the plasma compartment [50–52]. Indeed, the greater EGP rates in people with type 2 diabetes compared to healthy subjects have been questioned due to tracer protocol design. In our experience, using an adjusted prime and a 5–7-h continuous infusion of [U-^{13}C$_6$]-glucose or [6,6-^{2}H$_2$]-glucose, we can reproducibly demonstrate an isotopic steady state in essentially all subjects, and we consistently observe higher EGP values in type 2 diabetes compared to healthy subjects confirming published results.

While the primed-continuous infusion of a glucose tracer is the most commonly used method for the measurement of fasting EGP, and considered the gold standard, there may be some instances where a primed constant infusion is not desirable or possible. As an alternative, a bolus injection method has been validated against the primed-continuous infusion method [53]. By this method, a glucose tracer is administered as a bolus (7 mg/ kg body weight of [U-^{13}C$_6$]-glucose given over 1–3 min) and frequent blood samples are collected for 1–3 h. The decay of plasma glucose tracer enrichments is fit to a two- or three-exponential curve using a kinetic simulation module (e.g., SAAM II software [54]), and EGP is then calculated from the fit parameters. While published data are currently limited to healthy volunteers, we have seen very good agreement in patients with type 2 diabetes and impaired glucose tolerance as well (unpublished results).

Several endpoints can be calculated from the direct measurement of EGP. Hepatic insulin sensitivity has been calculated as the inverse of the product of EGP and fasting plasma insulin [55], while the metabolic clearance rate (MCR), which is a measurement of the ability of whole-body tissues to take up glucose in the fasting state, is calculated as EGP divided by glucose concentration.

Sources of Fasting EGP: Gluconeogenesis and Glycogenolysis

Several approaches have been described to measure the contribution of gluconeogenesis and glycogenolysis to fasting endogenous glucose production [3]. In this chapter we focus on the method described by Hellerstein et al. involving the infusion of $[2\text{-}^{13}C_1]$ glycerol and the use of MIDA [56, 57]. This method allows the calculation of gluconeogenesis from all three-carbon sources; lactate, amino acids, and glycerol. A primed-continuous infusion of $[2\text{-}^{13}C_1]$ glycerol is administered to label the precursor pool (hepatic triose phosphate) for glucose synthesis for several hours (see above), and samples are taken during the last 30–60 min. The $[2\text{-}^{13}C_1]$ glycerol can be infused with $[U\text{-}^{13}C_6]$-glucose or $[6,6\text{-}^2H_2]$-glucose for the simultaneous measurement of gluconeogenesis and endogenous glucose production. The principle of MIDA and its application for measuring biosynthesis of a variety of polymers (e.g., glucose) have been discussed in detail elsewhere [37, 58]. In brief, the technique consists of quantifying fractional abundances of different mass isotopomers (i.e., different isotopic isomers) in an intact polymer (e.g., glucose) that contains two or more repeats of a precursor monomeric subunit. Gluconeogenesis can be conceptualized as the polymerization synthesis of two triose-phosphate monomers. The fractional abundances of mass isotopomers (M0 for unlabeled glucose, M1 for singly labeled glucose, and M2 for doubly labeled glucose) in the polymer must then be accurately measured by GC/MS and compared with the natural fractional abundance of baseline values to calculate changes, or excesses, of mass isotopomeric species in the polymer. The precursor pool enrichment (i.e., the hepatic triose-phosphate isotope content, for glucose) can then be back-calculated from the pattern or distribution of mass isotopomeric excesses in the polymer (glucose), using formulae derived from the binomial or multinomial expansions, as described in detail elsewhere [57]. Once the precursor pool enrichment is established, the precursor/product relationship can be applied for calculation of the fraction of polymers that were derived from the endogenous biosynthetic pathway during the labeling period. In the case of gluconeogenesis, the ratio of excess doubly labeled glucose to excess single-labeled glucose species reveals the isotopic abundance of the true precursor pool, from which fractional gluconeogenesis can be calculated. Absolute flux through gluconeogenesis into plasma glucose can then be calculated as the fractional gluconeogenic contribution times the rate of fasting EGP. These two parameters can be assessed simultaneously, as described above. The absolute contribution of glycogenolysis to fasting EGP is calculated as the difference of rate of fasting EGP and rate of gluconeogenesis. Potential methodological problems have been addressed and discussed in detail by Neese et al. [57]. More complex stable isotope techniques like the secreted glucuronate technique have been described for the measurement of intrahepatic glycogen fluxes. This method has been described in detail elsewhere [57, 59].

Suppression of EGP During a Hypersulinaemic Euglycaemic Clamp

Hepatic insulin resistance is a key player of whole-body insulin resistance in people with type 2 diabetes [60]. Fasting rates of EGP are often elevated and suppression of glucose production during intestinal absorption of a meal is impaired in type 2 diabetes. The gold standard to determine hepatic insulin sensitivity is the measurement of partial suppression of EGP during a low-dose insulin infusion. Tracer methodology combined with the hyperinsulinaemic euglycaemic clamp allows the simultaneous measurement of fasting EGP, insulin-mediated suppression of hepatic glucose production (hepatic insulin sensitivity), and tissue glucose disposal (peripheral insulin sensitivity) independent of the effects of hyperglycaemia per se. Currently the best methodology to do this is the so-called hot GINF (glucose infusion) method proposed a few decades ago [61, 62]. The method is designed to keep the ratio of the glucose tracer to tracee in plasma constant during the fasting state and during the clamp to minimize errors (or negative values) in EGP measurements due to non-steady-state conditions. Ideally, deviations in circulating tracer enrichments should be kept to <20 % to avoid errors in the EGP results [63]. The method involves the administration of a glucose tracer as a primed-continuous infusion and as part of the exogenous glucose infusion (GINF) used during the clamp. The tracer enrichment of the GINF is calculated to be equal to the expected plasma tracer enrichment at the start of clamp. Originally a radioactive or hot glucose tracer was added to the exogenous glucose infusion, hence the name hot GINF. The continuous infusion of the glucose tracer is started before the clamp to determine fasting EGP as described above. Its rate is then reduced at the start of the clamp and after fasting EGP measures are completed to approximate the expected fall of EGP during the clamp (e.g., the infusion rate of the tracer is reduced to half the starting rate if a 50 % reduction of EGP is expected during the clamp). The anticipated fall in EGP during the clamp depends on several factors such as patient population (e.g., healthy subjects may have a greater suppression of EGP than subjects with type 2 diabetes under similar insulin conditions), clamp insulin infusion rates, and duration of the clamp. Pilot experiments are recommended to determine the optimal tracer design during the clamp if there is not prior experience with the patient population and method. An intrinsic limitation of this approach is therefore that the quantitative effects of an intervention on EGP have to be to some extent known in advance to apply the model. Examples of EGP measured during a

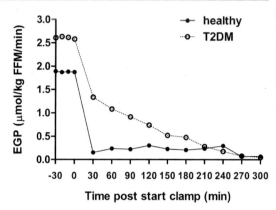

Fig. 3.3 Endogenous glucose production (EGP) measured after an overnight fast (from −30 to 0 min) and during a hyperinsulinemic isoglycemic clamp (from 0 to 300 min) in a healthy person and a person with type 2 diabetes (T2DM). Fasting EGP was measured with the isotope dilution methodology using a 5-h primed-continuous infusion of [6,6-^{2}H$_2$]-glucose. Suppression of EGP in response to insulin during the clamp was measured using the hot glucose infusion (hot GINF) protocol. During the clamp, insulin was infused at 40 mU/m^2/min which resulted in steady-state insulin concentration of approximately 50 μU/mL. *FFM* is fat free mass

clamp in a healthy subject and an individual with type 2 diabetes are shown in Fig. 3.3.

In order to perform hyperinsulinaemic euglycaemic clamps in subjects with type 2 diabetes, plasma glucose concentrations are typically lowered to euglycaemic levels by a low-dose overnight infusion of exogenous insulin prior to the clamp. Staehr et al. have shown that neither fasting EGP nor suppression of EGP or Rd during a hyperinsulinaemic euglycaemic clamp are affected by overnight normalization of plasma glucose levels; however, in their study, fasting glucose disposal rates were lowered by this procedure [64].

Measurement of Postprandial Glucose Fluxes During a Mixed Meal Test: The Dual Tracer Approach

Much of our knowledge about glucose metabolism is based on measurements performed in the fasting state or during nonphysiologic settings, such as intravenous glucose and insulin administration (glucose clamp) studies, as described above (also see Chap. 1). Although these measurements are important to understanding the

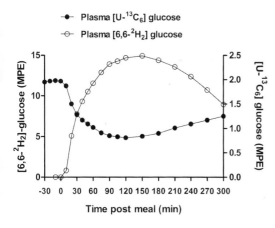

Fig. 3.4 Plasma glucose enrichments measured during a dual tracer test in a healthy subject. A 15-h primed-continuous infusion of [U-^{13}C$_6$] glucose (0.03 mg/kg body weight/min, prime 3 mg/kg body weight) was started at −300 min. A mixed meal was administered at 0 min and consisted of a glucose drink containing a total of 75 g of glucose of which 15 g was [6,6-^{2}H$_2$] glucose and foods containing fat and protein. *MPE* is molar percent excess

pathophysiology and treatment of type 2 diabetes, it should be recognized that humans spend most of their time in the postprandial (fed) state. The glucose response to a meal is a dynamic, non-steady-state process, and the determination of postprandial glucose fluxes is more challenging and complex than the fasting response. The dual glucose tracer method to assess glucose fluxes during the oral glucose tolerance test was first introduced by Steele et al. [65] and has been used and further adapted by others to study glucose responses to a mixed meal. The dual tracer method utilizes two distinct glucose tracers that can be differentiated analytically (e.g., [U-^{13}C$_6$] glucose and [6,6-^{2}H$_2$]). One is infused intravenously and the second is administered orally as part of the meal. An example of measured plasma glucose tracer enrichments during a dual glucose tracer test is shown in Fig. 3.4. Glucose fluxes are then calculated using Steele's non-steady-state one-compartment model [65]. The rate of appearance of total glucose (R$_a$T, labeled and unlabeled glucose from ingested, endogenous, and infused sources) is calculated from isotopic dilution of the infused glucose tracer. The rate of appearance of oral glucose (R$_a$O or often referred to as glucose absorption) is calculated from the rate of appearance of the ingested glucose tracer and the glucose tracer enrichment of the meal. EGP is then calculated by subtraction of R$_a$O and the infused glucose from R$_a$T. When using the dual tracer method, one has to recognize that the one-compartment model and its assumptions (e.g., a fixed value for the effective volume of distribution) may be inadequate for the measurement of glucose fluxes, especially when glucose concentrations and enrichments change rapidly. Investigators have tried to overcome this limitation by using more complex models [66, 67] or by minimizing the changes in tracer over time by changing the infusion rate of the intravenous tracer to mimic changes in EGP [68]. Additionally, a more complex triple-tracer approach was developed [69] to minimize changes in both meal and endogenous plasma tracer enrichments to provide model-independent estimates of glucose fluxes. These updated methods are experimentally and computationally complex, however, and require a priori knowledge of the changes in the glucose fluxes and have not consistently shown to outperform the dual tracer technique [70].

Glycolytic Disposal of an Oral Glucose Load

Glycolysis is the breakdown of glucose into pyruvate (aerobic glycolysis) or lactate (anaerobic glycolysis) in cells following glucose uptake and glucose phosphorylation, to provide substrates for energy production and energy storage (glycogenesis and lipogenesis). Glycolytic disposal in the postprandial state has been characterized in healthy subjects using sophisticated methods like the tritiated-glucose release of tritiated water technique [71]. Results from these studies show that glycolysis is an important route for glucose disposal and accounts for ~66 % of overall glucose disposal during a meal in healthy people [72]. In the presence of type 2 diabetes, however, glycolysis is significantly reduced [73], making glycolysis a potentially interesting target for the treatment of type 2 diabetes.

More recently, a simple method for the measurement of whole-body glycolytic disposal of oral glucose during an oral glucose tolerance test (OGTT) [14] and during a mixed meal [15] has been described. The method involves an oral glucose challenge containing deuterated glucose ([6,6-^{2}H$_2$]-glucose) with or without other foods, followed by the measurement of deuterated water in blood using a very sensitive infrared laser spectrophotometer. For [6,6-^{2}H$_2$]-glucose (which has deuterium label only on carbon 6), >90 % of the ^{2}H$_2$ atoms are only lost to tissue water during glycolytic metabolism to pyruvate and oxaloacetate; otherwise, the ^{2}H$_2$ atoms are non-labile and are retained in the glucose molecule [49], e.g., after phosphorylation and direct entry into tissue glycogen or partial glycolytic metabolism to the triose-phosphate level and recycling to the glucose-phosphate level. Using this method, Beysen et al. [14] and others [74] showed that the total flux of glucose through the glycolytic pathway in the postprandial state was similar in insulin-resistant and insulin-sensitive nondiabetic subjects but was confirmed to be reduced in subjects with type 2 diabetes (unpublished). When glycolysis was expressed per unit of plasma insulin exposure, however, glycolytic disposal of the oral glucose load was also impaired in the insulin-resistant nondiabetic subjects. These results indicate that insulin-mediated whole-body glycolytic disposal is a feature of insulin resistance but that, interestingly, the islet β-cell compensation in insulin-resistant nondiabetic subjects but not in type 2 diabetes is sufficient to overcome the insulin-resistant state of glycolytic flux and to normalize whole-body glycolytic rates. Whole-body glycolysis, corrected for ambient exposure to plasma insulin, as measured by this simple test (deuterated glucose disposal test or ^{2}H-GDT) was found to be a quantitative measure of insulin sensitivity, based on a high correlation of results from the ^{2}H-GDT to results obtained from the hyperinsulinaemic euglycaemic clamp, the gold standard for the measurement of insulin sensitivity. Results from the ^{2}H-GDT (^{2}H$_2$O production per unit of insulin) strongly ($r=0.95$, $P<0.0001$) correlated with the clamp results, whereas surrogate markers of insulin resistance (e.g., homeostasis model assessment (HOMA), fasting serum insulin, Matsuda index, etc.) correlated much less well [14]. The ^{2}H-GDT has been applied, for example, to investigate the mechanism of action of the glucose-lowering effect of colesevelam, a bile acid sequestrant. Colesevelam improved total glycolytic flux (total ^{2}H$_2$O produced) but not glycolysis per unit of insulin (^{2}H$_2$O per insulin AUC), indicating that colesevelam treatment resulted in an improved β-cell response without effects on insulin sensitivity.

Example of an Experimental Design Using Stable Isotopes for the Measurement of Glucose, Lipid and Bile Acid Pathways in Humans

Figure 3.5 shows an example of a stable isotope protocol to simultaneously measure glucose, lipid, and bile acid pathways. This experimental design was used to evaluate metabolic changes with colesevelam treatment in individuals with type 2 diabetes [15]. Multiple stable isotopes were used: [1-^{13}C$_1$]acetate (intravenous) for fractional DNL, cholesterol, and bile acid synthesis; [2-^{13}C$_1$]glycerol (intravenous) for gluconeogenesis; [U-^{13}C$_6$] glucose (intravenous) for EGP; and oral [6,6-^{2}H$_2$] glucose for glucose absorption and whole-body glycolysis. When designing an experimental stable isotope protocol such as this, great care needs to be taken to avoid isotopic interference and erroneous results. For example, the entry of ^{13}C from [U-^{13}C$_6$]glucose as a doubly labeled species into the triose-phosphate pool will contaminate measurement of gluconeogenesis based on the MIDA approach, which assumes that double-labeled glucose species derived from combination of two single-labeled triose-phosphate species. The result will be an underestimation of gluconeogenesis. Accordingly, a low tracer infusion rate for [U-^{13}C$_6$] glucose is used to minimize recycling of double-labeled ^{13}C$_2$-triose-phosphate species in liver when infused with [2-^{13}C$_1$]glycerol [75].

Translating Results into Clinical Practice

Systematic meta-analysis shows that currently approved oral glucose-lowering agents have similar effects on haemoglobin A$_{1C}$ (HbA$_{1c}$) [33]. On average, approximately a 1–1.25 % reduction in HbA$_{1C}$ has been observed, with most of the treatment effect evident by 3–6 months of initiation. Despite similar effects on glycemic controls, many of these drugs have distinct mechanism of action (MOA). Understanding the MOA of the different classes of oral glucose-lowering drugs will make

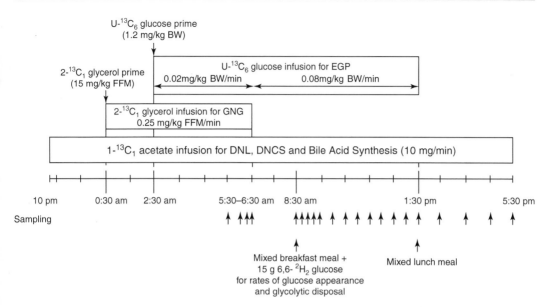

Fig. 3.5 Example of an experimental design using stable isotopes for the simultaneous measurement of glucose, lipid and bile acid pathways in humans. *BW* Body weight, *FFM* fat free mass, *DNL* de novo lipogenesis, *DNCS* de novo cholesterol synthesis, *GNG* gluconeogenesis, *EGP* endogenous glucose production

drug selection and disease management more successful. The use of stable isotope methods has been proven to be an excellent tool to investigate the MOA of drugs and may help in identifying responders vs. nonresponders to single-agent or combination therapy. Stable isotope technologies are also suitable for the investigation of the mechanism of adverse effects of glucose-lowering drugs. An example from our group is the application of stable isotope methods (see description of study design above) to elucidate the MOA of glucose-lowering of the bile acid sequestrant colesevelam [15]. We showed that the improvement in HbA$_{1C}$ (−0.6 % compared to placebo) was mediated through an increase in fasting plasma glucose clearance and an increase in glycolytic disposal of oral glucose but not by effects on intestinal glucose absorption. The improvements in glucose control were associated with increases in glucagon-like peptide (GLP)-1 and glucose-dependent insulinotopic peptide (GIP) concentrations. Colesevelam treatment also prevented increases in EGP and glycogenolysis, suggesting a predominant action of colesevelam on glucose homeostasis in the liver, distinct from the metabolic actions of metformin. Interestingly, every subject treated with colesevelam showed a significant increase in bile acid and cholesterol syntheses, confirming target engagement and inhibition of the cholesterol absorption pathway, but this did not always result in an improvement in glucose kinetics. These results not only indicate that drug compliance was excellent but that it may prove important to characterize the metabolic basis of responders vs. nonresponders to improve drug efficacy.

Stable isotope techniques have also been applied to better understand the differential metabolic effects of pioglitazone and rosiglitazone on hepatic glucose and lipid metabolism. Treatment with these two thiazolidinediones improves plasma glucose and HbA$_{1C}$ concentrations equally but differences in lipid metabolism have been observed [76]. Different effects on the regulation of hepatic metabolic pathways, for example, may be of relevance to the differences in cardiovascular disease outcomes that have been reported for these two thiazolidinediones [77, 78]. Using methods described above, it has been shown that hepatic DNL was reduced by 40 % with pioglitazone treatment, whereas no changes were seen with rosiglitazone treatment [36]. Moreover, fasting EGP improved with pioglitazone but not with rosiglitazone. Other studies have found effects on EGP with both treatments, but effects of pioglitazone on both EGP and hepatic lipid synthesis or DNL suggest greater activity of pioglitazone on liver metabolism in patients with type 2 diabetes. These results also highlight that even drugs within a given class of glucose-lowering agents cannot always be considered to have identical metabolic effects. Stable isotope methods have also been applied to investigate the MOA of recently approved sodium-glucose cotransporter 2 (SGLT2) inhibitors. SGLT2 inhibitors (e.g., canagliflozin and dapagliflozin) improve glucose control by increasing renal glucose excretion in the urine. Stable isotope methods revealed, however, that dapagliflozin [79] and empagliflozin [80] treatments increased EGP as a consequence of lower plasma glucose and insulin levels and higher glucagon levels. Results like these are helpful for clinicians to decide on an optimal treatment strategies for their patients and may want to consider using SGLT2 inhibitors together with therapies that suppress this increase in EGP (e.g., incretin or metformin therapy).

Conclusions

Assessment of glucose pathways such as EGP, glucose absorption, glucose disposal, glycolysis, and gluconeogenesis can provide critical information when assessing insulin-sensitizing and other classes of glucose-lowering drugs. With a wide range of tracers and methods available, small studies can be designed which give very comprehensive assessment of multiple pathways in a single study. On the other hand, oral and intravenous bolus methods can be easily applied to larger studies with minimal effort. Quantitative measurement of glucose metabolic pathways may enable the development of novel effective therapies and help open the door for personalized diabetes management.

Lipoprotein and Protein Metabolism

Introduction

In the study of cardio-metabolic disease, probably the most significant application of protein turnover measurements to date has been in the assessment of lipoprotein production and clearance. The production and catabolic rates for atherogenic apolipoprotein B (apo-B) containing lipoproteins, e.g., low-density lipoprotein (LDL), and anti-atherogenic high-density lipoprotein (HDL) have been determined for many disease states and treatments. In spite of this knowledge, there are still significant gaps in our understanding of the role of lipoprotein metabolism in diabetes and cardiovascular disease. New advances in tandem mass spectrometry (LC-MS/MS) have dramatically shifted the focus of protein metabolic studies away from the study of a single protein at a time, e.g., apo-B, toward the measurement of many dozens if not hundreds of proteins simultaneously (the "lipoproteome"). These developments promise to dramatically expand our understanding of protein regulation in dyslipidemia, atherosclerosis, and diabetes (also see Chap. 8).

Background

There is a long and very rich history of protein turnover being measured with stable isotopes. Indeed several textbooks have been written on the topic [2, 3, 9]. One of the biggest challenges that isotope methods for protein synthesis have had is the difficulty in determining the intracellular isotope enrichment of the labeled amino acids. This is because plasma amino acid enrichments do not reflect the intracellular pool, which is the source of label for protein synthesis. Much effort has gone into indirectly determining the intracellular pool enrichment though chemical and modelling approaches [2, 3, 9], although for lipoprotein metabolism, specifically apo-B metabolism, this has been less of an issue because of the availability of a precursor/product relationship within the plasma compartment for apo-B containing lipoprotein particles (see below).

Isotope tracer studies have been instrumental in shaping our understanding of lipoprotein metabolism. The study of lipoprotein metabolism using intravenous stable isotope-labeled amino acid has been successfully used to evaluate many metabolic diseases and therapies. As noted, there are several excellent reviews available that cover the use of these methods and the modelling principles involved [20, 54, 78, 82]. Lipoprotein metabolism is extremely complex, involving many different particle types, tissues, lipids, and clearance mechanisms.

Fortunately, in early clinical drug development, the critical questions about target engagement, treatment efficacy, or mechanism of action can be addressed with simplified clinical and analytical methods, depending on the hypothesis being tested. In the case of lipoprotein synthesis in the liver, two methods have been well validated and widely used. The bolus decay method combined with multi-compartment modelling is very well studied and has been applied successfully in many settings. A similar approach using a primed constant infusion has also been used successfully and can be combined with multi-compartment modelling or analyzed with simpler precursor/product calculations. Finally, deuterated water labeling has recently been applied to lipoprotein metabolism, [83] and although the advantages for these types of studies may be limited, a simple assessment of hepatic protein synthesis rates can be estimated with a single blood sample and no need for an intravenous infusion, making it attractive in some settings.

Key Methods

Regardless of the tracer method used for assessing lipoprotein metabolism, some general principles study design elements are important to take into consideration. Studies of lipoprotein metabolism require special attention to subject selection. Properly matching treatment and control groups for body composition, exercise habits, glucose tolerance, lipid-lowering medication, plasma cholesterol, triglyceride, and HDL and LDL apo-A and apo-B levels are all potentially important to ensure proper interpretation of results. Sex hormone status, hormone supplementation, alcohol intake, unusual dietary habits (e.g., low carbohydrate diet, vegan diet, etc.), and nutritional supplement use should also be considered. If medications are allowed, stable dose and laboratory values should be confirmed, and medication washout periods should be based on known pharmacokinetic/pharmacodynamic (PK/PD) parameters. If the study population has very high or very low plasma lipid values, genetic testing for known polymorphisms may also be warranted since mutations in lipoproteins and receptors (e.g., familial hypercholesterolemia) can significantly confound results if not taken into consideration.

Because much of the information regarding lipoprotein metabolism is related to the size and/or density of the lipoprotein particle, sample collection and storage are important to carefully control. Blood samples should be collected on ice, spun quickly, separated into aliquots, and frozen preferably at −80 °C. Particular care should be taken to avoid repeated freeze-thaw cycles. Generally 1 mL of plasma or serum is sufficient for isolation of lipoprotein particles and subsequent mass spectrometry. Sequential ultracentrifugation is commonly used to separate lipoproteins by density, followed by precipitation or isolation of individual proteins by polyacrylamide gel electrophoresis (PAGE). Isolated proteins are then hydrolyzed to amino acids. Following acid hydrolysis, amino acids are derivatized with pentafluorobenzyl bromide and leucine enrichments are measured by GC/MS.

Historically, these studies are performed in the fasted state, and a large literature concerning the effects of a variety of drugs and diet interventions is available. However, more recently, there has been a shift toward performing studies in a fed state, either a simulated "constant" fed state where subjects consume a small meal at regular intervals throughout the day [81, 84] or following a defined test meal [85]. Fasting apo-B metabolism has played an important role in elucidating the LDL-lowering mechanisms of statins [86–88], ezetimibe [89], ligands for peroxisome proliferator-activated receptors [90, 91], and niacin [92], among other drugs [88]. Because of this, fasting values provide a simple, steady-state condition to compare new therapeutic approaches to the standard of care. On the other hand, postprandial (fed) lipoprotein metabolism is emerging as a rich and important area for the study of atherosclerotic risk factors [85], particularly as related to the regulation of triglyceride and chylomicron metabolism. More studies are still needed to firmly establish which pathways are most important for reducing cardiovascular risk, however. In all studies of lipoprotein kinetics, accurate measurement of individual protein concentrations is extremely valuable. This is particularly important when performing studies in the fed state as the changes in concentration of each traced metabolite is used in the kinetic calculations.

Intravenous Bolus Method

Of the tracer methods available for determining apolipoprotein production and clearance rates, the intravenous bolus method is considered by many to be the "gold standard" approach, and indeed, it has been very thoroughly studied in many disease and treatment studies. The details of the method are available and published in several reviews [20, 93].

Method

A typical protocol will involve a single bolus of deuterated leucine ([5,5,5-^{2}H$_3$]leucine, also called d$_3$-leucine), 5 mg/kg of body weight administered intravenously within a 2-min period. Blood samples are taken immediately prior to and following the injection of the isotope at 5, 10, 20, 30, and 40 min and at 1.0, 1.5, 2.0, 2.5, 3.0, 4.0, 5.0, 6.0, 8.0, and 10.0 h. Sampling may continue at 2-h intervals depending on the turnover of the target particle. VLDL turnover may be complete by 12 h, whereas LDL and HDL apolipoproteins may require >18 h of sampling due to the relative half-lives of these apolipoproteins in the blood. Additional fasting blood samples can be collected at longer intervals, e.g., 24, 48, 72, and 96 h. Following determination of leucine enrichment in the apolipoproteins of interest, the data are modeled using SAAM II or similar multi-compartment modelling software. The compartmental model used and the specific parameters calculated should be selected based on the specific protocol and hypothesis being tested. Production and clearance rates of many individual lipoproteins can be determined with this method as well as the conversion rates from one particle to another.

Advantages/Disadvantages

The bolus method has some intrinsic advantages over other isotope labeling approaches. It is particularly useful to characterize the conversion of one particle into another, e.g., VLDL to intermediate-density lipoproteins (IDL) to LDL. This approach may also be desirable because it does not require a long intravenous infusion; data analysis does however require the use of relatively complex multi-compartment modelling and very frequent blood sampling. Blood volumes of at least 2 mL per time point are recommended for isolation of lipoprotein density fractions by ultracentrifugation. Plasma or serum samples are suitable for analysis. Until recently, the standard method for analysis of lipoprotein kinetics involved selective precipitation of apo-B from VLDL and LDL samples, and isolation of apo-A and other apolipoproteins by immunoaffinity precipitation or gel electrophoresis.

Primed Constant Infusion

A primed constant infusion of isotopically labeled leucine is a commonly utilized alternative to the bolus decay method. Operationally, it is very similar and can yield essentially the same types of kinetic results using multi-compartment models [20, 93] when frequent blood samples are obtained.

Method

A typical study design is as follows: subjects receive a primed constant infusion of d$_3$-leucine under fasted or fed conditions to determine the kinetics of LDL apo-B; [5,5,5-D3]L-leucine (10 μmol/kg body weight) is injected, intravenously, as a bolus followed by a continuous infusion (10 μmol/kg body weight/h) over a 15-h period. Blood samples are collected at 0, 30, 35, and 45 min and 1, 1.5, 2, 3, 4, 6, 9, 10, 12, and 15 h after the bolus. VLDL, IDL, and LDL are isolated by sequential ultracentrifugation. Blood samples (2–5 mL) for plasma or serum collection are drawn at each time points. Serum is collected immediately after centrifugation and stored at −70 °C as 1–2.5 mL serum or plasma aliquots in cryogenic vials. Lipoproteins are isolated and analyzed as described above.

Advantages/Disadvantages

The primed constant infusion method can be very useful in obtaining reasonable estimates of lipoprotein fractional synthesis rates with significantly fewer blood samples and modelling, which may be more compatible with early clinical

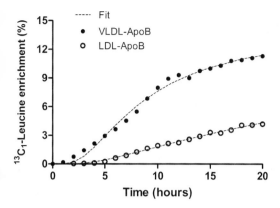

Fig. 3.6 Example of the use of a primed constant [1-^{13}C$_1$]-leucine infusion method for the measurement of very low-density lipoprotein (VLDL) apolipoprotein B (apo-B) and low-density lipoprotein (LDL) apo-B turnover in a healthy subject. The volunteer was confined to the Clinical Research Unit throughout the study under standardized conditions. The infusion was administered for 20 h, and fasting blood samples were obtained hourly for the assessment of ^{13}C-leucine enrichments in VLDL apo-B and LDL apo-B. The catabolic rates are 13.4 and 2.6 % per hour for VLDL apo-B and LDL apo-B, respectively, and the half-lives are 5 and 26 h for VLDL apo-B and LDL apo-B, respectively, for this subject

studies where blood volumes are limited and sampling protocols for safety and PK are involved. This modified approach utilizes the measured VLDL apo-B d$_3$-leucine enrichment as a surrogate for intrahepatic d$_3$-leucine, based on the assumption that VLDL apo-B is fully replaced when measured [94]. Once the precursor pool for hepatic lipoprotein synthesis is established, a simple precursor/product calculation can be used to determine the fractional synthesis rate of each lipoprotein of interest. This can be done, in principle, from a single blood sample. Confirming the complete replacement of VLDL is recommended, however, by taking several sequential samples and demonstrating plateau enrichment. As shown in Fig. 3.6, the VLDL apo-B reaches plateau enrichment by 20 h, which allows the % new LDL apo-B produced to be calculated as the ratio of d$_3$-leucine enrichment LDL apo-B to the VLDL apo-B. A primed constant infusion method is more frequently used in fed studies because the kinetics are simpler to calculate; however, the modelling parameters are similar. It is important to understand that in modelling studies of this type, the more frequent the sampling, the more accurate the fitting results are; therefore, reducing the number of samples collected should be balanced with the increased sample size likely required. In large studies it may be most practical and economical to study a greater number of subjects with fewer analyses per subject; however, this should be based on known intra-subject variability and good treatment effect estimates.

Recent Advances

LC-MS/MS methods are emerging as an exciting platform to perform kinetic analysis of many apolipoproteins and associated proteins at once [11, 22, 36, 83, 95]. This approach has been successfully used with a variety of LC-MS/MS instrument platforms. As an analytical modality, LC-MS/MS is compatible with any of the labeling protocols described above. While still early in its adoption, LC-MS/MS analysis of protein enrichment allows the simultaneous assessment of protein composition and turnover rates on lipoprotein particles. It is now well established that HDL, for example, can carry more than 100 different proteins which presumably impact its function as an anti-atherosclerotic particle [96–98]. Improved understanding of the relationship between the HDL-associated proteins and atherosclerotic risk will be valuable. Table 3.1 lists some simultaneously measured proteins on LDL and HDL and their half-lives as measured by LC-MS/MS.

Deuterated water labeling is also being used more frequently to assess human plasma protein metabolism [36]. Recent publications in mice demonstrate the feasibility of the approach and open the possibility to measuring the production and clearance of apolipoproteins without an intravenous infusion [83]. In fact, in some cases apolipoprotein kinetics could be obtained from dried blood spots from a finger stick, presenting the opportunity for essentially noninvasive measurements (i.e., no intravenous infusion, no blood draw). Needless to say, the possibility of a simple inexpensive labeling and a noninvasive sampling system would potentially allow the synthesis and degradation of apolipoproteins to be measured in thousands of subjects and could even be adapted into a diagnostic test based on flux rather than concentration of atherogenic particles. Currently, these methods could be applied using the same

Table 3.1 An example of the simultaneous measurement by LC-MS/MS of the fractional synthesis rates of multiple proteins in HDL and LDL fractions isolated by sequential ultracentrifugation from a healthy volunteer after a 20-h primed-continuous infusion of [U-^{13}C$_6$]-leucine

Protein	HDL			LDL		
	Mean (%)	SD (%)	Number of peptides	Mean (%)	SD (%)	Number of peptides
Apo-L1	2	1	3.3	22	6	1.2
Apo-A1	14	4	9.2	16	4	8.4
Apo-A2	14	4	2.2	13	3	2.1
Apo-A4	37	11	4.1	33	6	0.9
Apo-B	27	6	14.3	22	6	29.7
Apo-C2	51	17	3.9	44	9	6.7
Apo-C3	47	12	4.0	46	9	3.8
Apo-C4	53	12	1.2	50	10	1.6
Apo-E	80	19	7.8	89	10	14.4
Apo-M	5	1	4.1	16	4	1.7
PON1	5	2	4.1	–	–	–
Serum amyloid A	12	4	1.0	–	–	–

labeling paradigms as described above utilizing deuterated water. Careful monitoring of body water enrichments and some modelling is required to account for the changing body water during the loading phase, since this period will contribute to most of the label of apolipoproteins. Because this method can be combined with measurement of lipid fluxes simultaneously, it has enormous potential to inform early phase drug development in lipidology and cardiovascular disease.

Tissue and Whole-Body Protein Synthesis

The synthesis and degradation of proteins is critical to maintain cell viability, and alterations in protein homeostasis have been implicated in many diseases as well as the normal decline in cellular functions with age. Much of the early work studying protein turnover focused on protein balance in the whole body, with an emphasis on the assessment of adequate protein intake.

The application of LC-MS/MS to tracer studies of tissue protein metabolism has several important applications to the study of metabolic disease and development of new therapeutics. Loss of skeletal muscle mass with aging, for example, is a significant contributor to morbidity and mortality, particularly in patients with metabolic disease. The continued synthesis of skeletal muscle proteins is critical for maintenance of skeletal muscle mass; moreover, interventions aimed at improving metabolic health have significant beneficial impact on muscle mass and function. Examination of the dynamics of muscle proteome with deuterated labeling and LC-MS/MS can determine the fractional synthesis rate of glycolytic, mitochondrial, contractile, and ER proteins from a single 10-mg sample [22–24]. This approach can similarly be applied to adipose tissue samples or other tissues. The application of these methods to plasma proteins can be an effective method for biomarker discovery and can potentially be used to noninvasively monitor intracellular protein synthesis if there is sufficient transport of cellular proteins into the plasma. The ability to determine the synthesis of specific individual proteins within a cell allows improved understanding of the regulation or dysregulation of functional cellular components.

Deuterated water labeling has been critical for the development of methods to study skeletal muscle and adipose protein synthesis. Because of the ease of administration for long periods of time and the small physical sample requirements for LC-MS/MS analysis, large-scale studies evaluating changes in proteome turnover in cardiometabolic diseases are now possible. While still early in their development, the use of proteomic platforms with isotope labeling will have a significant impact on the breadth of drug targets and diseases that will ultimately be understood based on the changes in protein fluxes which are induced by disease and restored with effective therapies.

Translating Results into Clinical Practice

It is well established in the lipoprotein literature that statin treatment reduces LDL cholesterol levels by increasing the clearance of LDL particles through the upregulation of the LDL receptor in the liver [99]. This simple assessment is misleading, however, given the complex interactions between specific manifestations of cardio-metabolic disease, concurrent medications and lipoprotein metabolism. This makes generalizations regarding the effect of a treatment on lipoprotein metabolism and its relationship to improving traditional risk factors difficult. Based on the clinical experience with statin therapies, it is reasonable to predict that novel interventions, such as anti-PCSK9 therapies, which increase LDL clearance rates and lower LDL concentrations, will provide clinical benefit. Reductions in LDL that are a result of impaired hepatic production of apo-B-containing particles may provide LDL lowering; however, that may come with an increased risk of hepatic lipid accumulation. Early trials of apo-B antisense in humans suggest that this is not the case but larger and longer studies will be required to confirm this [100]. Recent trials using apo-C-III antisense provide some enticing data on the effect of reducing apo-C-III production. In human trials, inhibiting apo-C-III production reduced triglyceride levels and increased HDL cholesterol [101]. Preclinical studies also suggest that there may be potential for improvement in metabolic syndrome and atherosclerosis [102].

Conclusions

Using stable isotopes to assess the lipoprotein fluxes has been a critical element in our understanding and treatment of dyslipidemia and cardiovascular disease. Understanding the mechanisms of lipid lowering in early clinical studies will continue to be important in the evaluation of the potential safety and efficacy of novel agents. Continued development of novel tools and clinical studies examining the relationship between apolipoprotein fluxes and cardio-metabolic disease will continue to be essential in advancing novel treatments.

References

1. Buchanan JM. Biochemistry during the life and times of Hans Krebs and Fritz Lipmann. J Biol Chem. 2002;277(37):33531–6.
2. Waterlow JC. Protein turnover. Hammonds Plains: CABI; 2006; 315 p.
3. Wolfe RR, Chinkes DL. Isotope tracers in metabolic research: principles and practice of kinetic analysis. Hoboken: Wiley; 2005. 494 p.
4. Schoenheimer R, Rittenberg D. The study of intermediary metabolism of animals with the aid of isotopes. Physiol Rev. 1940;20:218–48.
5. Hellerstein MK, Murphy E. Stable isotope-mass spectrometric measurements of molecular fluxes in vivo: emerging applications in drug development. Curr Opin Mol Ther. 2004;6(3):249–64.
6. Turner SM, Hellerstein MK. Emerging applications of kinetic biomarkers in preclinical and clinical drug development. Curr Opin Drug Discov Devel. 2005;8(1):115–26.
7. Klein PD, Klein ER. Stable isotopes: origins and safety. J Clin Pharmacol. 1986;26(6):378–82.
8. Koletzko B, Sauerwald T, Demmelmair H. Safety of stable isotope use. Eur J Pediatr. 1997;156(1):S12–7.
9. Koletzko B, Demmelmair H, Hartl W, Kindermann A, Koletzko S, Sauerwald T, et al. The use of stable isotope techniques for nutritional and metabolic research in paediatrics. Early Hum Dev. 1998;53:S77–97.
10. Dufner D, Previs SF. Measuring in vivo metabolism using heavy water. Curr Opin Clin Nutr Metab Care. 2003;6(5):511–7.
11. Rachdaoui N, Austin L, Kramer E, Previs MJ, Anderson VE, Kasumov T, et al. Measuring proteome dynamics in vivo: as easy as adding water? Mol Cell Proteomics MCP. 2009;8(12):2653–63.
12. Jones PJ, Leatherdale ST. Stable isotopes in clinical research: safety reaffirmed. Clin Sci Lond Engl 1979. 1991;80(4):277–80.
13. Di Buono M, Jones PJ, Beaumier L, Wykes LJ. Comparison of deuterium incorporation and mass isotopomer distribution analysis for measurement of human cholesterol biosynthesis. J Lipid Res. 2000;41(9):1516–23.
14. Beysen C, Murphy EJ, McLaughlin T, Riiff T, Lamendola C, Turner HC, et al. Whole-body glycolysis measured by the deuterated-glucose disposal test correlates highly with insulin resistance in vivo. Diabetes Care. 2007;30(5):1143–9.
15. Beysen C, Murphy EJ, Deines K, Chan M, Tsang E, Glass A, et al. Effect of bile acid sequestrants on glucose metabolism, hepatic de novo lipogenesis, and cholesterol and bile acid kinetics in type 2 diabetes:

a randomised controlled study. Diabetologia. 2012;55(2):432–42.
16. Beysen C, Murphy EJ, Nagaraja H, Decaris M, Riiff T, Fong A, et al. A pilot study of the effects of pioglitazone and rosiglitazone on de novo lipogenesis in type 2 diabetes. J Lipid Res. 2008;49(12):2657–63.
17. Boren J, Taskinen M-R, Adiels M. Kinetic studies to investigate lipoprotein metabolism. J Intern Med. 2012;271(2):166–73.
18. Strawford A, Antelo F, Christiansen M, Hellerstein MK. Adipose tissue triglyceride turnover, de novo lipogenesis, and cell proliferation in humans measured with 2H2O. Am J Physiol Endocrinol Metab. 2004;286(4):E577–88.
19. Previs SF, McLaren DG, Wang S-P, Stout SJ, Zhou H, Herath K, et al. New methodologies for studying lipid synthesis and turnover: looking backwards to enable moving forwards. Biochim Biophys Acta. 2014;1842(3):402–13.
20. Barrett PHR, Chan DC, Watts GF. Thematic review series: patient-oriented research. Design and analysis of lipoprotein tracer kinetics studies in humans. J Lipid Res. 2006;47(8):1607–19.
21. Chan DC, Barrett PHR, Watts GF. Recent studies of lipoprotein kinetics in the metabolic syndrome and related disorders. Curr Opin Lipidol. 2006;17(1):28–36.
22. Gasier HG, Fluckey JD, Previs SF. The application of 2H2O to measure skeletal muscle protein synthesis. Nutr Metab. 2010;7:31.
23. Robinson MM, Turner SM, Hellerstein MK, Hamilton KL, Miller BF. Long-term synthesis rates of skeletal muscle DNA and protein are higher during aerobic training in older humans than in sedentary young subjects but are not altered by protein supplementation. FASEB J Off Publ Fed Am Soc Exp Biol. 2011;25(9):3240–9.
24. Scalzo RL, Peltonen GL, Binns SE, Shankaran M, Giordano GR, Hartley DA, et al. Greater muscle protein synthesis and mitochondrial biogenesis in males compared with females during sprint interval training. FASEB J Off Publ Fed Am Soc Exp Biol. 2014;28(6):2705–14.
25. Harwood Jr HJ. Treating the metabolic syndrome: acetyl-CoA carboxylase inhibition. Expert Opin Ther Targets. 2005;9(2):267–81.
26. Hellerstein MK, Schwarz JM, Neese RA. Regulation of hepatic de novo lipogenesis in humans. Annu Rev Nutr. 1996;16:523–57.
27. Lambert JE, Ramos-Roman MA, Browning JD, Parks EJ. Increased de novo lipogenesis is a distinct characteristic of individuals with nonalcoholic fatty liver disease. Gastroenterology. 2014;146(3):726–35.
28. Tuvdendorj D, Chandalia M, Batbayar T, Saraf M, Beysen C, Murphy EJ, et al. Altered subcutaneous abdominal adipose tissue lipid synthesis in obese, insulin-resistant humans. Am J Physiol Endocrinol Metab. 2013;305(8):E999–1006.
29. Hudgins LC, Parker TS, Levine DM, Hellerstein MK. A dual sugar challenge test for lipogenic sensitivity to dietary fructose. J Clin Endocrinol Metab. 2011;96(3):861–8.
30. Stanhope KL, Griffen SC, Bremer AA, Vink RG, Schaefer EJ, Nakajima K, et al. Metabolic responses to prolonged consumption of glucose- and fructose-sweetened beverages are not associated with postprandial or 24-h glucose and insulin excursions. Am J Clin Nutr. 2011;94(1):112–9.
31. Cramer CT, Goetz B, Hopson KLM, Fici GJ, Ackermann RM, Brown SC, et al. Effects of a novel dual lipid synthesis inhibitor and its potential utility in treating dyslipidemia and metabolic syndrome. J Lipid Res. 2004;45(7):1289–301.
32. Leitch CA, Jones PJ. Measurement of human lipogenesis using deuterium incorporation. J Lipid Res. 1993;34(1):157–63.
33. Hellerstein MK, Christiansen M, Kaempfer S, Kletke C, Wu K, Reid JS, et al. Measurement of de novo hepatic lipogenesis in humans using stable isotopes. J Clin Invest. 1991;87(5):1841–52.
34. Schoenheimer R. The dynamic state of body constituents. Cambridge, MA: Harvard University Press; 1946.
35. Busch R, Neese RA, Awada M, Hayes GM, Hellerstein MK. Measurement of cell proliferation by heavy water labeling. Nat Protoc. 2007;2(12):3045–57.
36. Price JC, Holmes WE, Li KW, Floreani NA, Neese RA, Turner SM, et al. Measurement of human plasma proteome dynamics with (2)H(2)O and liquid chromatography tandem mass spectrometry. Anal Biochem. 2012;420(1):73–83.
37. Hellerstein MK, Neese RA. Mass isotopomer distribution analysis at eight years: theoretical, analytic, and experimental considerations. Am J Physiol. 1999;276(6 Pt 1):E1146–70.
38. Chinkes DL, Aarsland A, Rosenblatt J, Wolfe RR. Comparison of mass isotopomer dilution methods used to compute VLDL production in vivo. Am J Physiol. 1996;271(2 Pt 1):E373–83.
39. Bederman IR, Reszko AE, Kasumov T, David F, Wasserman DH, Kelleher JK, et al. Zonation of labeling of lipogenic acetyl-CoA across the liver: implications for studies of lipogenesis by mass isotopomer analysis. J Biol Chem. 2004;279(41):43207–16.
40. Vedala A, Wang W, Neese RA, Christiansen MP, Hellerstein MK. Delayed secretory pathway contributions to VLDL-triglycerides from plasma NEFA, diet, and de novo lipogenesis in humans. J Lipid Res. 2006;47(11):2562–74.
41. Faix D, Neese R, Kletke C, Wolden S, Cesar D, Coutlangus M, et al. Quantification of menstrual and diurnal periodicities in rates of cholesterol and fat synthesis in humans. J Lipid Res. 1993;34(12):2063–75.
42. Siler SQ, Neese RA, Hellerstein MK. De novo lipogenesis, lipid kinetics, and whole-body lipid balances in humans after acute alcohol consumption. Am J Clin Nutr. 1999;70(5):928–36.
43. Schwarz JM, Neese RA, Turner S, Dare D, Hellerstein MK. Short-term alterations in carbohydrate energy intake in humans. Striking effects on hepatic glucose production, de novo lipogenesis, lipolysis, and whole-body fuel selection. J Clin Invest. 1995;96(6):2735–43.

44. Beysen C, Turner S, Carvajal-Gonzalez S, Buckeridge C, Hellerstein M, Esler W, et al. A new methodology for the reproducible measurement of hepatic de novo lipogenesis in humans. Diabetes. 2014;63(Suppl 1):A461.
45. Flannery C, Dufour S, Rabøl R, Shulman GI, Petersen KF. Skeletal muscle insulin resistance promotes increased hepatic de novo lipogenesis, hyperlipidemia, and hepatic steatosis in the elderly. Diabetes. 2012;61(11):2711–7.
46. Freckmann G, Hagenlocher S, Baumstark A, Jendrike N, Gillen RC, Rössner K, et al. Continuous glucose profiles in healthy subjects under everyday life conditions and after different meals. J Diabetes Sci Technol. 2007;1(5):695–703.
47. Steele R, Wall JS, De Bodo RC, Altszuler N. Measurement of size and turnover rate of body glucose pool by the isotope dilution method. Am J Physiol. 1956;187(1):15–24.
48. Gerich JE, Meyer C, Woerle HJ, Stumvoll M. Renal gluconeogenesis: its importance in human glucose homeostasis. Diabetes Care. 2001;24(2):382–91.
49. Katz J, Rognstad R. Futile cycles in the metabolism of glucose. Curr Top Cell Regul. 1976;10:237–89.
50. Rigalleau V, Beylot M, Laville M, Guillot C, Deleris G, Aubertin J, et al. Measurement of post-absorptive glucose kinetics in non-insulin-dependent diabetic patients: methodological aspects. Eur J Clin Invest. 1996;26(3):231–6.
51. Glauber H, Wallace P, Brechtel G. Effects of fasting on plasma glucose and prolonged tracer measurement of hepatic glucose output in NIDDM. Diabetes. 1987;36(10):1187–94.
52. Chen YD, Swislocki AL, Jeng CY, Juang JH, Reaven GM. Effect of time on measurement of hepatic glucose production. J Clin Endocrinol Metab. 1988;67(5):1084–8.
53. Hovorka R, Eckland DJ, Halliday D, Lettis S, Robinson CE, Bannister P, et al. Constant infusion and bolus injection of stable-label tracer give reproducible and comparable fasting HGO. Am J Physiol. 1997;273(1 Pt 1):E192–201.
54. Barrett PH, Bell BM, Cobelli C, Golde H, Schumitzky A, Vicini P, et al. SAAM II: Simulation, Analysis, and Modeling Software for tracer and pharmacokinetic studies. Metabolism. 1998;47(4):484–92.
55. Matsuda M, DeFronzo RA. Insulin sensitivity indices obtained from oral glucose tolerance testing: comparison with the euglycemic insulin clamp. Diabetes Care. 1999;22(9):1462–70.
56. Hellerstein MK, Neese RA, Linfoot P, Christiansen M, Turner S, Letscher A. Hepatic gluconeogenic fluxes and glycogen turnover during fasting in humans. A stable isotope study. J Clin Invest. 1997;100(5):1305–19.
57. Neese RA, Schwarz JM, Faix D, Turner S, Letscher A, Vu D, et al. Gluconeogenesis and intrahepatic triose phosphate flux in response to fasting or substrate loads. Application of the mass isotopomer distribution analysis technique with testing of assumptions and potential problems. J Biol Chem. 1995;270(24):14452–66.
58. Hellerstein MK, Neese RA. Mass isotopomer distribution analysis: a technique for measuring biosynthesis and turnover of polymers. Am J Physiol. 1992;263(5 Pt 1):E988–1001.
59. Hellerstein MK, Kaempfer S, Reid JS, Wu K, Shackleton CH. Rate of glucose entry into hepatic uridine diphosphoglucose by the direct pathway in fasted and fed states in normal humans. Metabolism. 1995;44(2):172–82.
60. Basu R, Basu A, Johnson CM, Schwenk WF, Rizza RA. Insulin dose-response curves for stimulation of splanchnic glucose uptake and suppression of endogenous glucose production differ in nondiabetic humans and are abnormal in people with type 2 diabetes. Diabetes. 2004;53(8):2042–50.
61. Steele R, Bishop JS, Dunn A, Altszuler N, Rathbeb I, Debodo RC. Inhibition by insulin of hepatic glucose production in the normal dog. Am J Physiol. 1965;208:301–6.
62. Cowan JS, Hetenyi Jr G. Glucoregulatory responses in normal and diabetic dogs recorded by a new tracer method. Metabolism. 1971;20(4):360–72.
63. Hother-Nielsen O. On the appropriate use of the primed-constant tracer infusion technique. Diabète Metab. 1994;20(6):568–70.
64. Staehr P, Hojlund K, Hother-Nielsen O, Holst JJ, Beck-Nielsen H. Does overnight normalization of plasma glucose by insulin infusion affect assessment of glucose metabolism in Type 2 diabetes? Diabet Med J Br Diabet Assoc. 2003;20(10):816–22.
65. Steele R, Bjerknes C, Rathgeb I, Altszuler N. Glucose uptake and production during the oral glucose tolerance test. Diabetes. 1968;17(7):415–21.
66. Mari A, Wahren J, DeFronzo RA, Ferrannini E. Glucose absorption and production following oral glucose: comparison of compartmental and arteriovenous-difference methods. Metabolism. 1994;43(11):1419–25.
67. Dalla Man C, Caumo A, Basu R, Rizza R, Toffolo G, Cobelli C. Minimal model estimation of glucose absorption and insulin sensitivity from oral test: validation with a tracer method. Am J Physiol Endocrinol Metab. 2004;287(4):E637–43.
68. Taylor R, Magnusson I, Rothman DL, Cline GW, Caumo A, Cobelli C, et al. Direct assessment of liver glycogen storage by 13C nuclear magnetic resonance spectroscopy and regulation of glucose homeostasis after a mixed meal in normal subjects. J Clin Invest. 1996;97(1):126–32.
69. Basu R, Di Camillo B, Toffolo G, Basu A, Shah P, Vella A, et al. Use of a novel triple-tracer approach to assess postprandial glucose metabolism. Am J Physiol Endocrinol Metab. 2003;284(1):E55–69.
70. Haidar A, Elleri D, Allen JM, Harris J, Kumareswaran K, Nodale M, et al. Validity of triple- and dual-tracer techniques to estimate glucose appearance. Am J Physiol Endocrinol Metab. 2012;302(12):E1493–501.
71. Rossetti L, Giaccari A. Relative contribution of glycogen synthesis and glycolysis to insulin-mediated glucose uptake. A dose-response euglycemic clamp study in normal and diabetic rats. J Clin Invest. 1990;85(6):1785–92.

72. Woerle HJ, Meyer C, Dostou JM, Gosmanov NR, Islam N, Popa E, et al. Pathways for glucose disposal after meal ingestion in humans. Am J Physiol Endocrinol Metab. 2003;284(4):E716–25.
73. Del Prato S, Bonadonna RC, Bonora E, Gulli G, Solini A, Shank M, et al. Characterization of cellular defects of insulin action in type 2 (non-insulin-dependent) diabetes mellitus. J Clin Invest. 1993;91(2):484–94.
74. Galgani JE, Ravussin E. Postprandial whole-body glycolysis is similar in insulin-resistant and insulin-sensitive non-diabetic humans. Diabetologia. 2012;55(3):737–42.
75. Christiansen MP, Linfoot PA, Neese RA, Hellerstein MK. Effect of dietary energy restriction on glucose production and substrate utilization in type 2 diabetes. Diabetes. 2000;49(10):1691–9.
76. Goldberg RB, Kendall DM, Deeg MA, Buse JB, Zagar AJ, Pinaire JA, et al. A comparison of lipid and glycemic effects of pioglitazone and rosiglitazone in patients with type 2 diabetes and dyslipidemia. Diabetes Care. 2005;28(7):1547–54.
77. Nissen SE, Wolski K. Effect of rosiglitazone on the risk of myocardial infarction and death from cardiovascular causes. N Engl J Med. 2007;356(24):2457–71.
78. Erdmann E, Dormandy JA, Charbonnel B, Massi-Benedetti M, Moules IK, Skene AM, et al. The effect of pioglitazone on recurrent myocardial infarction in 2,445 patients with type 2 diabetes and previous myocardial infarction: results from the PROactive (PROactive 05) Study. J Am Coll Cardiol. 2007;49(17):1772–80.
79. Merovci A, Solis-Herrera C, Daniele G, Eldor R, Fiorentino TV, Tripathy D, et al. Dapagliflozin improves muscle insulin sensitivity but enhances endogenous glucose production. J Clin Invest. 2014;124(2):509–14.
80. Ferrannini E, Muscelli E, Frascerra S, Baldi S, Mari A, Heise T, et al. Metabolic response to sodium-glucose cotransporter 2 inhibition in type 2 diabetic patients. J Clin Invest. 2014;124(2):499–508.
81. Welty FK, Lichtenstein AH, Barrett PH, Dolnikowski GG, Schaefer EJ. Human apolipoprotein (Apo) B-48 and ApoB-100 kinetics with stable isotopes. Arterioscler Thromb Vasc Biol. 1999;19(12):2966–74.
82. Foster DM, Barrett PH, Toffolo G, Beltz WF, Cobelli C. Estimating the fractional synthetic rate of plasma apolipoproteins and lipids from stable isotope data. J Lipid Res. 1993;34(12):2193–205.
83. Kasumov T, Willard B, Li L, Li M, Conger H, Buffa JA, et al. 2H2O-based high-density lipoprotein turnover method for the assessment of dynamic high-density lipoprotein function in mice. Arterioscler Thromb Vasc Biol. 2013;33(8):1994–2003.
84. Lichtenstein AH, Cohn JS, Hachey DL, Millar JS, Ordovas JM, Schaefer EJ. Comparison of deuterated leucine, valine, and lysine in the measurement of human apolipoprotein A-I and B-100 kinetics. J Lipid Res. 1990;31(9):1693–701.
85. Wong ATY, Chan DC, Pang J, Watts GF, Barrett PHR. Plasma apolipoprotein B-48 transport in obese men: a new tracer kinetic study in the postprandial state. J Clin Endocrinol Metab. 2014;99(1):E122–6.
86. Berthold HK, Mertens J, Birnbaum J, Bramswig S, Sudhop T, Barrett PHR, et al. Influence of simvastatin on apoB-100 secretion in non-obese subjects with mild hypercholesterolemia. Lipids. 2010;45(6):491–500.
87. Berglund L, Witztum JL, Galeano NF, Khouw AS, Ginsberg HN, Ramakrishnan R. Three-fold effect of lovastatin treatment on low density lipoprotein metabolism in subjects with hyperlipidemia: increase in receptor activity, decrease in apoB production, and decrease in particle affinity for the receptor. Results from a novel triple-tracer approach. J Lipid Res. 1998;39(4):913–24.
88. Parhofer KG, Barrett PHR. Thematic review series: patient-oriented research. What we have learned about VLDL and LDL metabolism from human kinetics studies. J Lipid Res. 2006;47(8):1620–30.
89. Telford DE, Sutherland BG, Edwards JY, Andrews JD, Barrett PHR, Huff MW. The molecular mechanisms underlying the reduction of LDL apoB-100 by ezetimibe plus simvastatin. J Lipid Res. 2007;48(3):699–708.
90. Ginsberg HN. Changes in lipoprotein kinetics during therapy with fenofibrate and other fibric acid derivatives. Am J Med. 1987;83(5B):66–70.
91. Watts GF, Barrett PHR, Ji J, Serone AP, Chan DC, Croft KD, et al. Differential regulation of lipoprotein kinetics by atorvastatin and fenofibrate in subjects with the metabolic syndrome. Diabetes. 2003;52(3):803–11.
92. Lamon-Fava S, Diffenderfer MR, Barrett PHR, Buchsbaum A, Nyaku M, Horvath KV, et al. Extended-release niacin alters the metabolism of plasma apolipoprotein (Apo) A-I and ApoB-containing lipoproteins. Arterioscler Thromb Vasc Biol. 2008;28(9):1672–8.
93. Parhofer KG, Hugh P, Barrett R, Bier DM, Schonfeld G. Determination of kinetic parameters of apolipoprotein B metabolism using amino acids labeled with stable isotopes. J Lipid Res. 1991;32(8):1311–23.
94. Reeds PJ, Hachey DL, Patterson BW, Motil KJ, Klein PD. VLDL apolipoprotein B-100, a potential indicator of the isotopic labeling of the hepatic protein synthetic precursor pool in humans: studies with multiple stable isotopically labeled amino acids. J Nutr. 1992;122(3):457–66.
95. Price JC, Khambatta CF, Li KW, Bruss MD, Shankaran M, Dalidd M, et al. The effect of long term calorie restriction on in vivo hepatic proteostatis: a novel combination of dynamic and quantitative proteomics. Mol Cell Proteomics MCP. 2012;11(12):1801–14.
96. Heinecke JW. The HDL, proteome: a marker–and perhaps mediator–of coronary artery disease. J Lipid Res. 2009;50(Suppl):S167–71.
97. Vaisar T, Pennathur S, Green PS, Gharib SA, Hoofnagle AN, Cheung MC, et al. Shotgun proteomics implicates protease inhibition and complement activation in the antiinflammatory properties of HDL. J Clin Invest. 2007;117(3):746–56.
98. Shah AS, Tan L, Long JL, Davidson WS. Proteomic diversity of high density lipoproteins: our emerging

understanding of its importance in lipid transport and beyond. J Lipid Res. 2013;54(10):2575–85.
99. Bilheimer DW, Grundy SM, Brown MS, Goldstein JL. Mevinolin and colestipol stimulate receptor-mediated clearance of low density lipoprotein from plasma in familial hypercholesterolemia heterozygotes. Proc Natl Acad Sci U S A. 1983;80(13):4124–8.
100. Reyes-Soffer G. Treatment with mipomersen reduces levels of ApoB-containing lipoproteins by increasing fractional removal of VLDL and LDL-apoB without reducing VLDL-apob secretion. ATVB 2014. Abstract 634.
101. Huff MW, Hegele RA. Apolipoprotein C-III: going back to the future for a lipid drug target. Circ Res. 2013;112(11):1405–8.
102. Graham MJ, Lee RG, Bell TA, Fu W, Mullick AE, Alexander VJ, et al. Antisense oligonucleotide inhibition of apolipoprotein C-III reduces plasma triglycerides in rodents, nonhuman primates, and humans. Circ Res. 2013;112(11):1479–90.

Imaging Techniques for the Assessment of Ectopic Fat in Liver and Skeletal Muscle

Gavin Hamilton, Michael S. Middleton, Elhamy R. Heba, and Claude B. Sirlin

Keywords

Magnetic resonance imaging (MRI) • Magnetic resonance spectroscopy (MRS) • Nonalcoholic fatty liver disease (NAFLD) • Proton density fat fraction (PDFF) • Intramyocellular lipid (IMCL)

Summary

Background

The increasing prevalence of obesity worldwide has prompted the development of noninvasive imaging techniques to monitor excessive accumulation of ectopic fat in liver and muscle. These methods may be applied to quantify liver, and skeletal muscle fat may be used to assess efficacy and safety endpoints in the development of new drugs for the treatment of nonalcoholic fatty liver disease (NAFLD) and related conditions such as type 2 diabetes.

Key Methods

Noninvasive Imaging Assessment of Liver Fat

Ultrasound (US)

Hepatic parenchymal imaging of liver fat using US currently is semiquantitative, difficult to interpret, and lacks reproducibility.

Computed Tomography (CT)

Non-contrast CT currently may have a limited role in the noninvasive assessment of liver fat when it is performed for other reasons such as evaluating coronary artery calcium or as part of a clinical CT abdomen examination or when magnetic resonance imaging (MRI) is contraindicated or not available. In such situations, non-contrast CT images of hepatic parenchyma could be evaluated for liver fat, but results may be difficult to interpret and, unless all CT exams performed on carefully calibrated scanners, may lack reproducibility.

Magnetic Resonance Spectroscopy (MRS)

The use of MRS to noninvasively assess liver fat has a limited role in drug development, mainly

G. Hamilton, PhD • M.S. Middleton, MD, PhD
E.R. Heba, MD • C.B. Sirlin, MD (✉)
Department of Radiology,
University of California, San Diego,
408 Dickinson St, San Diego, CA 92103, USA
e-mail: csirlin@ucsd.edu

due to challenges of implementation in multi-centre studies. However, it may be helpful in single-centre early exploratory or mechanistic studies.

Conventional Magnetic Resonance Imaging ((MRI) 2-Point Dixon Imaging)

Conventional 2-point Dixon MRI (i.e., double-echo imaging, usually at usually at in-phase (IP) and opposed phase (OP) echo time (TE) values, with a low flip angle to minimize T1 weighting, and analysis that accounts for interference effects between fat peaks) may play a role in drug development if acquisition parameters are rigorously standardized and limitations are understood. The most important limitation is that this kind of imaging neglects T2* effects and hence tends to underestimate liver fat content. However, so long as the study intervention does not affect T2* (e.g., by changing the degree of iron deposition in the liver from one time point to the next), 2-point Dixon MRI is likely to be accurate for assessing longitudinal *change* in liver fat content and hence may serve as a suitable biomarker for safety or efficacy in that setting.

Advanced Magnetic Resonance Imaging (MRI)

Advanced MRI (i.e., three or more echoes to permit T2* correction, low flip angle to minimize T1 weighting, and analysis that accounts for interference effects between fat peaks) can play an important role in drug development. These techniques provide an estimate of proton density fat fraction (PDFF), a biomarker of liver fat content, and are well suited for drug development trials where assessment of liver fat content is required, including those in which a baseline level of liver fat content is needed for study inclusion, and for studies in which drug efficacy, safety, and mechanism are being assessed. Importantly, MRI-estimated PDFF using advanced techniques is reproducible across scanner manufacturer and field strength which facilitates implementation in multicentre clinical trials. Moreover, comparison of different studies is reliable and meta-analysis of multiple studies is possible. Challenges facing advanced MRI estimation of PDFF are that it is not yet widely available, that care quality control is required, and that levels and changes of PDFF that are clinically and biologically meaningful have not been established. To improve availability, we recommend partnership with a team experienced in the acquisition and analysis of advanced MRI and centralized analysis of images. Analysis of PDFF levels and changes between treatment and placebo groups will require multidisciplinary input. Required numbers of subjects in clinical trials will likely strongly depend on the values of and changes in PDFF that are considered to be clinically significant.

Method	Measurement	Advantages	Disadvantages	Value in drug development decisions
Ultrasound (US)	Images based on frequency and strength (amplitude) of ultrasound signal and time it takes for that signal to return to transducer	Inexpensive, widely available	Inaccurate, imprecise, operator dependent	Low suitability for clinical trials requiring quantitative assessment of liver fat
Computer tomography (CT)	Images based on measuring x-ray attenuation	Widely available, moderate accuracy, high repeatability	Ionizing radiation, expensive, not always reproducible across different CT scanners	Limited suitability for clinical trials requiring quantitative assessment of liver fat
Magnetic resonance spectroscopy (MRS)	MR spectrum obtained from specified location in liver	Accurate, high repeatability, provides detailed spectral information for fat	Whole liver not assessed, analysis requires expertise, expensive, limited reproducibility across different MR scanners	Suitable for some single-centre cross-sectional and longitudinal studies where additional information to that available from MRI is being sought

Method	Measurement	Advantages	Disadvantages	Value in drug development decisions
Conventional magnetic resonance imaging (MRI)	MR T1-independent nominally out-of-phase and in-phase images obtained of liver	Whole liver imaging, widely available, good precision	Inaccurate, expensive, requires standardization	Suitable for some single and multicentre longitudinal studies requiring quantitative assessment of liver fat
Advanced magnetic resonance imaging (MRI)	MR T1-independent nominally alternately out-of-phase and in-phase images obtained of liver using three or more echoes	Whole liver imaging, accurate, precise, yields estimates of both PDFF and T2*	Not yet widely available, expensive, requires standardization	Suitable for single and multicentre cross-sectional and longitudinal studies requiring quantitative assessment of liver fat

Noninvasive Imaging Assessment of Skeletal Intramyocellular Lipid (IMCL)

Magnetic Resonance Spectroscopy (MRS)

As described above for MRS evaluation liver fat, MRS noninvasive assessment of IMCL may also have a limited role in drug development. Since MRI alone cannot assess IMCL and since MRS is the only way to assess IMCL noninvasively, if noninvasive assessment of IMCL is required, MRS is necessary. Hence, although there are limitations, MRS is feasible for single-centre trials where expertise in acquisition and analysis is available.

Conclusions

In the context of developing new drugs for nonalcoholic fatty liver disease (NAFLD) and related metabolic conditions (obesity, type-2 diabetes, cardiovascular disease, metabolic syndrome), advanced MRI currently stands out as the best method to assess liver fat. The advantages of whole-liver coverage, accuracy, precision, suitability for multi- as well as single-centre trials, and suitability for cross-sectional and longitudinal trials outweigh the disadvantages of cost and currently less-than-widespread availability. The various MRI scanner vendors are developing and can be expected in the future to support advanced MRI techniques. Future harmonization of acquisition and analysis techniques across MRI scanner vendors will result in advanced MRI becoming more widely available, and eventually results across sites, vendors, and time will be comparable. Conventional 2-point Dixon MRI is likely to remain useful in longitudinal trials.

Advanced ultrasound techniques are being developed to assess liver fat and, if validated as biomarkers of liver fat, may also become useful in clinical trials. CT is likely to be less useful than MRI but probably will continue to be of value on a limited basis when advanced MRI is not available or contraindicated. MRS is currently the only way to noninvasively assess IMCL, and so if that is required in single-centre or small multicenter trials, it may be of use. The use of MRS in large multicenter trials to assess IMCL is not feasible at this time.

Introduction

The global obesity epidemic is driving increasing rates of type 2 diabetes [1–3], nonalcoholic fatty liver disease (NAFLD) [4–6], and associated cardiometabolic disorders [6–9]. This urgent public health threat has prompted the development of noninvasive imaging techniques to monitor excessive accumulation of ectopic fat in liver and muscle. Ectopic fat is defined as the deposition of triglycerides within non-adipose tissue cells that normally contain only small amounts of fat [10]. Fat deposition in liver and/or muscle has adverse cardiometabolic consequences that arise through effects on aspects of local and systemic energy metabolism [11, 12]. In liver and muscle, triglyceride content usually correlates with whole-body and tissue-specific insulin sensitivity. Accumulation of fat in the abdominal viscera has an equal or more important role in the development of cardiometabolic risk compared with overall obesity [10].

NAFLD is a highly prevalent, and largely subclinical, disorder in which fat collects in hepatocytes in people who have limited alcohol consumption and who have no other condition causing steatosis [13]. NAFLD presents as a spectrum of disease, ranging from simple (or isolated) steatosis to nonalcoholic steatohepatitis (NASH), a more advanced form of the disease characterized by inflammation and cellular injury, and sometimes by fibrosis, as well as steatosis. NAFLD is associated with the metabolic syndrome, insulin resistance, and type 2 diabetes mellitus [9, 14]. NAFLD exacerbates insulin resistance in the liver and systemically [14]. Moreover, NAFLD generates an atherogenic lipid profile and other risk factors for cardiovascular disease [15, 16]. In a minority of affected subjects, NASH may progress ultimately to cirrhosis and hepatocellular carcinoma.

Intramyocellular lipid (IMCL) is fat that is deposited intracellularly within skeletal muscles. It also has been implicated in the pathogenesis of the metabolic syndrome [17]. Several studies have shown that increased IMCL is associated with decreased insulin sensitivity in individuals with obesity or type 2 diabetes [18, 19] and in the offspring of patients with type 2 diabetes [20, 21]. It has been hypothesized that defects in skeletal muscle mitochondrial function are associated with both decreased insulin resistance and accumulation of IMCL in skeletal muscle [22]. The thiazolidinedione class of glucose-lowering drugs, e.g., pioglitazone, may improve insulin sensitivity in subjects in part by reducing intracellular triglyceride content of skeletal muscle and liver [23].

NAFLD has emerged as a potential target for the prevention of type 2 diabetes, reflecting a potential bi-directional relationship between liver fat, insulin resistance, and the metabolic syndrome [9]. A range of non-pharmacological and pharmacological interventions has been evaluated for NAFLD and associated cardiometabolic risk factors. The latter include diet-induced weight reduction and physical exercise [24–26], bariatric surgery [25], metformin [27, 28], thiazolidinediones [23, 28, 29], omega-3 fatty acids [30], statins [31], and 11β-hydroxysteroid dehydrogenase type 1 inhibitors [32]. Noninvasive methods to quantify liver and skeletal muscle fat may be used to assess efficacy and safety endpoints in drug development (Table 4.1). In early-phase drug development, noninvasive methods can determine whether drugs have fat-lowering or fat-raising effects in liver and/or skeletal muscle. They can also determine the time course and duration of these effects. This information may be useful for go/no-go decisions. In late-phase drug development, noninvasive methods additionally may serve to measure surrogate or secondary biomarker endpoints in clinical trials for drugs intended to reduce ectopic fat accumulation.

Multiple imaging methods have been proposed to measure the amount fat in the liver [33, 34]. This chapter emphasizes magnetic resonance imaging (MRI) and magnetic resonance spectroscopy (MRS) methods as these are the most accurate and precise methods for liver fat quantification [35]. We also review ultrasound (US) and computed tomography (CT) and discuss relative strengths and weaknesses. For monitoring IMCL,

Table 4.1 Potential roles of liver and muscle fat imaging in cardiometabolic drug development

Screening of subjects to determine eligibility
To identify subjects with fatty liver, without fatty liver, and subjects spanning a spectrum of fat deposition severity
Endpoint in interventional clinical trials
Change in fat content in treatment vs. placebo groups. Imaging may be used to assess efficacy for drugs intended to lower liver fat, safety of drugs intended for other purposes that may cause fat accumulation as an unwanted effect, and interim analyses for clinical trials with vanguard design to determine whether to proceed or terminate early. Such data may inform go/no go decisions, design of larger studies, applications for Food and Drug Administration (FDA) approval, etc
Elucidation of mechanism
Serial analysis of fat accumulation in liver and extrahepatic fat depots may help elucidate mechanism of action of novel drugs for diabetes and related metabolic diseases

however, MRS is the only noninvasive method that has gained widespread acceptance [36].

History of Magnetic Resonance Imaging of Fat in Liver and Skeletal Muscle

A variety of MRI-, MRS-, CT-, and US-based approaches have been proposed to measure fat in the liver. As the leading methods for quantifying liver fat are MRI and MRS, we will briefly review only the history of MRI and MRS here.

MRI of liver fat began in 1984 when Dixon et al. proposed an MRI-based liver fat measurement technique; [37] to this day, MRI-based techniques to measure fat throughout the body are often referred to as Dixon imaging. In the 1990s, MRI-based quantification was extended to collect three echoes [38], and dual-echo techniques using gradient-recalled-echo (GRE) sequences were developed to allow single breath-hold fat assessment [39]. More complete understanding of the MR behavior of fat allowed development and refinement of advanced MRI methods to estimate proton density fat fraction (PDFF), a standardized biomarker un-confounded by biological, physical, or technical factors [40–42].

Liver and muscle MRS initially focused on ^{31}P and ^{13}C, but these techniques are not aimed at quantifying fat. ^{1}H MRS-based measurement of liver fat began in the 1990s when three landmark papers examined several confounding factors [43–45]. More recently, ^{1}H MRS was used to measure liver fat in over 2,000 subjects to investigate the prevalence of fatty liver at a population level [46]. Multi-TE ^{1}H MRS techniques have subsequently been developed that allow hepatic PDFF estimation in a single breath-hold [47, 48].

In 1993, Schick et al. [49] were the first to realize that there were two different types of fat in muscle; these were identified by Boesch et al. [50] as intramyocellular lipid (IMCL) and extramyocellular lipid (EMCL). It was recognized that skeletal muscle MRS was orientation-dependent [51] and that IMCL was important in providing an energy source in endurance exercise [52].

Noninvasive Liver Imaging Methods

Ultrasound

Perhaps the most common imaging modality to assess liver fat is conventional US, which is widely available and can be performed quickly, cheaply, and safely [53]. However, conventional US only produces a qualitative estimate of liver fat, relies on a subjective interpretation of features in the US image, and is both operator and machine dependent [54–56]. Thus estimates of liver fat derived from conventional US are semiquantitative and have lower repeatability and reproducibility than MRI or MRS and so are of limited value in assessing hepatic fat to inform drug development decisions. US is more reliable at identifying moderate-to-severe degrees of hepatic steatosis as confirmed by histology than are measurements of serum liver transaminase levels [15]. Advanced US methods are being investigated to provide quantitative estimates of liver fat [57]. However, these techniques are still in development and have only limited availability. While these techniques should provide more accurate estimates of liver fat than conventional US, only limited data are currently available on the accuracy and precision of these techniques. Hence, these investigational techniques currently have limited applicability in drug development.

Computed Tomography

Unenhanced CT evaluates liver fat by measuring x-ray attenuation; x-rays are attenuated less in fatty liver than in non-fatty liver [53]. While CT lacks the ease and portability of ultrasound, it is more widely available and more rapid than MR scans. Unlike US, x-ray attenuation is not subjective and can be measured precisely [58–60]. However x-ray attenuation is affected by several patient factors in addition to fat, reducing the accuracy and precision of liver fat estimation [58]. There may also be variability of attenuation values between CT scanners, particularly those produced by different manufacturers [61]. Finally, CT uses ionizing radiation, which limits its use in vulnerable groups such as children and pregnant women or in studies where multiple scans are required over time [62]. For these reasons CT has only limited applicability for liver fat quantification in drug development, and the use of CT for this purpose is not justified if MRI is available or unless CT of the liver is being performed anyway for other reasons.

Introduction to Magnetic Resonance Measurement Techniques

The two noninvasive MR-based techniques used to assess liver fat are ^{1}H (i.e., proton) MRS and MRI. Although the information that these techniques produces is different, the two approaches are similar; the same physics principles underlie and the same equipment is used for both techniques. The patient is placed in a strong magnetic field (called the "main" magnetic field), and then both water and fat molecules in the patient's body are excited with radiofrequency (RF) pulses. In MRI, gradients (additional magnetic fields of far smaller strength than the main magnetic field) and Fourier transformation are used to "encode" signals allowing images to be produced.

For MRS, gradients are used to locate (i.e., preferentially excite only) a region of interest, and then the Fourier transform of that signal produces a spectrum (which, as described further below, depicts the MR signal intensity transmitted from hydrogen protons in different chemical environments such as those in water molecules and those in the various moieties of triglyceride molecules). To the patient undergoing an MR examination, the difference between the two approaches may not be obvious, except that MRS sequences often are quieter than MRI sequences. Even though MRS measurements technically are not MRI per se, MRS examinations always require some imaging to allow accurate placement of the volume from which fat is being measured. Hence, the phrase "MRI" is often colloquially used to describe both MRI and MRS, even if the main outcome is an MRS measurement.

Most of the strengths and weakness of MRI apply equally to MRS. The lack of ionizing radiation in MR examinations safely permits repeat scanning and hence longitudinal monitoring. It also allows scanning of vulnerable groups, such as children and, if necessary, pregnant women. Given the increasing prevalence of obesity in children, with its downstream problems related to NAFLD, NASH, and other metabolic syndrome complications, the ability to scan children safely, accurately, and precisely to measure fat over time is a significant strength of both MRI and MRS.

A common contraindication to MR scanning is claustrophobia. MR systems are designed to achieve a highly uniform main magnetic field, which is required for both MRI and MRS. The most common scanner geometry that provides this is a long-cylinder (or long "bore") geometry. Modern MR systems generally have shorter bores than early scanners, decreasing claustrophobia-induced examination failure. Recent wider-bore MR systems have been designed which further reduce the incidence and severity of claustrophobic reactions and also increase the size of patients who can be scanned, which is of importance in conditions associated with obesity. Open systems have also been designed which further reduce claustrophobic reactions, but these systems operate at lower fields strengths and have poorer uniformity than equivalent smaller-bore systems. As yet the advanced MRI and MRS methods detailed in this chapter have not been validated in open systems. Other contraindications to MR scanning arise from the interaction of the (necessary) magnetic field or RF pulses, with metallic "foreign bodies" in the patient being scanned. Many objects implanted for clinical purposes such pacemakers, metallic cardiac valves, and some surgical clips exclude patients from undergoing an MR scan. Also metal that has entered the body accidentally may be of concern, particularly metal fragments in the orbits since the MRI magnet can exert a pull on these tiny metal fragments potentially leading to serious injuries. For this reason, screening is required beforehand, generally in the form of a questionnaire to ensure that patients can safely be scanned.

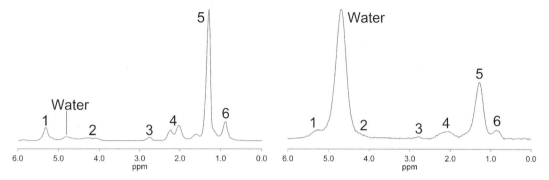

Fig. 4.1 Typical in vivo adipose MR spectrum (*left*) and liver MR spectrum (*right*). Both spectra acquired at 3T with the STEAM sequence, TR=3,500 ms and TE=10 ms. The peak assignments are shown in Table 4.2

Both MRS and MRI exploit differences in the resonance frequency of hydrogen nuclei in water and fat molecules to measure fat signal quantitatively. Typical MR spectra from adipose and liver tissue are shown in Fig. 4.1, displaying the separate frequencies, or chemical shifts, of the various water and fat peaks. The resonant frequency of each hydrogen nucleus is determined by the magnetic field it "experiences." The frequency position of a particular peak, or chemical shift, is determined by the amount of electron shielding it experiences. Both protons in water molecules experience the same amount of shielding and hence the same magnetic field, so there is only one water spectral peak. Different hydrogen nuclei in fat molecules experience slightly different levels of shielding and hence experience different magnetic fields, resulting in a fat spectrum that has several peaks [63]. Individual fat peaks will have a complex shape due to j-coupling, but a discussion of this affect is beyond the scope of this chapter [47]. While the individual main fat peaks can be partially discerned in pure fat tissue, there is insufficient spectral resolution at clinical field strengths (1.5 T and 3 T) to delineate all of the liver fat peaks in vivo [63].

The resonant frequency of each MR spectral peak (fat, water, and other) could be, but rarely is, given as its actual resonant frequency (near 63 MHz for 1.5 T scanners and near 127 MHz for 3 T scanners). However, it is useful and is common practice to indicate the position of each spectral peak in parts-per-million (ppm), which is independent of the strength of the main magnetic field. By convention, spectral peak frequencies are measured with respect to a reference material (tetramethylsilane (TMS)), which is assigned a frequency of 0 ppm. In vivo, there will be no TMS present, and so the water spectral peak acts as a surrogate reference. Water has a chemical shift (i.e., spectral peak position) of 4.7 ppm at 37 °C. Different types of fat will have slightly different spectra, depending on the amount of saturated, monounsaturated, and polyunsaturated fat they contain. Several studies have shown that MRS and MRI both can be used to determine "type" of fat – i.e., the degree and type of unsaturation of fat [63–65]. However, description of the details of these more advanced methods is beyond the scope of this chapter; we will focus here only on MR measurement of fat content.

MRI and MRS both measure the amount of fat by referencing the MR signal from fat to the MR signal from water. To be of utility, the fat and water signal values are converted to a value which is independent of possible confounding effects present in both MRI and MRS, some of which arise from and can be avoided or corrected for by judicious choice of MR scanner settings. When placed in a magnet field, hydrogen nuclei align with the main magnetic field to create longitudinal magnetization (M_z). This magnetization is not detectable when a patient is just placed in the main magnetic field, so an "excitation" RF pulse at the resonant frequency of the hydrogen nuclei is applied which transfers energy to (excites) M_z, rotating it into the transverse plane where it begins to process (rotate), as shown in Fig. 4.2.

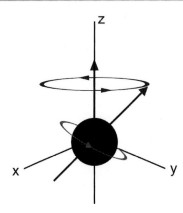

Fig. 4.2 Diagrammatic representation of a precessing hydrogen nucleus following a radio frequency (RF) pulse. The magnetization is no longer purely in the *z* direction, and the proportion of magnetization in the *x-y* plane is detectable by the MR system

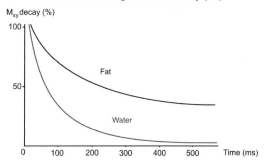

Fig. 4.3 T2 relaxation fat and water in liver. The different T2 decay rates for liver water and fat are evident in this figure, with water having a shorter T2 than fat. Hence in the liver, signal from water decays more rapidly than that from fat

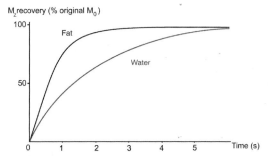

Fig. 4.4 T1 relaxation of fat and water in liver. Water has longer T1 than fat and hence it takes water longer for longitinidal magnetiztion to recover

The magnitude of the magnetization in the *x-y* plane is called M_{xy}. When excited into the *x-y* plane, the precession frequency of the magnetization vector as it rotates at the resonant frequency is given by the Larmour equation:

$$V = \gamma \cdot B_0$$

where ν is the Larmour (resonant, precession) frequency, γ is the gyromagnetic ratio (which is different for each type of nucleus), and B_0 is the main magnetic field that each atomic nucleus experiences (i.e., after shielding).

The signal radiated by the excited protons will exponentially decay with a (transverse) rate of decay (or relaxation) given by T2, as described in the equation:

$$M_{xy} = M_{xy}(0)\exp\left(\frac{-TE}{T2}\right)$$

where $M_{xy}(0)$ is the initial transverse magnetization before it starts to decay, the echo time (TE) is the time between the RF pulse and the signal acquisition, and T2 is the time for M_{xy} to decay to $1/e$ of its initial value (Fig. 4.3). In MRS, we have to correct for T2 decay, but in the MRI sequences discussed in this chapter, this decay is described by T2*, rather than T2, which accounts for additional sources of relaxation that protons typically experience during imaging. MR images require numerous excitations, often hundreds to thousands, and the amount of M_z (i.e., ready to be tipped again into the *x-y* place to give more signal) after an excitation is given by the equation:

$$M_z = M_z(0)\left(1 - \exp\left(\frac{-TR}{T1}\right)\right),$$

where TR is the time between acquisitions and T1 is the time required for M_z to recover to $(e-1)/e$ of its original value (Fig. 4.4).

Water and fat have different values of T1, T2, and T2*. These values will vary from patient to patient and also are dependent on the field strength of the MR scanner [66]. Thus different sequences with different TR and TE values may give different estimates of the fat content. Choosing sequence parameters that minimize T1 and T2 weighting, or acquiring data such that these parameters can be corrected, can avoid or correct for these patient-related differences. This chapter will discuss several of these, as well as other confounding factors, and discuss how to produce an estimate of fat that is independent of field strength and scanner platform.

MRS Liver Fat Measurement Techniques

MRS is widely considered to be the most accurate, noninvasive method to estimate hepatic PDFF [53]. As shown in Fig. 4.1, MRS at 1.5 and 3 T can directly identify the main spectral peaks in fat and water. The amount of signal associated with a spectral peak is related to the area under the peak. Thus, if there were no confounding effects, summing the areas under all the spectral fat peaks and also measuring the area under the water peak would produce an estimate of the ratio of fat-to-water signal, which is related to how much fat is present. However, as stated above, these signals can be confounded by several factors. To produce a repeatable, reproducible estimate of amount of fat, independent of confounding factors, specialized acquisition, and analysis procedures are required. As a first step, MR images of the liver are acquired to allow a volume of the liver to be selected. Normally, images are acquired in more than one plane to assist in selecting an MRS volume of interest, also known as a "voxel." The MRS voxel, generally a $2 \times 2 \times 2$ cm cube, is manually placed in liver parenchyma, using the localizing MR images, to avoid liver edges, large vessels, and large bile ducts as shown in Fig. 4.5. Shimming, a series of short tuning scans, is then performed to achieve a maximally homogeneous magnetic field across the MRS voxel. After successful shimming, an MRS sequence is performed.

There are two main MRS sequences used to measure liver fat. These are PRESS (point resolved spectroscopy) [67] and STEAM (stimulated echo acquisition mode) [68, 69]. There are advantages to both these sequences. PRESS provides twice the signal to noise obtainable from STEAM, but STEAM is capable of a shorter echo time (TE) [70]. Both sequences have been used to measure hepatic PDFF, but as discussed later in this section, STEAM is preferable to PRESS for liver fat quantification. When measuring liver fat using MRS, no water or fat saturation should be used [35]. Also, spatial saturation bands should be disabled. Spatial saturation bands remove all signals from a selected volume band and are used in spectroscopy to remove possible contamination from outside the voxel but can also introduce an unequal response across the spectrum within the selected MRS voxel [71]. While previous studies have used free breathing and multiple averages, there is

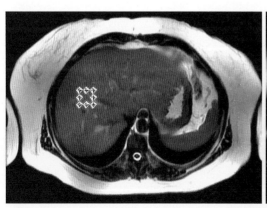
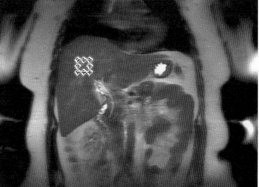

Fig. 4.5 Liver MRS voxel selection in a typical subject as shown on axial (*left*) and coronal (*right*) images. The MRS voxel position is selected to avoid major blood vessels, bile ducts and the edge of the liver

sufficient signal to noise to accurately measure liver in a single breath-hold.

As discussed previously, water and fat have different T1 and T2 values, and these vary between individuals. In MRS, to remove T1-induced variability (mainly of water), TR >3,000 ms is chosen. This TR is sufficient to minimize/avoid the natural variability in T1 between individuals, while still allowing multiple spectra to be acquired in a single breath-hold. This long TR also minimizes the effect of the water and fat having different T1 values.

There are two ways to correct for T2 variability between individuals. The simplest is to collect spectra at as short a TE as possible. This minimizes differences in the amount of decay that occurs due to intersubject variability in T2 values. STEAM has a shorter minimum TE than PRESS and so avoids T2 variability better than PRESS. Mean values of T2 for water and fat, taken from literature, are then used to correct approximately for the T2 decay that does occur. A more advanced solution is to collect single-average spectra at multiple TE values [47, 48]. With a TR of 3,500 ms, spectra at five different TE values can be comfortably collected in a single breath-hold. This allows the areas of fat and water peaks to be calculated by fitting the T2 decay equation:

$$S = S_0 \exp\left(\frac{-TE}{T2}\right)$$

Here S is the area under the spectral peak curve, and S_0 is the T2-corrected peak area (i.e., the area under the curve that would be present at TE=0 ms).

The range of TE values for multi-TE T2 measurement must carefully be chosen, as at longer TE values the decay of fat is no longer purely exponential due to j-coupling. This again suggests the use of the STEAM sequence, which is capable of shorter TEs [72]. A typical liver MRS multi-TE acquisition is shown in Fig. 4.6. However, acquisition of spectra at multiple TE values in a single breath-hold requires a specialized version of MRS sequence. For some scanners, the ability to run these specialized sequences may require a research agreement with the scanner manufacturer.

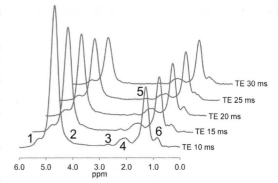

Fig. 4.6 Typical in vivo liver multi-TE MRS acquisition. Spectra acquired at 3T with the STEAM sequence, TR 3,500 ms. The peak assignments are shown in Table 4.1. The difference in the change in peak area of the water and fat peaks with increasing TE shows the differing T2s of fat and water

Virtually all liver MRS is effectively limited to single-voxel acquisition. Thus MRS cannot readily provide information about the spatial distribution of fat in the liver. Liver fat distribution can be heterogeneous, and it is possible that the MRS voxel location is not indicative of the liver as a whole. This may pose a challenge in longitudinal studies, as care must be taken to co-localize the MRS voxel in follow-up scans to a similar location as was selected in the initial study. Otherwise spatial variation in the liver may be mistaken for a change in liver fat over time. There are multi-voxel MRS sequences available that cover large volumes of the liver, providing information on the spatial distribution of fat. However, the large volume reduces the uniformity of magnetic field within the volume, producing poor quality spectra. Also multi-voxel sequences are time consuming and beyond the range of single breath-hold techniques. Thus, they are highly susceptible to artifacts introduced by patient breathing, such as contamination of fat signal from surrounding adipose tissue [35, 66].

Automated, reliable, online analysis methods of spectral analysis are not yet available, so spectral analysis must be performed offline with specialized software by experienced personnel [73]. Spectral tools available from MR scanner manufacturers generally are suitable for viewing spectra, but not optimally suited to estimate hepatic PDFF. However there are a number of advanced tools that incorporate prior knowledge of the structure of the spectrum into fitting algorithms [74, 75]. These tools require initial input from a physicist with advanced knowledge of fat-related MRS to set up so-called "prior knowledge" constraints for analysis of fat spectra. This prior knowledge is generated from a number of factors, including biochemical data and MR scanner parameters. Further, these tools are generally designed for research rather than clinical use, and even when prior knowledge has been set up, an experienced user is still needed to analyze the spectra. Finally on many MR scanners, the raw MR data required for MRS analysis is not automatically archived but instead is stored in temporary files that require a research agreement with the scanner manufacturer to access.

As discussed above, for maximum utility, hepatic fat estimates should be independent of measurement technique. Previous studies have measured just the area of the main CH_2 peak at 1.3 ppm (peak 5, Fig. 4.1) [76, 77]. However, this provides an estimate that is not directly comparable to the fat estimate provided by MRI (see next section). Also, as shown in Figs. 4.1 and 4.6, the fat peaks at 2.1 ppm and 0.9 ppm (peaks 4 and 6) partially overlap the main fat peak 5. This overlap changes with field strength, and it is more difficult to differentiate these peaks at lower field strengths. Thus, measurement of peak 5 (only) may be dependent on spectral analysis technique and on field strength, which limits reproducibility. An alternative strategy is to sum all fat signals between 0 and 3 ppm, treating these peaks as a single peak, assuming a single value of T2 for correction. The difference in T2 between the fat peaks is smaller than the difference between water and fat, justifying this assumption. This removes the problem of differentiating the individual peaks, giving a more robust and reproducible estimate. Two of the fat peaks, at 4.2 and 5.3 ppm (peaks 1 and 2), have similar/close frequencies to the water peak and, in in vivo liver spectra, cannot be clearly differentiated from the water peak (see Figs. 4.1 and 4.6). To provide a fat estimate that is comparable to that obtainable from MRI, the contribution of these fat peaks must be distinguished from the water peak. The spectrum from fat, including the contributions from these peaks, has been calculated from in vivo measurements, which showed that an estimated 8.6 % of total fat in included in the "water" signal, allowing correction for those contributions [63]. Finally, assuming fat and water signals have been corrected for confounding factors, the fat fraction signal is expressed as PDFF, given by

$$PDFF = \text{total fat signal} / (\text{total fat signal} + \text{total water signal})$$

If confounding factors have not been fully accounted for, then the estimate obtained will be just an (uncorrected) signal fat fraction, and not the PDFF, and that estimate will not be independent of measurement technique [35]. If confounding factors have been avoided or corrected, as noted above, then the effects of scanner and patient-dependent parameters will have been mostly removed from the estimate. Thus, PDFF is essentially un-confounded by biological, physical, and technical factors [42]. PDFF is not a direct measure of the mass of fat with respect to the total mass of liver tissue, as there is a fraction of material, such as protein, which is not detected by MRS (or MRI). However it has been shown that PDFF is highly correlated to biochemically measured fat [41]. Thus, PDFF provides a reliable, meaningful, and standardized estimate of hepatic steatosis, which are key elements in the validation of a biomarker.

While MRS can accurately and precisely estimate hepatic PDFF, it cannot provide information about the spatial distribution of PDFF, and it requires advanced technical support to acquire and analyze spectra. For this reason there are few sites with sufficient experience of liver MRS that can adequately estimate PDFF using MRS. Thus the use of MRS for hepatic PDFF quantification for drug development is not advised if the advanced MRI techniques detailed below are available.

Conventional MRI Liver Fat Measurement Techniques

MRI uses chemical shift-based techniques to estimate the amount of fat in the liver. These techniques seek to separate MR signal acquired with a GRE sequence into its water and fat components by acquiring images using two or more echo times (TEs) after signal excitation. These techniques do not rely on water or fat suppression to measure the amount of fat. This chapter will focus only on magnitude-based approaches of MRI quantification of liver fat. There are advanced complex-based techniques available that measure both the magnitude and phase of MRI signal [78]. However, most of the issues with magnitude-based chemical shift MRI are equally applicable to complex-based chemical shift MRI, and other than a short section detailing the differences and possible advantages of complex MRI, all our discussion will apply to magnitude-based MRI.

To understand how MRI measures fat, we need to explore in some detail the underlying physics of MRI. The frequency of each spectral peak we measure indicates how fast protons in fat and water molecules precess while within the main magnetic field. For example, focusing on just the water peak at 4.7 ppm and the main fat peak at 1.3 ppm, these peaks are separated by approximately 434 Hz at 3 T. Protons in the 1.3 ppm methylene (-CH$_2$-) peak precess at the lower frequency, which is 434 Hz lower than that of protons in the water molecule at 3 T. This means that every 1/434th of a second, or each 2.3 ms, 1.3 ppm methylene protons will precess once (i.e., 2π radians) less than water protons. So, at 3 T, those two sets of protons will be "aligned," or in-phase (IP), at 0 ms, 2.3 ms, 4.6 ms, 6.9 ms …, and at points exactly halfway between those values (i.e., at 1.15 ms, 3.45 ms, 5.75 ms …,) signal from those water and fat protons will be out of phase or opposed phase (OP). At 1.5 T, the IP and OP echo times double those at 3 T.

MRI cannot directly measure signal contributions from individual spectral peaks but rather measures the sum of the all the adding and cancelling signals from all of the water and fat protons. The portion of the change in signal as TE increases that is due to interaction of fat and water protons is often referred to fat-water interference. If we ignore all other confounders such as T2* decay, and we assume that all fat signal comes from the 1.3 ppm peak (which it does not) and that all water signal comes from the 4.7 ppm peak, the IP signal will be given by $S_{IP} = S_{water} + S_{fat}$, where S_{water} and S_{fat} are the signals from the water and fat peaks respectively, as simplified above. When those two idealized peaks are OP, water and fat signal cancels and the OP signal is given by $S_{OP} = S_{water} - S_{fat}$, assuming water is the dominant signal.

This is the approach taken by the most common conventional MRI-based approach of measuring liver fat [79, 80]. Just two echoes are collected, generally at the shortest IP and OP times available to the scanner, to maximize signal to noise and to reduce the effect of T2* decay. Because just two echoes are measured, this technique is general referred to as a "dual-echo" technique. The spectral complexity of fat is ignored, and as noted above, it is assumed that the entire fat signal is located at single peak at 1.3 ppm. All other confounders are also ignored. Ideally the first OP and IP images are acquired (1.15 and 2.3 ms at 3 T; 2.3 and 4.6 ms at 1.5 T). However, technical scanner limitations may preclude collecting images at these TEs, and thus longer or shorter TEs may be used. In this simplified case, it is clear that rearranging the two equations above yields the following equations:

$$S_{water} = \frac{S_{IP} + S_{OP}}{2}$$

$$S_{fat} = \frac{S_{IP} - S_{OP}}{2}.$$

With further rearrangement of terms, the (uncorrected) signal fat fraction (FF=fat/(fat+water)) is given by

$$FF = \frac{S_{IP} - S_{OP}}{2S_{IP}}$$

One limitation of this technique is that it cannot differentiate whether water and fat has the larger signal. Hence this technique and magnitude-based MRI imaging techniques in general are limited to measuring signal fat fractions of approximately <50 % signal ratio.

There are two major limitations to this conventional technique. The first is the assumption that all the fat in the liver resonates at 1.3 ppm. Studies have shown in the liver only 70 % of the total fat signal is allocated at the 1.3 ppm peak

[63]. The other fat peaks are at different frequency locations, meaning they precess at different rates, and hence, the IP and OP times for these peaks with reference to water will be different from those for the main CH_2 peak at 1.3 ppm. Thus the assumption that the fat signal is out of phase at the OP TE (e.g., 1.15 ms at 3 T) is invalid. Similarly the assumption that all the fat will be back in phase at the IP TE is also invalid.

Secondly, there is no attempt to correct for the effects of $T2^*$. It is known that $T2^*$ will vary between individuals due to number of biological factors [81]. This means that FF estimates will be affected by subject-dependent factors. As discussed above, different scanners will use different choices of IP and OP echo times due to scanner limitations. The lack of $T2^*$ correction means that different scanners may produce considerably different signal FF estimates. Lack of correction for the fat spectrum and for $T2^*$ results in FF estimates which are inaccurate and imprecise due to both patient and technical factors. Thus, signal FF estimates produced by these techniques are only semiquantitative. For these reasons, the use of the conventional MRI approach should be avoided for drug development decisions if more advanced techniques (discussed below) are available.

Advanced MRI Liver Fat Measurement Techniques

Advanced MRI techniques in many ways use the same approach as conventional MRI, in that MRI signal is sampled at nominally OP and IP TEs. However, careful selection of acquisition parameters and collection of images at more than two echo times provides an accurate and precise quantitative PDFF estimate that is independent of subject and technical factors, as opposed to uncorrected FF estimates from conventional techniques that are less reproducible. The three major confounding factors in estimating PDFF are T1 decay, $T2^*$ decay, and the complexity of the fat spectrum [35]. Fat quantification error is introduced when sequence parameters result in MR images that are T1-weighted. As well as introducing subject-dependent confounders, the shorter T1 of fat compared to water will introduce T1 bias into uncorrected FF estimates. Since MRI requires many acquisitions to produce an image (usually with TR values in the 100–200 ms range), the requirement to acquire all images in a single breath-hold means that using a long TR to avoid T1 weighting is not an option; a sequence with TR = 3,000 ms would take 5–6 min to acquire, well beyond breath-hold capacity. However, T1 weighting can be reduced by using low flip angle excitations (the flip angle being a measure of strength of the RF pulse) [81]. The exact flip angle required depends on the TR, with smaller flip angles needed for shorter TRs.

As discussed previously, fat has a complex spectrum that consists of multiple spectral components or peaks. The degree to which these peaks go in and out of phase with increasing TE depends on their spectral peak frequency location. However, since the liver fat spectrum has been determined from in vivo MRS experiments (Table 4.2) [63], that spectrum can be used to calculate the amplitude of each of the fat peaks at any TE. Thus the amount of fat signal that is still present when the TE is nominally out of phase can be calculated, as can the fat signal that has not re-phased when an image with nominally in-phase TE is acquired. The simple IP/OP equations no longer apply and more advanced mathematical models must be used to fit the measured signal to the theoretical models to provide

Table 4.2 The assignments of fat peaks in the MR spectrum

Peak	Location (ppm)	Assignment	Observed ppm	% total fat signal
1	5.29	-CH=CH-	5.3	3.7
	5.19	-CH-O-CO-		1.0
Water	4.70	H_2O	4.7	–
2	4.20	$-CH_2$-O-CO-	4.2	3.9
3	2.75	$-CH=CH-CH_2-CH=CH-$	2.75	0.6
4	2.24	$-CO-CH_2-CH_2-$	2.1	5.8
	2.02	$-CH_2-CH=CH-CH_2-$		6.2
5	1.60	$-CO-CH_2-CH_2-$	1.3	5.8
	1.30	$-(CH_2)_n-$		64.2
6	0.90	$-(CH_2)_n-CH_3$	0.9	8.8

The magnitude of the individual fat peaks in liver, taken from Hamilton et al. [39], is also shown an estimated PDFF. These spectral correction techniques can be applied for sequences of only two echoes, but as noted in the following paragraph, they work better for sequences of three or more echoes which can also account for T2* effects. T2* correction is necessary for accurate and precise MRI PDFF estimation since if T2* decay is not included in the signal analysis model, fat estimation algorithms will incorrectly separate water and fat signals. Think of T2* decay as the rate of decrease in signal with increasing TE that would occur if there were no fat-interference effects. In conventional dual-echo sequences, T2* cannot be measured as there is no way to know how much T2* contributes to the observed change of signal from the first to the second echo. However, there are techniques which attempt to model T2* decay as part of the algorithm to measure fat fraction which fits the in-phase/out-of-phase behavior.

These approaches can be used to partially improve the accuracy of dual-echo techniques. If a dual-echo acquisition is acquired with low flip angle, and the images are analyzed with a full-fat spectrum model that may include some population-based T2* correction, then the resulting FF estimate will be more accurate but still partially confounded by intersubject T2* variability. Dual-echo techniques are less accurate than MRS and the advanced multi-echo MRI techniques described below. For drug development, dual-echo techniques may be of limited use for cross-sectional studies, though they may be useful for longitudinal studies if advanced methods are not available on the assumption that T2* is not likely to change significantly for any given subject over the time course of longitudinal observation and PDFF estimation. To fully correct for T2* decay, MR images need to be collected at more than two echoes. Multi-echo (i.e., more than two-echo) techniques allow subject-specific estimation of T2* decay [40, 81, 82]. T2* measurement can be performed with as few as three echoes, but the most common advanced methods use six echoes. The larger number of echoes may allow more accurate estimation of PDFF. In theory, these methods could allow T2* of fat and water to measured separately, but the common assumption

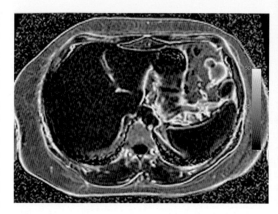

Fig. 4.7 Proton density fat fraction (PDFF) map from a subject with 'normal' liver fat levels (PDFF ~ 1.5 %)

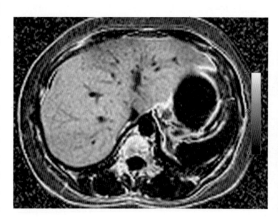

Fig. 4.8 Proton density fat fraction (PDFF) map from a subject with elevated liver fat levels (PDFF ~ 39 %)

made by these techniques is that water and fat have the same T2*, which is justified as long as T2* is significantly less than T2.

Figures 4.7 and 4.8 show PDFF maps derived from two subjects. In Fig. 4.7, the subject has a "normal" level of fat in the liver (PDFF ~1.5 %) and the liver appears dark on the PDFF map. In Fig. 4.8, the subject has an elevated level of fat in the liver (PDFF ~39 %) and hence the liver appears bright on the PDFF map. On both images adipose tissue appears dark since, as discussed above, magnitude-based MRI methods are restricted to FF and PDFF values of less than 50 %.

Multi-echo, chemical-shift MRI can estimate PDFF from most or all of the liver in a single breath-hold. If low flip angle is used, and fitting algorithms are used that include the fat spectral model and T2* estimation, then PDFF values will not be significantly confounded by biological, physical, and technical factors. Hence, as discussed in the MRS section, MRI-estimated PDFF is also a reliable, meaningful, and standardized measure of hepatic steatosis. PDFF values given by these advanced MRI techniques closely match those provided by MRS [40], though unlike MRS, they can provide information about the spatial distribution of fat. MRI PDFF sequences also do not require the level of advanced technical support required by MRS.

Complex-based MRI techniques work in a similar fashion to magnitude-based MRI methods to estimate PDFF [83–85]. However instead of measuring just the magnitude of the MR signal, they measure both magnitude and phase. They are limited by the same considerations as magnitude-based MRI; a low flip angle is used, and fitting algorithms are used that include the fat spectral model and allow measurement of T2*. However by measuring phase, these techniques can measure PDFF values from 0 to 100 %. This is not of prime importance in liver as it only in rare cases that PDFF exceeds 50 %. In these cases, PDFF values will only be just above 50 %, and magnitude-based MRI methods will give PDFF values just below 50 %. Whether the PDFF is slightly above or below 50 % will not make a difference in clinical decisions. However, for imaging elsewhere in the body, outside the liver, complex-based MRI methods are able to differentiate very high fat adipose tissue from the majority of low fat tissues. Thus these techniques can produce accurate and precise fat-water maps. This is important when mapping the overall fat distribution in the body.

Advanced MRI techniques can accurately estimate PDFF in the liver and provide information about the spatial distribution of fat. However, while these techniques are more widely available than MRS, the technology is not yet universally available or readily implementable on all scanners. Since PDFF is a standardized, reproducible biomarker of liver fat content, advanced MRI techniques may provide valuable information in development of drugs that may alter liver fat content.

MRS Skeletal Muscle Fat Measurement Techniques

Using MRS to estimate IMCL in skeletal muscle requires different acquisition parameters and analysis techniques than are used to estimate liver PDFF. Another difference is that liver fat accumulates only inside liver hepatocyte cells, but muscle fat accumulates inside skeletal muscle cells (IMCL) and in between skeletal muscle cells (EMCL) [50].

Muscle spectra normally are collected in the leg, usually in a calf muscle. A typical muscle spectrum is shown in Fig. 4.9. Instead of the single set of fat peaks seen in the liver, two overlapping sets of fat peaks are observed – one for IMCL and one for EMCL. There are also detectable signals from metabolites in the muscle: choline (Cho) and creatine (Cr) [86]. The IMCL fat peaks occur at the same locations as the fat peaks we see in liver. However there is also present in the muscle skeletal spectrum a set of "shifted" fat peaks associated with EMCL. IMCL is located as droplets inside the cell and provides an energy store during endurance exercise [50, 52]. and EMCL is located in layers outside cells, within muscle and is visible in MR images as "streaky" fat deposits in muscle. This layered structure of EMCL is responsible for the shifted fat peaks as these layers lie at an angle to the main magnetic field [49, 50, 87]. The interaction of magnetic field and muscle structure may not give rise to separate peaks in muscle groups outside the leg. Usually it is only possible to clearly distinguish two main skeletal muscle fat CH_2 peaks, at approximately at 1.3 ppm for IMCL, and 1.5 ppm for EMCL. Hence, IMCL "content" is commonly expressed as the ratio of the area under the IMCL 1.3 ppm CH_2 peak to the area under the water peak. Unfortunately, the most challenging subjects in which to obtain an IMCL measurement are obese patients, who may be of most interest for metabolic syndrome-related conditions. To accurately measure IMCL, good separation from the EMCL peak is required, but in obese patients, there is usually abundant streaky fat (i.e., EMCL), making it more difficult to distinguish

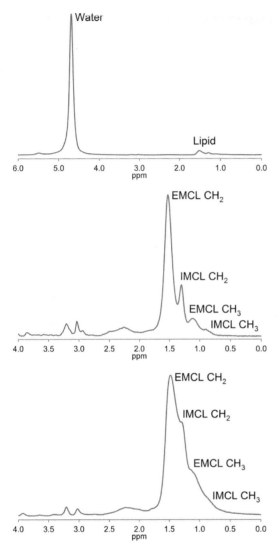

Fig. 4.9 Typical in vivo muscle MR spectrum (*top*) acquired at 3 T with PRESS, TR=3,000 ms, TE=30 ms. Focusing on the fat region of the spectrum (*middle*), the two sets of fat peaks associated with EMCL and IMCL become apparent. In the *bottom spectrum*, the amount of EMCL was far greater than the *middle spectrum*, obscuring the IMCL peak

the smaller ICML peak from the larger, close-by EMCL peak (see Fig. 4.9).

MRS can provide an estimate of IMCL content but is less well suited to measure EMCL content. IMCL signal (relative to water signal) should be similar throughout typical calf muscles, and so a shift in voxel position within calf muscle should not change the amount of IMCL detected. EMCL on the other hand is localized to discrete "structures" or collections, consistent with its streaky appearance on MR images. Figure 4.10 shows EMCL in a skeletal calf muscle as bright streaks in grey muscle. The IMCL, being located diffusely through the muscle, cannot be identified in this image. As can be seen Fig. 4.10, a small change in voxel position may increase or decrease the presence of streaky EMCL fat within the MRS voxel, resulting in a different measured value for EMCL. Hence, MR imaging is probably a better way to evaluate EMCL than MRS. The advanced complex-based MRI methods discussed earlier are well suited to measure the volume of EMCL fat. However, such analysis is beyond the scope of this chapter. Another difference between liver and muscle fat is the amount of fat. In liver, we see PDFF values from 0 to 50 %. In muscle, the range of IMCL is an order of magnitude smaller than that (roughly 0–5 %). Thus, small changes in the amount of IMCL may be significant.

Due to the requirement to clearly differentiate the (1.3 ppm) IMCL from the (1.5 ppm) EMCL peak, and accurately measure low levels of IMCL, appropriate sequence parameters are required, different from those used to estimate hepatic PDFF. In muscle, the PRESS sequence is generally preferred as it has intrinsically double the signal to noise compared to STEAM. This does mean that a longer minimum TE must be used. Similar to liver MRS, a long TR of 3,000 ms or greater is chosen to minimize T1 weighting. However, the requirement to accurately measure IMCL means that we do not collect spectra at multiple TEs; instead we collect spectra with many averages at a single TE. The size of the voxel is limited by muscle size and is often rectangularly shaped (e.g., 15×15×30 mm).

High-resolution localizing images should be performed prior to muscle MRS to allow the EMCL fat depots to be identified. Effort should be made to select a voxel location that minimizes EMCL presence in the MRS voxel on these high-resolution images. Large EMCL depots and adipose tissue should be avoided. Generally a sequence lasting several minutes is used to generate a sufficiently high quality spectrum. To

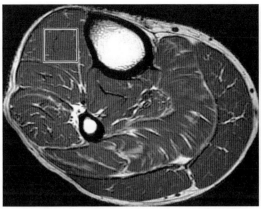 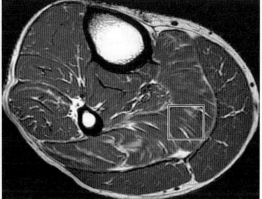

Fig. 4.10 Skeletal calf muscle MRS voxel selection in tibialis (*left*) and soleus (*right*) in a typical subject as shown on axial high-resolution localization image. EMCL appears as bright streaks in the muscle. The amount of EMCL seen in the muscle spectrum will change depending on voxel position. Selecting a voxel position within the muscle group with as little EMCL as possible allows better identification of IMCL. In this case, the tibialis voxel selection contains less EMCL compared to soleus

minimize T2 weighting, the minimum TE value available to PRESS is used. Then, either T2 decay is corrected for by values taken from literature, or a rapid multi-TE MRS sequence is used to measure water T2 allowing subject-specific T2 correction.

Different muscle groups have different levels of IMCL, and it has not been established that all muscle groups act equally in response to any particular drug. So, muscle spectra often are acquired in two different muscle groups. In calf muscle MRS, for example, generally the tibialis and soleus muscles are selected [77]. The same limitations seen in liver MRS analysis apply also to muscle MRS analysis. Analysis of spectra must be performed offline with specialized software by experienced personnel. Analysis of muscle spectra is particularly challenging, since the IMCL peak is close to, and often overlaps a larger EMCL peak. Generally muscle group-specific prior knowledge is used in the specialized MRS analysis software, but there is currently no standardization of techniques used to analyze muscle spectra. This may introduce variability due to difference in analysis technique. Finally, the ratio of the area of the IMCL CH_2 peak to the area under the water peak does not share the robustness of hepatic PDFF estimation. The use of differing acquisition and analysis techniques means that measurement of skeletal muscle IMCL levels is less generalizable than PDFF measurement in the liver.

While MRS can accurately measure IMCL levels, doing so requires advanced technical support in both the acquisition and the analysis of the spectra. For this reason, there are few sites with sufficient experience of muscle MRS to accurately and precisely measure IMCL levels. Thus, while the use of MRS to measure IMCL may be of relevance in drug development, it use is limited to smaller-scale clinical trials in centres with appropriate expertise. In such trials muscle, MRS may inform decisions on whether drugs may alter ectopic fat content in skeletal muscle independently of effects on liver fat, and measurement of skeletal muscle IMCL may help to elucidate pathogenesis.

Translation to Clinical Practice

For estimation of hepatic PDFF, the authors advocate the use whenever possible of advanced MRI techniques. PDFF estimation of hepatic steatosis is a generalizable, standardized measurement that is probably reproducible across sites and scanner manufacturers, models, and software and is expected to be independent, within reasonable limits, of MRI technologists, most technical scan acquisition factors, and subject factors (age, sex, race/ethnicity, body habitus, concomitant metabolic, or other disorders). This facilitates implementation in multicentre trials as well as pooling of or comparison with results from different studies. Use of less advanced methods to quantify liver fat will be less generalizable. Expected PDFF results in clinical practice are expected to mirror results that have been observed in clinical trials. Namely, a drug that in clinical trials reduces hepatic PDFF as estimated by MRI will be expected to have the same effect in clinical practice. If hepatic FF is estimated with non-standardized techniques, then translation of results to clinical practice becomes less predictable.

Muscle MRS is still a research tool. There is no equivalent of PDFF for muscle MRS. Most muscle MRS studies are carried out at single sites, and depending on acquisition and analysis techniques, different groups may produce different estimates of IMCL. For IMCL measurement to become clinically relevant, standardized tools and techniques for the acquisition and analysis of muscle spectra need to be validated to ensure that IMCL estimates are sufficiently accurate and precise for their intended purposes.

References

1. Kahn BB, Flier JS. Obesity and insulin resistance. J Clin Invest. 2000;106(4):473–81.
2. DeFronzo RA. Insulin resistance, lipotoxicity, type 2 diabetes and atherosclerosis: the missing links. The Claude Bernard Lecture 2009. Diabetologia. 2010;53(7):1270–87.
3. Caprio S. Development of type 2 diabetes mellitus in the obese adolescent: a growing challenge. Endocr Pract. 2012;18(5):791–5.
4. Karlas T, Wiegand J, Berg T. Gastrointestinal complications of obesity: non-alcoholic fatty liver disease (NAFLD) and its sequelae. Best Pract Res Clin Endocrinol Metab. 2013;27(2):195–208.
5. Hui E, Xu A, Bo Yang H, Lam KS. Obesity as the common soil of non-alcoholic fatty liver disease and diabetes: role of adipokines. J Diabetes Investig. 2013;4(5):413–25.
6. Birkenfeld AL, Shulman GI. Nonalcoholic fatty liver disease, hepatic insulin resistance, and type 2 diabetes. Hepatology. 2014;59(2):713–23.
7. Byrne CD, Olufadi R, Bruce KD, Cagampang FR, Ahmed MH. Metabolic disturbances in non-alcoholic fatty liver disease. Clin Sci (Lond). 2009;116(7):539–64.
8. Oni ET, Agatston AS, Blaha MJ, Fialkow J, Cury R, Sposito A, et al. A systematic review: burden and severity of subclinical cardiovascular disease among those with nonalcoholic fatty liver; should we care? Atherosclerosis. 2013;230(2):258–67.
9. Yki-Jarvinen H. Non-alcoholic fatty liver disease as a cause and a consequence of metabolic syndrome. Lancet Diabetes Endocrinol. 2014. doi: 10.1016/S2213-8587(14)70032-4. Epub ahead of print.
10. Lettner A, Roden M. Ectopic fat and insulin resistance. Curr Diab Rep. 2008;8(3):185–91.
11. Hardy OT, Czech MP, Corvera S. What causes the insulin resistance underlying obesity? Curr Opin Endocrinol Diabetes Obes. 2012;19(2):81–7.
12. Shimabukuro M, Kozuka C, Taira S, Yabiku K, Dagvasumberel M, Ishida M, et al. Ectopic fat deposition and global cardiometabolic risk: new paradigm in cardiovascular medicine. J Med Invest. 2013;60(1–2):1–14.
13. Schwenger KJ, Allard JP. Clinical approaches to non-alcoholic fatty liver disease. World J Gastroenterol. 2014;20(7):1712–23.
14. Marchesini G, Bugianesi E, Forlani G, Cerrelli F, Lenzi M, Manini R, et al. Nonalcoholic fatty liver, steatohepatitis, and the metabolic syndrome. Hepatology. 2003;37(4):917–23.
15. Targher G, Byrne CD. Clinical review: nonalcoholic fatty liver disease: a novel cardiometabolic risk factor for type 2 diabetes and its complications. J Clin Endocrinol Metab. 2013;98(2):483–95.
16. Ballestri S, Lonardo A, Bonapace S, Byrne CD, Loria P, Targher G. Risk of cardiovascular, cardiac and arrhythmic complications in patients with non-alcoholic fatty liver disease. World J Gastroenterol. 2014;20(7):1724–45.
17. Perseghin G. Muscle lipid metabolism in the metabolic syndrome. Curr Opin Lipidol. 2005;16(4):416–20.
18. Pan DA, Lillioja S, Kriketos AD, Milner MR, Baur LA, Bogardus C, et al. Skeletal muscle triglyceride levels are inversely related to insulin action. Diabetes. 1997;46(6):983–8.
19. Petersen KF, Shulman GI. Pathogenesis of skeletal muscle insulin resistance in type 2 diabetes mellitus. Am J Cardiol. 2002;90(5A):11G–8.
20. Perseghin G, Scifo P, De Cobelli F, Pagliato E, Battezzati A, Arcelloni C, et al. Intramyocellular triglyceride content is a determinant of in vivo insulin resistance in humans: a 1H-13C nuclear magnetic resonance spectroscopy assessment in offspring of type 2 diabetic parents. Diabetes. 1999;48(8):1600–6.
21. Jacob S, Machann J, Rett K, Brechtel K, Volk A, Renn W, et al. Association of increased intramyocellular lipid content with insulin resistance in lean nondiabetic offspring of type 2 diabetic subjects. Diabetes. 1999;48(5):1113–9.
22. Kelley DE, He J, Menshikova EV, Ritov VB. Dysfunction of mitochondria in human skeletal muscle in type 2 diabetes. Diabetes. 2002;51(10):2944–50.

23. Teranishi T, Ohara T, Maeda K, Zenibayashi M, Kouyama K, Hirota Y, et al. Effects of pioglitazone and metformin on intracellular lipid content in liver and skeletal muscle of individuals with type 2 diabetes mellitus. Metabolism. 2007;56(10):1418–24.
24. Bradford V, Dillon J, Miller M. Lifestyle interventions for the treatment of non-alcoholic fatty liver disease. Hepat Med. 2014;6:1–10.
25. Rabl C, Campos GM. The impact of bariatric surgery on nonalcoholic steatohepatitis. Semin Liver Dis. 2012;32(1):80–91.
26. Lim EL, Hollingsworth KG, Aribisala BS, Chen MJ, Mathers JC, Taylor R. Reversal of type 2 diabetes: normalisation of beta cell function in association with decreased pancreas and liver triacylglycerol. Diabetologia. 2011;54(10):2506–14.
27. Mazza A, Fruci B, Garinis GA, Giuliano S, Malaguarnera R, Belfiore A. The role of metformin in the management of NAFLD. Exp Diabetes Res. 2012;2012:716404.
28. Ozturk ZA, Kadayifci A. Insulin sensitizers for the treatment of non-alcoholic fatty liver disease. World J Hepatol. 2014;6(4):199–206.
29. Mahady SE, Webster AC, Walker S, Sanyal A, George J. The role of thiazolidinediones in non-alcoholic steatohepatitis – a systematic review and meta analysis. J Hepatol. 2011;55(6):1383–90.
30. Scorletti E, Bhatia L, McCormick KG, Clough GF, Nash K, Calder PC, et al. Design and rationale of the WELCOME trial: a randomised, placebo controlled study to test the efficacy of purified long chain omega-3 fatty treatment in non-alcoholic fatty liver disease. Contemp Clin Trials. 2014;37(2):301–11.
31. Eslami L, Merat S, Malekzadeh R, Nasseri-Moghaddam S, Aramin H. Statins for non-alcoholic fatty liver disease and non-alcoholic steatohepatitis. Cochrane Database Syst Rev. 2013;(12):CD008623.
32. Ratziu V. Targeting non-alcoholic fatty liver disease through 11-βHSD1 inhibition. Lancet Diabetes Endocrinol. 2014;2:354–6.
33. Schwenzer NF, Springer F, Schraml C, Stefan N, Machann J, Schick F. Non-invasive assessment and quantification of liver steatosis by ultrasound, computed tomography and magnetic resonance. J Hepatol. 2009;51(3):433–45.
34. Lee SS, Park SH. Radiologic evaluation of nonalcoholic fatty liver disease. World J Gastroenterol. 2014;20(23):7392–402.
35. Reeder SB, Cruite I, Hamilton G, Sirlin CB. Quantitative assessment of liver fat with magnetic resonance imaging and spectroscopy. J Magn Reson Imaging. 2011;34(4):729–49.
36. Machann J, Stefan N, Schick F. (1)H MR spectroscopy of skeletal muscle, liver and bone marrow. Eur J Radiol. 2008;67(2):275–84.
37. Dixon WT. Simple proton spectroscopic imaging. Radiology. 1984;153(1):189–94.
38. Glover GH. Multipoint Dixon technique for water and fat proton and susceptibility imaging. J Magn Reson Imaging. 1991;1(5):521–30.
39. Fishbein MH, Gardner KG, Potter CJ, Schmalbrock P, Smith MA. Introduction of fast MR imaging in the assessment of hepatic steatosis. Magn Reson Imaging. 1997;15(3):287–93.
40. Yokoo T, Shiehmorteza M, Hamilton G, Wolfson T, Schroeder ME, Middleton MS, et al. Estimation of hepatic proton-density fat fraction by using MR imaging at 3.0 T. Radiology. 2011;258(3):749–59.
41. Hu HH, Li Y, Nagy TR, Goran MI, Nayak KS. Quantification of absolute fat mass by magnetic resonance imaging: a validation study against chemical analysis. Int J Body Compos Res. 2011;9(3):111–22.
42. Reeder SB, Hu HH, Sirlin CB. Proton density fat-fraction: a standardized MR-based biomarker of tissue fat concentration. J Magn Reson Imaging. 2012;36(5):1011–4.
43. Longo R, Ricci C, Masutti F, Vidimari R, Crocé LS, Bercich L, et al. Fatty infiltration of the liver. Quantification by 1H localized magnetic resonance spectroscopy and comparison with computed tomography. Invest Radiol. 1993;28(4):297–302.
44. Thomsen C, Becker U, Winkler K, Christoffersen P, Jensen M, Henriksen O. Quantification of liver fat using magnetic resonance spectroscopy. Magn Reson Imaging. 1994;12(3):487–95.
45. Longo R, Pollesello P, Ricci C, Vidimari R, Crocé LS, Bercich L, et al. Proton MR spectroscopy in quantitative in vivo determination of fat content in human liver steatosis. J Magn Reson Imaging. 1995;5(3):281–5.
46. Szczepaniak LS, Nurenberg P, Leonard D, Browning JD, Reingold JS, Grundy S, et al. Magnetic resonance spectroscopy to measure hepatic triglyceride content: prevalence of hepatic steatosis in the general population. Am J Physiol Endocrinol Metab. 2005;288(2):E462–8.
47. Hamilton G, Middleton MS, Bydder M, Yokoo T, Schwimmer JB, Kono Y, et al. Effect of PRESS and STEAM sequences on magnetic resonance spectroscopic liver fat quantification. J Magn Reson Imaging. 2009;30(1):145–52.
48. Pineda N, Sharma P, Xu Q, Hu X, Vos M, Martin DR. Measurement of hepatic lipid: high-speed T2-corrected multiecho acquisition at 1H MR spectroscopy–a rapid and accurate technique. Radiology. 2009;252(2):568–76.
49. Schick F, Eismann B, Jung WI, Bongers H, Bunse M, Lutz O. Comparison of localized proton NMR signals of skeletal muscle and fat tissue in vivo: two lipid compartments in muscle tissue. Magn Reson Med. 1993;29(2):158–67.
50. Boesch C, Slotboom J, Hoppeler H, Kreis R. In vivo determination of intra-myocellular lipids in human muscle by means of localized 1H-MR-spectroscopy. Magn Reson Med. 1997;37(4):484–93.
51. Kreis R, Boesch C. Spatially localized, one- and two-dimensional NMR spectroscopy and in vivo application to human muscle. J Magn Reson B. 1996;113(2):103–18.
52. Boesch C, Decombaz J, Slotboom J, Kreis R. Observation of intramyocellular lipids by means of

1H magnetic resonance spectroscopy. Proc Nutr Soc. 1999;58(4):841–50.
53. Charatcharoenwitthaya P, Lindor KD. Role of radiologic modalities in the management of non-alcoholic steatohepatitis. Clin Liver Dis. 2007;11(1):37–54, viii.
54. Graif M, Yanuka M, Baraz M, Blank A, Moshkovitz M, Kessler A, et al. Quantitative estimation of attenuation in ultrasound video images: correlation with histology in diffuse liver disease. Invest Radiol. 2000;35(5):319–24.
55. Saadeh S, Younossi ZM, Remer EM, Gramlich T, Ong JP, Hurley M, et al. The utility of radiological imaging in nonalcoholic fatty liver disease. Gastroenterology. 2002;123(3):745–50.
56. Mottin CC, Moretto M, Padoin AV, Swarowsky AM, Toneto MG, Glock L, et al. The role of ultrasound in the diagnosis of hepatic steatosis in morbidly obese patients. Obes Surg. 2004;14(5):635–7.
57. Barry CT, Mills B, Hah Z, Mooney RA, Ryan CK, Rubens DJ, et al. Shear wave dispersion measures liver steatosis. Ultrasound Med Biol. 2012;38(2):175–82.
58. Limanond P, Raman SS, Lassman C, Sayre J, Ghobrial RM, Busuttil RW, et al. Macrovesicular hepatic steatosis in living related liver donors: correlation between CT and histologic findings. Radiology. 2004;230(1):276–80.
59. Kodama Y, Ng CS, Wu TT, Ayers GD, Curley SA, Abdalla EK, et al. Comparison of CT methods for determining the fat content of the liver. AJR Am J Roentgenol. 2007;188(5):1307–12.
60. Lee SW, Park SH, Kim KW, Choi EK, Shin YM, Kim PN, et al. Unenhanced CT for assessment of macrovesicular hepatic steatosis in living liver donors: comparison of visual grading with liver attenuation index. Radiology. 2007;244(2):479–85.
61. Birnbaum BA, Hindman N, Lee J, Babb JS. Multidetector row CT attenuation measurements: assessment of intra- and interscanner variability with an anthropomorphic body CT phantom. Radiology. 2007;242(1):109–19.
62. Fazel R, Krumholz HM, Wang Y, Ross JS, Chen J, Ting HH, et al. Exposure to low-dose ionizing radiation from medical imaging procedures. N Engl J Med. 2009;361(9):849–57.
63. Hamilton G, Yokoo T, Bydder M, Cruite I, Schroeder ME, Sirlin CB, et al. In vivo characterization of the liver fat (1)H MR spectrum. NMR Biomed. 2011;24(7):784–90.
64. Ren J, Dimitrov I, Sherry AD, Malloy CR. Composition of adipose tissue and marrow fat in humans by 1H NMR at 7 Tesla. J Lipid Res. 2008;49(9):2055–62.
65. Bydder M, Girard O, Hamilton G. Mapping the double bonds in triglycerides. Magn Reson Imaging. 2011;29(8):1041–6.
66. Hu HH, Kan HE. Quantitative proton MR techniques for measuring fat. NMR Biomed. 2013;26(12):1609–29.
67. Bottomley PA. Spatial localization in NMR spectroscopy in vivo. Ann N Y Acad Sci. 1987;508:333–48.
68. Granot J. Selected volume excitation using stimulated echoes (VEST): applications to spatially localized spectroscopy and imaging. J Magn Reson Imaging. 1986;70:488–92.
69. Frahm J, Merboldt K-D, Hänicke W. Localized proton spectroscopy using stimulated echoes. J Magn Reson Imaging. 1987;72:502–8.
70. Keevil SF. Spatial localization in nuclear magnetic resonance spectroscopy. Phys Med Biol. 2006;51(16):R579–636.
71. Middelton M, Hamilton G, Sirlin CB. Effect of saturation bands on quantitative liver fat proton MR spectroscopy. In: Proceedings of the RSNA Annual Meeting, Chicago; 2011.
72. De Graff R, Rothman DL. In vivo detection and quantification of scalar coupled 1H NMR resonances. Concepts Magn Reson. 2001;13:32–76.
73. in 't Zandt H, van Der Graaf M, Heerschap A. Common processing of in vivo MR spectra. NMR Biomed. 2001;14:224–32.
74. Vanhamme L, Sundin T, Hecke PV, Huffel SV. MR spectroscopy quantitation: a review of time-domain methods. NMR Biomed. 2001;14(4):233–46.
75. Mierisova S, Ala-Korpela M. MR spectroscopy quantitation: a review of frequency domain methods. NMR Biomed. 2001;14(4):247–59.
76. Szczepaniak LS, Babcock EE, Schick F, Dobbins RL, Garg A, Burns DK, et al. Measurement of intracellular triglyceride stores by H spectroscopy: validation in vivo. Am J Physiol. 1999;276(5 Pt 1):E977–89.
77. Thomas EL, Potter E, Tosi I, Fitzpatrick J, Hamilton G, Amber V, et al. Pioglitazone added to conventional lipid-lowering treatment in familial combined hyperlipidaemia improves parameters of metabolic control: relation to liver, muscle and regional body fat content. Atherosclerosis. 2007;195(1):e181–90.
78. Reeder SB, Pineda AR, Wen Z, Shimakawa A, Yu H, Brittain JH, et al. Iterative decomposition of water and fat with echo asymmetry and least-squares estimation (IDEAL): application with fast spin-echo imaging. Magn Reson Med. 2005;54(3):636–44.
79. Kawamitsu H, Kaji Y, Ohara T, Sugimura K. Feasibility of quantitative intrahepatic lipid imaging applied to the magnetic resonance dual gradient echo sequence. Magn Reson Med Sci. 2003;2:47–50.
80. Qayyum A, Goh JS, Kakar S, Yeh BM, Merriman RB, Coakley FV. Accuracy of liver fat quantification at MR imaging: comparison of out-of-phase gradient-echo and fat-saturated fast spin-echo techniques-initial experience. Radiology. 2005;237:507–11.
81. Bydder M, Yokoo T, Hamilton G, Middleton MS, Chavez AD, Schwimmer JB, et al. Relaxation effects in the quantification of fat using gradient echo imaging. Magn Reson Imaging. 2008;26(3):347–59.
82. Yokoo T, Bydder M, Hamilton G, Middleton MS, Gamst AC, Wolfson T, et al. Nonalcoholic fatty liver disease: diagnostic and fat-grading accuracy of low-flip-angle multiecho gradient-recalled-echo MR imaging at 1.5 T. Radiology. 2009;251(1):67–76.

83. Yu H, Shimakawa A, McKenzie CA, Brodsky E, Brittain JH, Reeder SB. Multiecho water-fat separation and simultaneous R2* estimation with multifrequency fat spectrum modeling. Magn Reson Med. 2008;60(5):1122–34.
84. Yu H, Shimakawa A, Hines CD, McKenzie CA, Hamilton G, Sirlin CB, et al. Combination of complex-based and magnitude-based multiecho water-fat separation for accurate quantification of fat-fraction. Magn Reson Med. 2011;66(1):199–206.
85. Meisamy S, Hines CD, Hamilton G, Sirlin CB, McKenzie CA, Yu H, et al. Quantification of hepatic steatosis with T1-independent, T2-corrected MR imaging with spectral modeling of fat: blinded comparison with MR spectroscopy. Radiology. 2011;258(3):767–75.
86. Boesch C, Machann J, Vermathen P, Schick F. Role of proton MR for the study of muscle lipid metabolism. NMR Biomed. 2006;19(7):968–88.
87. Szczepaniak L, Dobbins RL, Stein DT, McGarry JD. Bulk magnetic susceptibility effects on the assessment of intra- and extramycellular lipids in vivo. Magn Reson Med. 2001;47:607–10.

Positron-Emission Tomography and Computed Tomography Measurement of Brown Fat Thermal Activation: Key Tools for Developing Novel Pharmacotherapeutics for Obesity and Diabetes

5

Monte S. Buchsbaum and Alex DeCastro

Keywords

Adipose tissue • Fluorodeoxyglucose • Temperature homeostasis • Obesity • Diabetes

Summary

Background

Unlike white adipose tissue, brown adipose tissue is a heat-generating fat that burns energy and may have beneficial effects on obesity. Activation of brown fat by cold room temperatures increases glucose uptake that can be imaged using positron-emission tomography with 18F-deoxyglucose (FDG-PET). Brown fat is an important contributor to body energy consumption. The volume of brown fat is greater in children and young adults as well as in lean adults; in general, these groups are less likely to be obese or to have type 2 diabetes. Brown and white fat can be separated in computed tomography (CT) images by their Hounsfield unit values and together with FDG-PET provide an index of energy consumption valuable in understanding the effects of new glucose-lowering and anti-obesity drugs.

Key Methods

This chapter reviews the methods for the segmentation of brown and white fat, the coregistration to FDG-PET, and the effects of room temperature on metabolic rate.

M.S. Buchsbaum, MD (✉)
Department of Psychiatry and Radiology, University of California, San Diego, San Diego, CA, USA
e-mail: Monte.buchsbaum@gmail.com

A. DeCastro, MS
Department of Psychiatry, University of California, San Diego, San Diego, CA, USA

Method	Measurement	Advantages	Disadvantages	Value in drug development decisions
Thorax computed tomography (CT)	Yields Hounsfield unit images which can be segmented into types of fat, muscle, air, and bone; tissue volume in mm³ assessed	1. Absolute units can be calibrated against water standard 2. Integral to PET scanners	Some radiation exposure	Medium
Fluorodeoxyglucose positron-emission tomography (FDG-PET)	Metabolic rate in fat and muscle	1. Standardized metabolic measurement conditions 2. Yields absolute metabolic rate in micromoles/100 g tissue/min	Radiation exposure Complex quantification	High
Metabolic quantification from aortic blood	Absolute metabolic rate, relative metabolic rate, standard uptake value (SUV), and ratio (SUVR) can be obtained to follow therapeutic trial	Arterial or arterialized blood samples not required	Limited to thorax scanning	High

Conclusions

The combination of FDG-PET and CT provides a tool for assessing brown and white fat metabolic activity and volume. These measurements can be used to assist in the monitoring of pharmacological interventions thereby informing the development of novel agents for obesity and diabetes.

Introduction

While increased body fat is associated with type 2 diabetes, the location and tissue type of fat are important aspects of the physiological concomitants of obesity. The location of fat in the truncal region in comparison to leg fat is an indicator of both the metabolic syndrome and mortality, even after statistical adjustment for body mass index (BMI) and waist circumference [1]. Visceral adipose tissue volume assessed by computed tomography (CT) scans is more highly associated with the metabolic syndrome than abdominal subcutaneous adipose tissue [2] and using specific regional fat location has been found to enhance the correlation between fat volume and response to experimental obesity interventions [3]. Adipose tissue type is also an important factor. White adipose tissue is involved in energy storage, while brown adipose tissue is thermogenic and may be an especially advantageous target for treatment intervention [4]. Brown and white fat can be regionally parcelled with x-ray computed tomography and the metabolic correlates of thermogenesis quantitatively assessed with positron-emission tomography as reviewed below. Thus, regional and adipose tissue type assessment of fat tissue for pharmaceutical trials of drugs which affect obesity and diabetes can be an important contributor to documenting drug activity, interpreting individual differences in drug efficacy, and characterizing the physiological effects of new compounds. This chapter reviews the imaging-based assessment of the metabolic rate of brown fat during thermogenesis. 18F-deoxyglucose (FDG) uptake measurement with positron-emission tomography (PET) and coregistered x-ray CT provides a methodology for this assessment.

Drug Action, Energy Expenditure, Thermogenesis, and Brown Fat

Increases in energy expenditure without corresponding caloric intake are associated with weight reduction. Drug treatment for obesity might reduce appetite, diminish food absorption, alter circadian rhythms, or enhance locomotor activity among multiple mechanisms, but enhancing energy expenditure is an attractive mechanism for drug action. As noted by Arch and Trayhurn in their reviews, thermogenesis may be an appropriate target in antidiabetic [5] and anti-obesity drug discovery [6, 7]. Targeting brown adipose tissue is an appealing therapeutic strategy because activation of brown adipocytes has the potential to safely improve metabolic control independent of defects in insulin production or sensitivity [8]. There may be as much as 0.2–1 % of body weight as brown fat [9] and capable of using as much as 20 % of caloric expenditure for cold exposure [9] (see review [10]). To advance new drug development, increasingly detailed assessments of body tissue function is necessary to capture relevant physiology, to increase tissue specificity, and to understand individual differences in response. Individual, personalized approaches to drug development may be especially important in conditions such as obesity where subtypes and mechanisms may differ widely. In obesity, degrees of insulin resistance, hyperlipidemias, genetic subtypes, and activity levels differ widely and may impact responsiveness to particular pharmacological interventions [11]. A drug to increase thermogenesis may not be found efficacious in individuals without a brown fat deficit in activity or volume, just as an anti-amyloid drug for Alzheimer's disease may not be efficacious in a patient without excess brain amyloid.

Brown Fat Thermogenesis and Autonomic Regulation

The contribution of brown fat to thermal homeostasis begins with skin warm and cold receptors which stimulate neurons in the dorsal horn. These carry thermal information into a network of GABAergic and glutamatergic neurons in the preoptic area and the dorsomedial hypothalamus. Sympathetic activation of brown fat is then the output of this complex and multitransmitter circuit; for details see the insightful and detailed review of Tupone et al. [12]. Brown fat metabolic rates in rats [13–15] were measured with FDG-PET. To provide a quantitative measure, these and other investigators use the standard uptake value which is computed as the average FDG uptake within a volume of interest (in kBq/ml) divided by the administered amount of FDG (in MBq) multiplied by the body weight (in Kg). This corrects the observed uptake counts per unit volume for the amount of tissue in the whole body and the amount of FDG given. The standard uptake value (SUV) activity was enhanced fivefold in brown fat in response to treatment with the B-3 adrenoreceptor selective agonist CL316243 and to a lesser extent (twofold) in white fat and muscle. No significant differences were found in other body tissues. Of further interest is that in the rat the distribution of adrenergically activated fat was in the same infrascapular region that brown fat is found in man. The mechanism of thermogenesis, including the role of uncoupling protein-1, which is a unique marker for brown adipose tissue, is reviewed elsewhere [16–20].

Computed Tomography Quantitated Imaging of Body Tissue

Estimates of human body fat may be approximated by BMI, the ratio of height and weight; by skinfold thickness, anthropometric measurements, and electrical impedance; and by whole body counting techniques, but these techniques lack adipose tissue type specificity and anatomical exactness. In order to assess both brown and white fat in the infrascapular [21] regions, x-ray attenuation can be used as a potential differentiator to assess both brown fat and white fat. CT imaging was invented by Godfrey Hounsfield and Allan Cormack who combined electrical engineering and mathematical reconstruction algorithms to make the first CT scanner [22]. The initial clinical success of the first CT scanner was detecting a tumor in a patient in 1971, and CT scanners were subsequently widely adopted across the world. These images are quantitative, with type of fat tissue, muscle, bone, and air having different values. Hounsfield unit ratings are standardized with a value of 0 for distilled water and −1,000 for air. Fat typically has values from −250 to −50, muscle from 10 to 200, other soft tissue 150–300, and bone 700–300. The modern CT scanner produces a series of contiguous slice images, typically a matrix of 256 by 256 values for each horizontal slice of the body and 40–100 slices with each picture element or voxel containing a value for Hounsfield value. While quite narrow ranges of values can be obtained from pure postmortem materials or water-filled phantoms, in life, individual tissues have varied content of fat, water, blood, bone, marrow, and other tissue constituents so that neighboring voxels may have a range of values (Figs. 5.1 and 5.2). A low level of noise persists with water phantoms showing means close to 0 with a standard deviation (SD) in the 2–3 Hounsfield range. Nevertheless, tissues can be identified and the volumes of different tissues determined using computer programs.

Interestingly, Hounsfield, an electrical engineer, used the inference that if a computer could identify printed characters, it could be used to compute the slice images [22]. However, early CT-based anatomical quantitative volumetric image analysis of the brain based on values of water was pioneered by two psychologists with Eve Johnstone's [21] measurement of brain ventricular enlargement in schizophrenia and Terry Jernigan's semi-automated brain cerebrospinal fluid quantification with numerical illustrations (presented at the 64th Annual Meeting of the Radiological Society of North America, November 26, 1978 and submitted as a paper on November 30, 1978) [23]. Jernigan's paper includes statistical images showing the proportion of patients with CSF for each voxel and is the earliest voxel-by-voxel statistical brain image derived from CT so far located. The first quantitative voxel-value-based study of muscle (cited in the historical review of skeletal mass assessment [24]) was the work of J. A. Bulcke (submitted to the journal *Neuroradiology* on October 31, 1978, 1 month earlier than the Jernigan submission) [25]. Bulcke and coworkers gives means, standard deviations, and scatterplots for Hounsfield units in several muscles with the sternocleidomastoid muscle showing mean Hounsfield value = 68, SD = 16. This study relied on hand-drawn edges and does not present

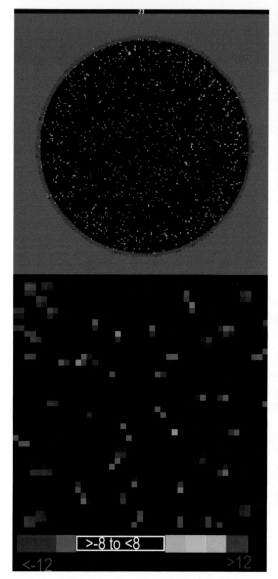

Fig. 5.1 Cylindrical water phantom for CT calibration shows values close to zero. Above: Display thresholded so that values from −8 to +8 are black and values below −8 and above +8 are shown on the *lower color bar*. *Below*: Magnified phantom to show scatter of values outside −8–8 limit. The mean value was 0.93 SD = 3.1 Hounsfield units and the modal value 0.07. The values show calibration deviates approximately only one part in 2000 from the data range from air to bone

a statistical image, so the Jernigan paper remains the first to use computer algorithms for CT volumetric tissue analysis, a use apparently first anticipated by Hounsfield. However, the earlier 1978 study by Haggmark may deserve partial

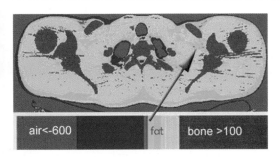

Fig. 5.2 Axial CT image of the thorax showing tissues with Hounsfield number with discrete color bands. This illustration was created with Brainflow (Brainflow visualization program, http://code.google.com/p/brainflow/). The color bar extends from −600 to +600. *Blue-green*, *aqua*, *green*, and *yellow-green narrow color bands* correspond to −140 to −120, −120 to −100, −100 to −80, and −80 to −60 Hounsfield units, respectively. Air (lung) is less than −600 (*cerise*) and bone (*red*) >100

credit as the earliest voxel-based tissue CT volumetric study although they used printed pictures from the scanner and an Aristo planimeter to quantify area rather than computation from the actual digital record [26]. Similar methods were used to quantify photomicrographs of tissue cultures with a Keuffel and Esser polar planimeter [27] in one of the earliest quantitative tissue studies.

Qualitative and Quantitative CT-Based Anatomical Tissue Segmentation

Brown fat is located primarily in the neck and upper thorax. Visual inspection identified brown fat clusters in the supraclavicular region in 100 % of 38 lean women [28], in 70 % of 27 subjects [18], in 52 % of 31 unselected patients [29], and in 6.8 % of 4,842 patients [30]. Since brown fat is more metabolically active than white fat, especially if the patient was cold during the FDG uptake period, regions of brown fat, active muscle, and/or cancer-related metastatic regions have been found to be a potential source of ambiguity in FDG-PET scan evaluation of metastatic disease of the upper thorax and neck. The range of brown fat-positive patients reported on visual inspection range suggests the need for quantitative criteria based on anatomical and functional imaging. This may be especially important in pharmacological treatment studies of elderly men, patients with obesity, and/or patients with diabetes where brown fat may be less visually prominent.

The earliest quantitative image analysis of fat located is that of Borkan [31]. Eight men had their total fat area and total tissue area measured by examining abdominal image voxels; a bimodal distribution was observed with a peak at −110 interpreted as fat, a point of rarity at −50, and a second peak at 20, interpreted as lean tissue. Subcutaneous and abdominal fat was first differentiated by Grauer and coworkers with a wide Hounsfield unit bands for fat of −10 to −200 [32].

The introduction of FDG-PET with integral CT scanning made the evaluation of the Hounsfield unit values for areas of high uptake possible. Cohade [33] is the earliest located report demonstrating that patients displaying focally located regions of increased FDG uptake had CT density in the fat range (mean −76, SD = 24, 2SD range −124 to −48) and they hypothesized these to be foci of brown fat. In a similar approach [34], regions of high SUV on FDG-PET were defined as brown fat if the CT Hounsfield values were between −250 and −50. Criteria for brown fat based on both CT and FDG SUV were Hounsfield 30 to −150 and FDG uptake of >1.5 SUV [35] and Hounsfield −100 to −10 and SUV >1.0 [30]. Segmentation of a CT image into bands of Hounsfield values is shown in Fig. 5.2.

Season, Thermal Accommodation, and Brown Fat FDG Imaging

Since brown fat is thermogenic, one might hypothesize an increase in volume and/or activity during winter months. In individuals who had two FDG-PET scans months apart with one scan showing high SUV PET uptake (>3) and one scan with low SUV PET uptake (<2), a difference of Hounsfield units was found with predominantly winter month scans showing Hounsfield values of −71, SD = 18, and predominantly summer months showing a value of −104, SD = 17 [36], in Fukuoka (27 °C in August and 5 °C in December). However, the CT and FDG images were not reported as coregistered. Since the FDG regions of interest were selected as high on one occasion and low on a second (from a pool of 1,384 scans, 73 showed visually identified BAT and 23 had two scans, one high and one low), the FDG change cannot be unambiguously interpreted. Significantly, more subjects showed cold-activated brown fat (as determined by two trained observers) in winter- than summer-scanned patients [29] in Sapporo (26 °C in August and 0 °C in January). Brown fat was more likely to be visualized in patients scanned in winter than in summer in Los Angeles [37] suggesting a chronic effect of low-temperature exposure even in a narrow range of exposure (29.4 °C in August and 19.2 °C in December). Lean men exposed to 10 °C in water-cooled suits for 4 weeks of acclimation [35] showed an increase in tissue oxidative metabolism index ([11C] acetate k) in cervicothoracic brown fat before and after acclimation. Similarly, quantitative FDG showed an increase of approximately 40 nmoles/ml/min after acclimation but this was not statistically significant.

Brief Exposure to Cold and Warm Environments

Saito [29] acquired FDG-PET on eight subjects who showed clear FDG uptake following cold exposure (19 °C for 2 h) and rescanned them following warm exposure (27 °C) but does not report means or statistical tests comparing the experimentally exposed subjects. Virtanen [38] found marked increase in glucose metabolic rate assessed quantitatively using FDG-PET (Patlak-Gjedde method [39]) in five subjects exposed to cold (17–19 °C) and warm (ambient scanner temperature). Supraclavicular regions outlined on CT scan by visual inspection were associated with higher metabolic rates on the coregistered PET scan following cold exposure. However, associated Hounsfield unit values were not used to segment tissue in individuals who had two FDG-PET scans months apart with one scan showing high SUV PET uptake (>3) and one scan with low SUV PET uptake (<2); a difference of Hounsfield units was found with predominantly winter month scans showing Hounsfield values of −71, SD = 18, and predominantly summer months showing a value of −104, SD = 17 [36]. Again, however, CT and FDG images were not reported as coregistered. Since the FDG regions of interest were selected as high on one occasion and low on a second (from a pool of 1,384 scans, 73 showed visually identified BAT and 23 had two scans, one high and one low), the FDG change cannot be easily interpreted. Saito [29] found a seasonal effect with higher prevalence of brown fat in winter was found although not statistically tested.

Brown Fat, Age, and Sex

While not based on CT quantification, 162 healthy volunteers had FDG-PET/CT and were divided into BAT positive ($n=67$) and BAT negative ($n=95$). The BAT-positive subjects were significantly younger and showed lower BMI, subcutaneous fat, and abdominal fat [40]. Similarly, brown fat activity was greater in younger adults [29] and higher in women than men [29], and men showed more marked age decline in brown fat than women [41].

Histopathological and Genetic Validation of PET/CT Brown Fat Imaging

In an important validation step, histological examination of the biopsy of the fat tissue in three subjects with regions of high FDG uptake revealed cells characteristic of brown fat [38]. In other biopsy studies [34, 42], patients with a upper thorax tumors with high FDG uptake were found to have a hibernoma (brown fat tumor) so named because of the role of brown fat in hibernating animals. High FDG SUV masses with CT values in the adipose tissue range appear typical of hibernomas [43]. The presence of brown fat-specific protein uncoupling protein-1 (UPC1) in brown adipose islands of tissue from the neck of patients undergoing surgery also supports the supposition that the active FDG uptake spots in the neck are consistent with brown fat [44]. In a third biopsy study, brown and white fat in the supraclavicular region were biopsied, and UCP1 was identified in brown but not in white fat [41]. Lastly, while not a quantitative study, coregistered and fused PET/CT scans on 199 subjects were divided by visual inspection into brown fat positive ($n=88$) and brown fat negative (111), and genotyping showed that among older subjects, UCP1 A/G substitutions were associated with diminished chance of being brown fat positive [45].

Animal Studies

Early experiments in marmot [46] identified the thermogenesis in brown fat as important in maintaining a steady temperature in hibernation. This stimulated basic research on the neural mechanisms of control of brown fat metabolism. In rats with brown fat activated with amoxetine, the traced activated area had a mean Hounsfield unit value of approximately −200 to −180 with more negative values in white fat [14]. Much higher Hounsfield unit values were found in rats [36] examined after 4 h of exposure to 4 °C (−12, SD=22) and 23 °C (−28, SD=9.6). However, these values were obtained from a visually placed FDG-PET image circular region of interest and are not reported to be coregistered between warm and cold, or use exactly the same region of interest location.

Image Analysis and Brown Fat

The studies reviewed above clearly demonstrate that islands of high metabolic activity in the neck and upper thorax are associated with cold-activated adipose tissue and that biopsy studies indicate brown adipose tissues in these areas. These studies have sometimes used a CT Hounsfield level for identifying brown fat, but the same CT template for cold and warm conditions with algorithmically defined brown fat has not been carried out. Bias associated with outlining regions on the FDG scan to select brown fat areas confounds region selection with activity, and studies with very wide ranges of Hounsfield units do not clearly use an objective measure to separate brown and white. Studies in which visual observation of both PET and CT was used to define brown fat also lack independence of region of interest selection and may bias the results toward a higher brown fat than white fat result and also bias Hounsfield unit determination. A study in which the images from a group of subjects are exposed to both cold and warm conditions with the PET images coregistered to a single CT with regions of interest based purely on defined computer algorithms applied to Hounsfield unit images has not been reported. In such a study, the voxels associated with specific narrow Hounsfield values can be selected, and their FDG metabolic rate and SUV can be assessed and statistical analysis performed. Below, pilot data are presented [47] that address these issues and apply variations of image coregistration methods in brain imaging to the multiple coregistration problems.

Key Methods in Tissue Segmentation Study

Subjects

As a prelude to an early phase interventional study of a new drug with putative effects on BAT metabolism, Buchsbaum et al. [47] studied a group of insulin-resistant subjects ($n=9$, mean ± SD homeostasis model assessment (HOMA-IR) = 5.2 ± 2.5) and overweight healthy volunteers ($n=2$) with fluorodeoxyglucose positron-emission tomography and x-ray computed tomography (FDG-PET/CT) of the thorax (C6-T8) to assess the glucose metabolic rate (GMR) of brown and white fat. Of these, eight of the insulin-resistant subjects also underwent imaging of the upper leg. Subjects were exposed to a 90-min period of either cold (67–68 °F; 19–20 °C) or warm (72–73 °F; 22–23 °C) temperature on separate days and then moved to the PET/CT scanner, which was kept at the same temperature for FDG uptake. The initial high-resolution warm 200 MA CT was used to coregister the cold and warm PET scans. All scans were converted to .nii format using PMOD (PMOD Technologies, Zurich, Switzerland). Segmented CT masks of 7 Hounsfield unit (HU) bands, −600 to −160 (mainly lung), −160 to −120, −120 to −80, −80 to −40, −40–0, 0–100 (muscle), and 100–600 (bone and some muscle), were computed. GMR was quantified as micromoles glucose/100 g/min using an arterial input function from the aorta image as used in one other study [35]. The FDG-PET scans for the cold and warm sessions were both registered to the initial CT so that the same CT anatomical scan Hounsfield values could be applied to both the cold and warm conditions. All scans were then visually reviewed for registration quality. Thus, all measurements were automated and did not depend on visual interpretation. Cold minus warm GMR values were obtained at 47 thoracic levels, and we summarized the 47 levels into five slices (slice 0–9, 10–19, 20–29, 30–39, and 40–46). The uppermost group had more anatomical variability due to variations in the length of the neck and flexion of the neck, and so the analysis focused on slices from the superiormost slice which included the shoulder to the inferiormost slice passing through the superior portions of the heart. Since the bed appears in cross section in CT but not the PET scan, CT was masked with PET values >0 to remove the bed.

FDG Quantification

Images were quantified using the time-activity curves from each voxel and from a region of interest in the aorta using PMOD software. A lumped constant of 1.14 was used following an earlier report in the quantification equation [39]. This forms a rectangular cube of body metabolic rate measurements approximately 128 by 128 by 47 for each of the four adjacent neck/thorax levels. Thus, the data set is the 3D xyz spatial matrix of metabolic rate measurements in micromoles glucose/100 g/min, with expected values in the range of 1–10 µmol/100 g/min across all adipose tissue voxels.

Glucose Metabolic Rate Following Cold and Warm Exposure

Whole Slice Glucose Metabolic Rate (Micromoles Glucose/100 g/min)

Metabolic rate was significantly greater in voxels in the fat range than in other tissue at the Hounsfield levels less than −160 and greater than 100 (Fig. 5.3). The wider spread of values from −160 to 0 was consistent with the earlier studies, and

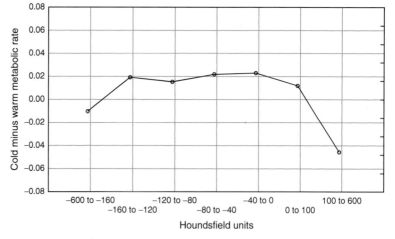

Fig. 5.3 Metabolic rate in micromoles/100 g/min in FDG-PET voxels in entire thorax coregistered to CT scan at selected bands of Hounsfield units. The Hounsfield unit by environmental temperature interaction was significant ($F = 2.45$, $df = 6, 60$, $p = 0.035$)

large standard deviations were found. The cold vs. warm effect significantly varied across Hounsfield unit bands, and this was confirmed with a 3-factor repeated measures analysis of variance (ANOVA) (cold/warm × Hounsfield unit band × thorax level) and with a temperature by Hounsfield unit interaction (see Fig. 5.3). Examination of the SUV in a narrow analysis with bands 20 units wide found a peak cold minus warm effect at −140 to −100, but the cold minus warm effect was not significant ($F=2.48$, df-1, 10, $p=0.15$) and the Hounsfield unit by cold/warm interaction was also not significant ($F=0.89$, $p=0.51$).

Clustering Voxels of Similar Values

First, the voxels associated with the bed had to be removed from the image. This was done by masking the CT with FDG-PET scan since the bed was inactive. Next, the AFNI (analysis of functional neuroimages, http://afni.nimh.nih.gov/pub/dist/doc/program_help/) routine 3dmerge -1clust_order command was used on the CT scan for each Hounsfield unit range. We used the command as "3dmerge -1clust_order 1.5 500 –prefix output file input file." This forms clusters with a connection distance of 1.5 mm and excludes clusters less than 500 mm³. This is illustrated in number 3 in Fig. 5.4, for a −140 to −90 Hounsfield unit band. All neighboring voxels with values in this band were assigned a value of 1, and all voxels outside this range were assigned a value of 0. The clusters were then ranked for size, and each of the largest 16 clusters was assigned a color. The cluster mask was then applied to the cold minus warm PET scan .nii images, and the mean metabolic rate, SUV, and volume in mm³ for each cluster were determined. Each individual-colored cluster size image (#4 in Fig. 5.4) was then examined, and supraclavicular clusters in the same two positions on the right and left were selected and their volumes organized into right and left body columns in a spreadsheet for statistical analysis. This step

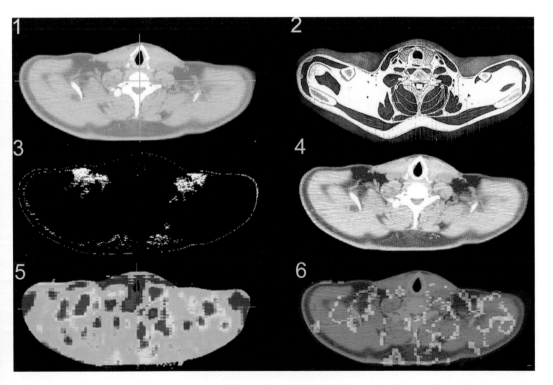

Fig. 5.4 Clustering methods for contiguous pixels. (*1*) CT scan of upper thorax. (*2*) Frozen section human atlas [48]. (*3*) CT mask with white (value = 1) for contiguous pixels in the −140 to −90 range and black (value = 0) elsewhere. (*4*) Clusters superimposed in color on CT image with pixel clusters ranked for size with *violet, blue, light blue*...for clusters of size rank 1, 2, 3.... (*5*). FDG-PET. (*6*) PET fused with CT image

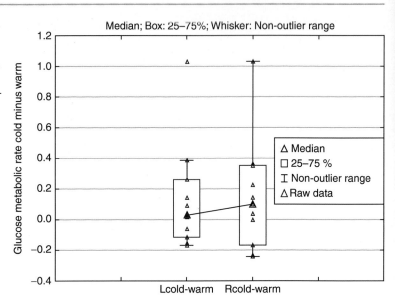

Fig. 5.5 Cold minus warm metabolic rate in Hounsfield unit clusters in left and right supraclavicular area. Note wide range of activation values with skewed distribution demonstrating the range from little environmental temperature change to large FDG uptake increases with cold exposure. Median values are above zero

was necessary because small changes in volume resulted in a different order for the clusters.

Individual cluster values showed a wide variability (Fig. 5.5), but most individuals had cold values greater than warm values, some to a marked extent of two- to fourfold increases.

To provide a test of reliability, the correlation between glucose metabolic rate in the left and right clusters for Hounsfield range −120 to −70, $n=11$, was examined. The metabolic rate increases with cold exposure compared to warm exposure, left vs. right correlation was highly reliable ($r=0.96$, df=9, $p<0.001$), and cluster volume was less reliable ($r=0.39$). For the higher Hounsfield range, the metabolic rate change left vs. right correlation was also highly significant (0.99), and the cluster volume right vs. left correlation was also highly significant ($r=0.90$, df=9, $p<0.001$).

Total Fat Volume and Distribution of Fat Hounsfield Units

For examination of the computations, we [47] made the simple approximation of a typical man's thorax as a rectangle 500×250 mm. For ten typical slices that were 3.27 mm thick, we then estimated the approximate order of magnitude to be 4,087,500 mm². We then counted (see section "R language usage especially suitable for tissue segmentation") the number of CT voxels meeting the two criteria: (1) Hounsfield >−10,000 and <10,000 and (2) PET metabolic >0 found 1,072,044 which corresponds to 3,505,584 mm³ indicating that we had an appropriate unit estimation. Next, the number of mm³ between −120 and −40 Hounsfield units was evaluated and found to be 669,372 or about 19 % of the volume to be in the fat range, consistent with other estimates.

R Language Usage Especially Suitable for Tissue Segmentation

Code is presented to show compact features of R for CT tissue segmentation.

We used the CT volume containing 47 slices as a .nii file and package neuroim for reading .nii files.

```
install.packages("neuroim", repos="http://R-Forge.R-project.org")
install.packages("C:/adata/neuroim_0.0.1.zip", repos=NULL, source=TRUE)   #final load which worked
vol <- loadVolume("ct.nii")
```

For this example, we formed a three-dimensional array containing the inferior ten slices from the 47-slice ct.nii as ct09 and a CT mask as ctmask09 (0 for negative PET and 1 for positive PET) to remove the bed based on PET values. Then, the compact R commands yielded the number of voxels meeting the criteria of a valid CT voxel and valid PET voxel (being inside the body).

```
    prune=ct09[((ct09>=(-10000))
& (ct09<=(10000))) &
((ctmask09>0.5)&(ctmask09<3))]
    > length(prune)
    [1] 1072064
    > print( 1072044*3.27)
    [1] 3,505,584 mm3
```

Next, we obtained the number of CT voxels in the designated volume in the fat range of −120 to −40 using the conjunction grammar to place the voxels meeting the criteria into the variable "prune." Then the "length" function determined the number of voxels (1×1×3.27 mm).

```
    > prune=ct09[((ct09>=(-120))
& (ct09<(-40))) & ((ctmask09>0.5)&
(ctmask09<3))]
    > length(prune)
    [1] 204701
    > print(204701*3.27)
    [1] 669372.3 mm3
```

Lastly, we examined the quantiles related to the Hounsfield units, filling array "band2" with sequential proportion values and then applying it to the array containing the CT values.

```
    > band2=c(.1,  .2,  .25,  .30,
.35, .40, .45, .5, .6, .7, .8, .9)
    > quantile(prune, band2)
    10% 20% 25% 30% 35% 40% 45% 50
% 60% 70% 80% 90%
    -105  -95  -91  -87  -83  -80
-76  -73  -67  -60  -54  -47
```

Hounsfield unit levels at each decile are shown between −120 and −40 indicating that about half of the voxels fell between the 20th percentile (−95) and the 70th percentile (−60).

Leg Metabolic Activity

The lower leg was scanned immediately following the completion of the 67-min thorax scan in eight subjects. Since we had only the FDG blood uptake curve for the thorax and did not have one for minutes 67–72 for the leg, we developed a linear regression line between metabolic rate values in the entire upper section of the thorax and the raw FDG counts and then applied this transformation to the legs as an approximation. Based on the location of the edges of the tibia and fibula on CT, we stereotaxically located (Fig. 5.6) four spherical regions of interest (tibialis anterior, soleus, gastrocnemius, and subcutaneous fat) 8 mm in diameter (calling the R neuroim subroutine RegionSphere (FDG-PET-inputfile-name.nii, xyz-location, radius-mm)). These regions were chosen to differ in fast twitch (tibialis anterior, gastrocnemius/mixed) and slow twitch (soleus). Leg muscles were significantly more active in the warm condition than in the cold condition (environmental temperature main effect $F=10.6$, df=1, 7, $p=0.014$) in temperature condition by tissue type 2-way repeated measures ANOVA). Muscles and subcutaneous fat had differing metabolic rates (2-way repeated measures ANOVA, main effect of tissue type $F=23.9$, df=3, 21, $p<0.0001$; Fig. 5.7). However, the tissue type × temperature interaction was not significant ($f=1.00$, df=3. 21, $p=0.41$). A larger number of regions of interest on the vertical axis (along the length of the tibia) and refined stereotaxic placement may yield significant results. A limitation of the method is that the soleus and gastrocnemius are close together, sometimes referred to as the triceps surae [48, 49]. However, the finding that the leg metabolic rate was not greater during the cold condition indicates that shivering was probably not common during our cold exposure [9].

Discussion

Hounsfield Unit Values of Fat and Other Tissues

A salient test of the concept that absolute Hounsfield unit values are associated with brown rather than white fat requires the assumption that only brown fat will show a change in metabolic rate. A significant Hounsfield unit by temperature exposure condition interaction would strongly support the concept. This is confirmed for

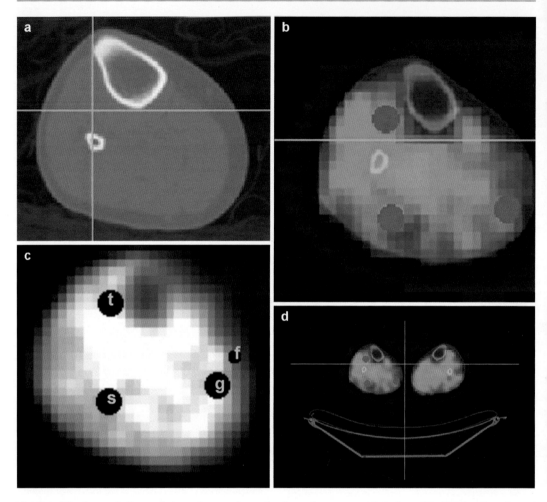

Fig. 5.6 Muscle metabolic rate in lower leg muscles and subcutaneous fat. *Top row*: *Left*, Atlas [48] from human frozen section. *Middle*, CT image at approximately the same level showing cursor placed so as to touch the lateral edge of the tibia and posterior edge of the tibia. This provided one of the stereotaxic points used to locate the circular region of interest. *Right*, FDG-PET image of the legs. *Bottom row*: *Left*, Leg CT. *Middle*, Coregistered FDG-PET with circular stereotaxic regions of interest on gray scale. *Right*, Merged image of CT and PET. This R program used Brainflow routines loadVolume (nii.filename), and RegionSphere (nii.imagename, image x,y,z, and diameter in pixels) to obtain values

metabolic rate, with a peak from −160 to −40, but the curve has a relatively flat shape without a narrow peak of width 20–40 Hounsfield units. Thus, the Buchsbaum et al. data [47] is most similar to Cypess [34] who defined it as brown fat if the CT Hounsfield values were between −250 and −50. It is also similar to [33] demonstrating that patients displaying focally located regions of increased FDG uptake had CT density in the fat range (mean −76, SD = 24, 2SD range −124 to −48). It should be noted that the Hounsfield unit values in these studies come from examining areas of thermal response on the FDG-PET visually, rather than including all Hounsfield units of a particular range. Thus, the fact that our Hounsfield regions statistically confirmed approximately as wide a band as in those studies is of interest since our data was not biased by FDG-PET selection. Our metabolic rates in micromoles/100 g/min (see Fig. 5.6) were similar to those observed elsewhere (see Fig. 5.1b [50]). It should also be noted that the clustering technique used here (see

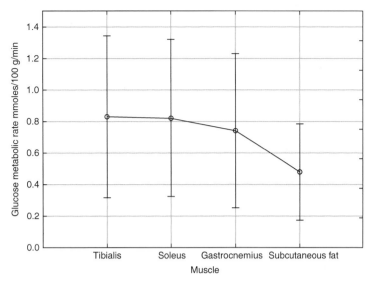

Fig. 5.7 Approximate metabolic rate in lower leg muscles and subcutaneous fat

Fig. 5.4, image 4) is strikingly similar to the areas identified as showing increased tissue glucose uptake by Ouellet in their Fig. 5.2 and in the supplement.

Brown fat volumes and brown fat activation are highly variable from subject to subject in our data and are noted by others (e.g., [9]). Understanding this variability is key to selecting specific drugs for exploiting brown fat as a modulator of diabetes and obesity.

Brown Fat by CT Hounsfield Units vs. Brown Fat by FDG-PET Activation

The Buchsbaum et al. [47] pilot study showed that both of the two overweight but not insulin resistant subjects showed positive values for the cold minus warm clusters while four of nine insulin-resistant subjects had small negative values. Our overall percentage of individuals with activatable brown fat is 64 %, between the 70 % percentage [18] and 52 % found [29] found elsewhere. This suggests that Hounsfield-identified fat in the brown fat range may not necessarily be thermoactivated, may take a stronger environmental thermal stimulus, or may require pharmacological treatment to become activated. The exact correspondence of thermogenic brown fat and a specific Hounsfield band may also be diluted by the presence of beige adipocytes which may appear within white adipose tissue and develop from different progenitor cells [16, 17]. It is possible that brown, beige, and white adipose tissue may each respond to separate pharmacological effects. The curve seen in Fig. 5.3 might become more narrowly peaked in response to the action of a drug which affected only thermogenic brown fat or more broad and flat if beige and/or white fat was affected. Volume change in subpopulations of adipose cells might also be detected by changes in Hounsfield intensity maps or the size, location, and shape of contiguous clusters of Hounsfield unit range voxels.

Brown Fat Metabolism, Brain Metabolism, Obesity and Depression

It has recently been reported that brown fat metabolic rate assessed by FDG-PET in the thorax under cold conditions is correlated with glucose metabolism in the cerebral cortex and subcortical regions including the frontal lobe, thalamus, and cingulate [50]. This correlation was observed only in lean individuals but not observed in obese individuals or for white adipose tissue metabolic rate. Significant negative correlations between BMI and glucose metabolic rate in the prefrontal cortex and cingulate gyrus, but not other areas, have been observed [51]. Obese individuals have higher rates of depression [52]. Patients with morbid obesity who are candidates for stomach surgery have a high incidence of psychiatric illness, predominately depression [53–56], but the relationship between antidepressant use, weight loss success, and depressive symptom change before and after surgery remains unknown [56]. The finding that affective disorder may be characterized by both weight loss and weight gain and that antidepressant drugs may be associated with weight loss (e.g., bupropion, fluoxetine [57, 58]) and gain (e.g., paroxetine, amitriptyline) is a further contradiction [58]. Further understanding of the interaction between brown fat metabolic rate, obesity, and depression may provide more specific treatments for depression in the obese and the effect of mood-regulating drugs on weight.

Conclusions

Our data demonstrate that automated algorithms can detect the metabolic increase due to cold exposure in thermogenic tissue in the upper thorax in man using combined FDG-PET and CT. Earlier brown adipose tissue studies have demonstrated that FDG uptake is increased by exposure to cold temperatures and cold seasonal effects. These studies noted the visibility of tissue areas that were associated with CT Hounsfield image units in a broad range (−200 to −20) but did not statistically compare the increase in uptake as a function of coregistered Hounsfield unit ranges. Our investigator-initiated program extended these findings with analysis of variance confirmation of differential thermogenesis in tissues with different mean Hounsfield unit values. We also demonstrated the application of brain-imaging-derived clustering techniques for identifying specific regions of thermosensitive adipose tissue based entirely on algorithmic identification of contiguous Hounsfield unit areas. This assay complements the simple measurements of weight or BMI, more specific metabolic assessments of blood insulin measurement and the glucose tolerance test, as well as the sophisticated hyperinsulinemic clamp.

The applications for the therapeutics of diabetes are of great potential as individual differences in the multifactorial contributions to diabetes are identified. Translational research on diabetes and obesity and development of new pharmacological treatments can only move forward by using the most specific assessments of glucose metabolic change. If a new investigational drug were to only affect insulin sensitivity, then a trial in which the diabetes of only half the subjects had reduced insulin sensitivity, then the power of the trial to detect efficacy would be greatly reduced or insufficient. Similarly, if a new drug targeted brown fat thermogenesis, younger female subjects who already had greater amounts of brown fat might show less efficacy than older male subjects with compromised activity and volume of brown fat. Salient biomarkers can save efficacious drugs from discard by identifying the individual subjects for which the new drug is needed and clinically valuable.

The potential applications in clinical research include (1) metabolic characterization of individuals with thermogenically unresponsive adipose tissue in the brown Hounsfield unit range; (2) wider mapping of the thermal response range in both adipose and muscle tissue; (3) determination of the relationship between body temperature/change with thermal exposure, diurnal temperature rhythms, basal metabolic rate, and FDG adipose metabolism; (4) quantitative mapping of regional obesity by Hounsfield units (abdominal, leg, upper thorax) and its relationship to insulin disorders; (5) the effect of weight loss on adipose tissue Hounsfield characterization and metabolic responsiveness to thermal conditions; and (6) the relation of regional brain appetite areas to metabolism in Hounsfield unit-characterized adipose tissue.

There is wide agreement that obesity is complex with many physiological mechanisms at its root. To paraphrase Tolstoy's memorable first line in the novel Anna Karenina [59], every obese person is obese in their own way. As drugs with more specific anti-obesity mechanisms are developed, the detailed assessment of every aspect of a patient's pathophysiology will become increasingly important.

Acknowledgements The authors thank Andrew Krentz, Linda Morrow, and Marcus Hompesch for their support and useful advice at varied stages of the preparation of this chapter. Gisela Peterson and Laurel Glockler provided careful data organization support. George Madirossian provided assistance with scanner calibration and phantoms, Tim Erickson with electronic records, and Steven Hardy with file organization and scanner operation. Didier Laurent made useful suggestions for the data analysis.

References

1. Wilson JP, Kanaya AM, Fan B, Shepherd JA. Ratio of trunk to leg volume as a new body shape metric for diabetes and mortality. PLoS One. 2013;8(7):e68716. PubMed PMID: 23874736, Pubmed Central PMCID: 3707853.
2. Kuk JL, Church TS, Blair SN, Ross R. Does measurement site for visceral and abdominal subcutaneous adipose tissue alter associations with the metabolic syndrome? Diabetes Care. 2006;29(3):679–84. PubMed PMID: 16505526.
3. Brown RE, Kuk JL, Lee S. Measurement site influences abdominal subcutaneous and visceral adipose tissue in obese adolescents before and after exercise. Pediatr Obes. 2014. PubMed PMID: 24729534.
4. Schulz TJ, Tseng YH. Brown adipose tissue: development, metabolism and beyond. Biochem J. 2013;453(2):167–78. PubMed PMID: 23805974, Pubmed Central PMCID: 3887508.
5. Arch JR. Thermogenesis and related metabolic targets in anti-diabetic therapy. Handb Exp Pharmacol. 2011;203:201–55. PubMed PMID: 21484574.
6. Arch JR, Trayhurn P. Detection of thermogenesis in rodents in response to anti-obesity drugs and genetic modification. Front Physiol. 2013;4:64. PubMed PMID: 23580228, Pubmed Central PMCID: 3619105.
7. Clapham JC, Arch JR. Targeting thermogenesis and related pathways in anti-obesity drug discovery. Pharmacol Ther. 2011;131(3):295–308. PubMed PMID: 21514319.
8. Peirce V, Vidal-Puig A. Regulation of glucose homoeostasis by brown adipose tissue. Lancet Diabetes Endocrinol. 2013;1(4):353–60. PubMed PMID: 24622420.
9. Ouellet V, Labbe SM, Blondin DP, Phoenix S, Guerin B, Haman F, et al. Brown adipose tissue oxidative metabolism contributes to energy expenditure during acute cold exposure in humans. J Clin Invest. 2012;122(2):545–52. PubMed PMID: 22269323, Pubmed Central PMCID: 3266793.
10. Cypess AM, Kahn CR. The role and importance of brown adipose tissue in energy homeostasis. Curr Opin Pediatr. 2010;22(4):478–84. PubMed PMID: 20489634, Pubmed Central PMCID: 3593062.
11. Sims EA. Storage and expenditure of energy in obesity and their implications for management. Med Clin North Am. 1989;73(1):97–110. PubMed PMID: 2643011.
12. Tupone D, Madden CJ, Morrison SF. Autonomic regulation of brown adipose tissue thermogenesis in health and disease: potential clinical applications for altering BAT thermogenesis. Front Neurosci. 2014;8:14. PubMed PMID: 24570653, Pubmed Central PMCID: 3916784.
13. Mirbolooki MR, Constantinescu CC, Pan ML, Mukherjee J. Quantitative assessment of brown adipose tissue metabolic activity and volume using 18F-FDG PET/CT and β3-adrenergic receptor activation. EJNMMI Res. 2011;1(1):30. PubMed PMID: 22214183, Pubmed Central PMCID: 3250993.
14. Mirbolooki MR, Constantinescu CC, Pan ML, Mukherjee J. Targeting presynaptic norepinephrine transporter in brown adipose tissue: a novel imaging approach and potential treatment for diabetes and obesity. Synapse. 2013;67(2):79–93. PubMed PMID: 23080264, Pubmed Central PMCID: 3808851.
15. Mirbolooki MR, Upadhyay SK, Constantinescu CC, Pan ML, Mukherjee J. Adrenergic pathway activation enhances brown adipose tissue metabolism: a [(1)(8)F]FDG PET/CT study in mice. Nucl Med Biol. 2014;41(1):10–6. PubMed PMID: 24090673, Pubmed Central PMCID: 3840120.
16. Lidell ME, Betz MJ, Dahlqvist Leinhard O, Heglind M, Elander L, Slawik M, et al. Evidence for two types of brown adipose tissue in humans. Nat Med. 2013;19(5):631–4. PubMed PMID: 23603813.
17. Lidell ME, Betz MJ, Enerback S. Two types of brown adipose tissue in humans. Adipocyte. 2014;3(1):63–6. PubMed PMID: 24575372, Pubmed Central PMCID: 3917936.
18. Orava J, Nuutila P, Lidell ME, Oikonen V, Noponen T, Viljanen T, et al. Different metabolic responses of human brown adipose tissue to activation by cold and insulin. Cell Metab. 2011;14(2):272–9. PubMed PMID: 21803297.
19. Orava J, Nuutila P, Noponen T, Parkkola R, Viljanen T, Enerback S, et al. Blunted metabolic responses to cold and insulin stimulation in brown adipose tissue of obese humans. Obesity. 2013;21(11):2279–87. PubMed PMID: 23554353.
20. Enerback S. Brown adipose tissue in humans. Int J Obes. 2010;34 Suppl 1:S43–6. PubMed PMID: 20935666.
21. Johnstone EC, Crow TJ, Frith CD, Husband J, Kreel L. Cerebral ventricular size and cognitive impairment in chronic schizophrenia. Lancet. 1976;2(7992):924–6. PubMed PMID: 62160.
22. Raju TN. The Nobel chronicles. 1979: Allan MacLeod Cormack (b 1924); and Sir Godfrey Newbold Hounsfield (b 1919). Lancet. 1999;354(9190):1653.

23. Jernigan TL, Zatz LM, Naeser MA. Semiautomated methods for quantitating CSF volume on cranial computed tomography. Radiology. 1979;132(2):463–6. PubMed PMID: 461809.
24. Heymsfield SB, Adamek M, Gonzalez MC, Jia G, Thomas DM. Assessing skeletal muscle mass: historical overview and state of the art. J Cachex Sarcopenia Muscle. 2014;5:9–18. PubMed PMID: 24532493.
25. Bulcke JA, Termote JL, Palmers Y, Crolla D. Computed tomography of the human skeletal muscular system. Neuroradiology. 1979;17(3):127–36. PubMed PMID: 450236.
26. Haggmark T, Jansson E, Svane B. Cross-sectional area of the thigh muscle in man measured by computed tomography. Scand J Clin Lab Invest. 1978;38(4):355–60. PubMed PMID: 684368.
27. Buchsbaum R. Size of explant and volume of medium in tissue cultures [Ph.D.]. Chicago: The University of Chicago; 1932.
28. Pasanisi F, Pace L, Fonti R, Marra M, Sgambati D, De Caprio C, et al. Evidence of brown fat activity in constitutional leanness. J Clin Endocrinol Metab. 2013;98(3):1214–8. PubMed PMID: 23393181.
29. Saito M, Okamatsu-Ogura Y, Matsushita M, Watanabe K, Yoneshiro T, Nio-Kobayashi J, et al. High incidence of metabolically active brown adipose tissue in healthy adult humans: effects of cold exposure and adiposity. Diabetes. 2009;58(7):1526–31. PubMed PMID: 19401428, Pubmed Central PMCID: 2699872.
30. Ouellet V, Routhier-Labadie A, Bellemare W, Lakhal-Chaieb L, Turcotte E, Carpentier AC, et al. Outdoor temperature, age, sex, body mass index, and diabetic status determine the prevalence, mass, and glucose-uptake activity of 18F-FDG-detected BAT in humans. J Clin Endocrinol Metab. 2011;96(1):192–9. PubMed PMID: 20943785.
31. Borkan GA, Gerzof SG, Robbins AH, Hults DE, Silbert CK, Silbert JE. Assessment of abdominal fat content by computed tomography. Am J Clin Nutr. 1982;36(1):172–7. PubMed PMID: 7091027.
32. Grauer WO, Moss AA, Cann CE, Goldberg HI. Quantification of body fat distribution in the abdomen using computed tomography. Am J Clin Nutr. 1984;39(4):631–7. PubMed PMID: 6711470.
33. Cohade C, Osman M, Pannu HK, Wahl RL. Uptake in supraclavicular area fat ("USA-Fat"): description on 18F-FDG PET/CT. J Nucl Med. 2003;44(2):170–6. PubMed PMID: 12571205.
34. Cypess AM, Lehman S, Williams G, Tal I, Rodman D, Goldfine AB, et al. Identification and importance of brown adipose tissue in adult humans. N Engl J Med. 2009;360(15):1509–17. PubMed PMID: 19357406, Pubmed Central PMCID: 2859951.
35. Blondin DP, Labbe SM, Christian Tingelstad H, Noll C, Kunach M, Phoenix S, et al. Increased brown adipose tissue oxidative capacity in cold-acclimated humans. J Clin Endocrinol Metab. 2014;99:E438–46. jc20133901. PubMed PMID: 24423363.
36. Baba S, Jacene HA, Engles JM, Honda H, Wahl RL. CT Hounsfield units of brown adipose tissue increase with activation: preclinical and clinical studies. J Nucl Med. 2010;51(2):246–50. PubMed PMID: 20124047.
37. Hu HH, Chung SA, Nayak KS, Jackson HA, Gilsanz V. Differential computed tomographic attenuation of metabolically active and inactive adipose tissues: preliminary findings. J Comput Assist Tomogr. 2011;35(1):65–71. PubMed PMID: 21245691. Pubmed Central PMCID: 3074500.
38. Virtanen KA, Lidell ME, Orava J, Heglind M, Westergren R, Niemi T, et al. Functional brown adipose tissue in healthy adults. N Engl J Med. 2009;360(15):1518–25. PubMed PMID: 19357407.
39. Virtanen KA, Peltoniemi P, Marjamaki P, Asola M, Strindberg L, Parkkola R, et al. Human adipose tissue glucose uptake determined using [(18)F]-fluoro-deoxy-glucose ([(18)F]FDG) and PET in combination with microdialysis. Diabetologia. 2001;44(12):2171–9. PubMed PMID: 11793018.
40. Yoneshiro T, Aita S, Matsushita M, Okamatsu-Ogura Y, Kameya T, Kawai Y, et al. Age-related decrease in cold-activated brown adipose tissue and accumulation of body fat in healthy humans. Obesity. 2011;19(9):1755–60. PubMed PMID: 21566561.
41. Pfannenberg C, Werner MK, Ripkens S, Stef I, Deckert A, Schmadl M, et al. Impact of age on the relationships of brown adipose tissue with sex and adiposity in humans. Diabetes. 2010;59(7):1789–93. PubMed PMID: 20357363, Pubmed Central PMCID: 2889780.
42. Sachpekidis C, Roumia S, Schwarzbach M, Dimitrakopoulou-Strauss A. Dynamic (18) F-fluorodeoxyglucose positron emission tomography/CT in hibernoma: enhanced tracer uptake mimicking liposarcoma. World J Radiol. 2013;5(12):498–502. PubMed PMID: 24379937. Pubmed Central PMCID: 3874507.
43. Agrawal A, Kembhavi S, Purandare N, Shah S, Rangarajan V. Report of two cases of fluorodeoxyglucose positron emission tomography/computed tomography appearance of hibernoma: a rare benign tumor. Indian J Nucl Med. 2014;29(1):40–2. PubMed PMID: 24591783. Pubmed Central PMCID: 3928751.
44. Zingaretti MC, Crosta F, Vitali A, Guerrieri M, Frontini A, Cannon B, et al. The presence of UCP1 demonstrates that metabolically active adipose tissue in the neck of adult humans truly represents brown adipose tissue. FASEB J. 2009;23(9):3113–20. PubMed PMID: 19417078.
45. Yoneshiro T, Ogawa T, Okamoto N, Matsushita M, Aita S, Kameya T, et al. Impact of UCP1 and beta3AR gene polymorphisms on age-related changes in brown adipose tissue and adiposity in humans. Int J Obes. 2013;37(7):993–8. PubMed PMID: 23032405.
46. Smith RE, Hock RJ. Brown fat: thermogenic effector of arousal in hibernators. Science. 1963; 140(3563):199–200. PubMed PMID: 13989560.
47. Buchsbaum M, Morrow L, Meyers D, Krentz A, Peterson G, Swan T, et al. Brown adipose tissue metabolic activity assessed with FDG-PET/CT correlates with BMI and glucose. Diabetologia. 2013;56.

48. Eycleshymer AC, S DM. A cross-section anatomy. New York: D. Appleton and Company; 1911.
49. Gray H. Anatomy of the human body. Philadelphia: Lea & Febiger; 1959.
50. Orava J, Nummenmaa L, Noponen T, Viljanen T, Parkkola R, Nuutila P, et al. Brown adipose tissue function is accompanied by cerebral activation in lean but not in obese humans. J Cereb Blood Flow Metab. 2014;34:1018–23. PubMed PMID: 24667912.
51. Volkow ND, Wang GJ, Telang F, Fowler JS, Goldstein RZ, Alia-Klein N, et al. Inverse association between BMI and prefrontal metabolic activity in healthy adults. Obesity. 2009;17(1):60–5. PubMed PMID: 18948965. Pubmed Central PMCID: 2681079.
52. de Wit L, Luppino F, van Straten A, Penninx B, Zitman F, Cuijpers P. Depression and obesity: a meta-analysis of community-based studies. Psychiatry Res. 2010;178(2):230–5. PubMed PMID: 20462641.
53. Sarwer DB, Cohn NI, Gibbons LM, Magee L, Crerand CE, Raper SE, et al. Psychiatric diagnoses and psychiatric treatment among bariatric surgery candidates. Obes Surg. 2004;14(9):1148–56. PubMed PMID: 15527626. eng.
54. Rosenberger PHHK, Grilo CM. Psychiatric disorder comorbidity and association with eating disorders in bariatric surgery patients: a cross-sectional study using structured interview-based diagnosis. J Clin Psychiatry. 2006;67(7):6.
55. Lier HO, Biringer E, Stubhaug B, Tangen T. Prevalence of psychiatric disorders before and 1 year after bariatric surgery: the role of shame in maintenance of psychiatric disorders in patients undergoing bariatric surgery. Nord J Psychiatry. 2013;67:89–96. PubMed PMID: 22587601. ENG.
56. Cunningham JL, Merrell CC, Sarr M, Somers KJ, McAlpine D, Reese M, et al. Investigation of antidepressant medication usage after bariatric surgery. Obes Surg. 2012;22(4):530–5. PubMed PMID: 21901283. eng.
57. Anderson JW, Greenway FL, Fujioka K, Gadde KM, McKenney J, O'Neil PM. Bupropion SR enhances weight loss: a 48-week double-blind, placebo-controlled trial. Obes Res. 2002;10(7):633–41. PubMed PMID: 12105285. eng.
58. Serretti A, Mandelli L. Antidepressants and body weight: a comprehensive review and meta-analysis. J Clin Psychiatry. 2010;71(10):1259–72. PubMed PMID: 21062615. eng.
59. Tolstoy L. Anna Karenina. Ebook: Gutenberg Project; 1998.

Assessment of Body Composition

Mark Punyanitya and Paul R. Clark

Keywords

Adipose tissue • Body composition • Dual-energy X-ray absorptiometry • Computed tomography • Magnetic resonance imaging • Muscle tissue • Organ volume • Segmentation

---

Summary

Background

The assessment of body composition for research began in the late 1800s with basic investigations of the human body for fat, protein, salt, and water content, while the early 1900s moved into more specific quantifications on the atomic, chemical, and molecular level for the whole body. With advances in science and technology, the 1960s and 1970s saw development of the three-compartment model and the introduction of new methods and devices, such as bioimpedance analysis and dual-photon absorptiometry. With increased clinical adoption of medical imaging in the 1980s, body composition assessment expanded from single and multiple slices to whole body imaging, as well as from computed tomography (CT) to magnetic resonance imaging (MRI). In the 1990s, continued refinement and cross-validation of different research methodologies led to the commercial development of bioimpedance analysis (BIA), air displacement plethysmography (BOD POD), and dual-energy X-ray absorptiometry (DXA) systems with widespread clinical, consumer, and research utilization.

Key Methods

Body composition imaging has been utilized for over 35 years in scientific research, but has yet to be implemented as a routine clinical measurement. Frequently designated as "non-standard of care", body composition imaging can be classified as a highly technical imaging technique. Since the average imaging technologist does not frequently perform these types of specialized scans in routine clinical practice, there is a

---

M. Punyanitya, MA, MS (✉)
Image Reading Center, Inc., New York, NY, USA
e-mail: mark@imagereadingcenter.com

P.R. Clark, PhD(Dist), BE(Hons)
MagnePath Pty. Ltd., Perth, Australia

need for comprehensive training where emphasis is placed on a number of factors including adherence to a specified acquisition protocol, maximum reproducibility and minimum variability between timepoints, and strict accountability for documentation and transfer of source data. The most accurate and precise use of these imaging techniques in translational research requires an evaluation of the type and maintenance of equipment to be utilized, the experience and training of imaging technologists who will perform the scan, and the protocol to be utilized for acquiring the images and managing the data. The key methods are organized by imaging modality and typically selected based on the prioritization of logistical concerns versus scientific need. The less complicated methods will be more readily available and can be implemented in a more scalable manner, but only provide a limited number of results. The more advanced techniques require higher end scanners and additional equipment, which are most often located at academic medical centres or large imaging facilities, but are able to produce additional results which are not directly available from other modalities.

Image Acquisition

Method	Measurement	Advantages	Disadvantages	Value in drug development decisions
DXA	Density of whole body tissue to determine the separate composition of fat tissue, lean soft tissue, and bone mineral content/density	Short scan time (5–10 min); open table configuration; user-friendly software; easy to standardize	X-ray exposure; table weight limit (~300 lb; ~136 kg); table scan limit (~60 cm width); cannot separate different types of adipose tissues; technologists may be unfamiliar as this is not usual standard of care	Suggested by FDA (Food and Drug Administration) in Draft Guidance as general safety assessment for reduction in fat content not lean-body mass
CT	Density of various tissues in order to produce anatomical images for the assessment of normal and abnormal body structures	Cross-sectional imaging; larger bore size (70–90 cm); higher table weight limit (~400–450 lb; ~182–2,014 kg)	X-ray exposure; technologists typically rotate between modalities; more difficult to standardize	Should be used for direct VAT* measurement, rather than waist circumference, as a surrogate measure
MRI	Water content of various tissues in order to produce anatomical and dynamic images for the assessment of normal and abnormal body structures and function	Cross-sectional imaging; no X-ray exposure; higher table weight limit (~350 lb; ~159 kg); technologists are more consistent	Smaller bore sizes (60–70 cm); claustrophobia risk; smaller field of view (~50 cm); longer scan times (~30 min); more difficult to standardize	Should be used for direct VAT measurement, rather than waist circumference, as a surrogate measure

VAT visceral adipose tissue

Image Analysis

Method	Measurement	Advantages	Disadvantages	Value in drug development decisions
DXA	Separation of anatomical regions of interest to quantify fat tissue, lean soft tissue, and bone mineral content/density	Auto-analysis features available; manual analysis procedures are software driven; easy to develop a protocol	Site technologists are not typically familiar with body composition scan, as they are not standard of care; sites often perform local image analysis according to their established procedures and independent of other sites	FDA Draft Guidance suggests centralized process can better provide verifiable and uniform training, management, and performance

Method	Measurement	Advantages	Disadvantages	Value in drug development decisions
CT	Quantification of internal organs or tissue volumes, as well as some qualitative measurements	Thresholding by Hounsfield units; some automated segmentation available; can be performed on existing PACS/workstations	Analysis by CT technologists is inefficient and often interrupted by scanning responsibilities; clinical software is typically for routine measurements, not rigorous analysis	FDA Draft Guidance suggests centralized process can better provide verifiable and uniform training, management, and performance
MRI	Quantification of internal organ or tissue volumes, as well as a range of dynamic, functional, and qualitative measurements	Wider range of acquisition protocols allow for a larger number of quantitative and qualitative analyses	Images are more varied and complicated to analyse; fewer options for automated analysis; strict protocols must be followed in order to reduce individual analyst bias	FDA Draft Guidance suggests centralized process can better provide verifiable and uniform training, management, and performance

PACS picture archiving and communications system

Conclusions

Body composition imaging is more technical than general clinical imaging and should be constrained to a rigorous protocol in order to provide reproducibility and scalability for translational research. Since image acquisition and processing technologies are rapidly evolving, researchers and scientists should thoroughly evaluate logistical concerns and scientific needs before selecting an imaging modality. As with any scientific methodology, the quality and validity of results are only as good as the source data; therefore, engineers, physicists, and technologists should be included in discussions with clinical researchers in order to address technical issues that must be resolved for use in translational research. Body composition imaging has long been utilized for obesity/diabetes research and drug development and is expanding into other disease and therapeutic areas. Broader implementation will increase the familiarity and quality of these techniques while building a solid foundation for new investigations.

Introduction

The Pathophysiology of Obesity or Diabetes

Adipose tissue mass and function are closely associated with health-related conditions such as impaired insulin sensitivity, metabolic syndrome [1], and type 2 diabetes [2]. The utilization of medical imaging has allowed for a better understanding of the effects of obesity and diabetes and has also increased our understanding of the mechanism of these conditions. Hyperglycaemia, impaired postprandial insulin secretion, elevated fasting plasma insulin levels, increased fatty acids and triglycerides, and insulin resistance are associated with adiposity but more specifically, with certain patterns of adipose tissue and fat distribution.

The measurement of visceral adipose tissue (VAT) by computed tomography (CT) and magnetic resonance imaging (MRI) has allowed for the breakdown of abdominal adiposity into separate VAT and subcutaneous adipose tissue (SAT) compartments, but also for further subdivision into more detailed and distinct anatomical depots [3]. As a single depot, VAT is strongly associated with insulin resistance of skeletal muscle, as well as with dyslipidaemia, and increased risks for hypertension and glucose intolerance [4]. Differences in the amount of VAT have been determined to account for a significant amount of the variability in the severity of insulin resistance and also have a stronger correlation than fat mass [5] (Fig. 6.1).

The high resolution of cross-sectional imaging has allowed for the identification of an established fascial plane that separates SAT into deep and superficial layers, which are known to have distinct histological properties. The deep SAT layer has been shown to have an association with

Fig. 6.1 (a) CT image acquisition. (b) CT Analysis for SAT and VAT. (c) MRI image acquisition. (d) MRI analysis for muscle, SAT, and VAT

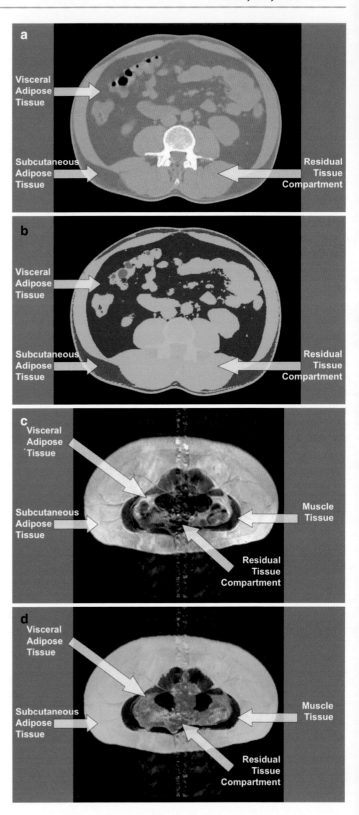

Fig. 6.2 (a) CT image of abdomen. (b) CT analysis for deep and superficial SAT

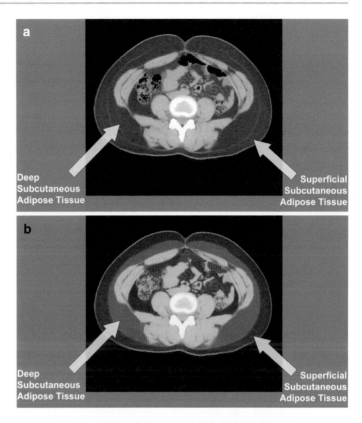

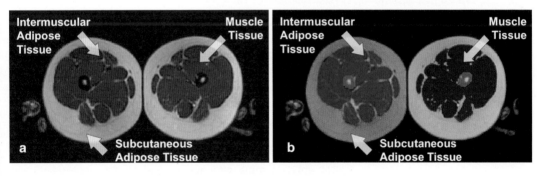

Fig. 6.3 (a) CT image of thigh. (b) CT analysis for muscle, IMAT, and SAT

insulin resistance that is similar to VAT, which the superficial SAT layer has a weaker association [6] (Fig. 6.2).

Intermuscular adipose tissue (IMAT) has also been identified as adipose tissue located beneath the muscle fascia and combined with contiguous depots of adipose tissue between muscle bundles [7]. IMAT has been show to be significantly correlated with insulin resistance in middle-age [8] and older adults [1, 9]. Continued interest is focused on the qualitative analysis of other tissue or organ composition, such as skeletal muscle and liver, where higher fat content has been identified in obesity and type 2 diabetes (Fig. 6.3).

The Development of Pharmacological Agents

Drug distribution within the body is dependent on a number of factors including blood flow, body composition, fluid distribution, and protein/

tissue binding. It is possible for drug distribution to shift as protein concentration and body composition changes occur. Once in the blood, circulation throughout the body can be affected by regional flow in the central compartment of high metabolic rate organs (brain, heart, kidney, and liver) and the peripheral compartment of less well-perfused organs (adipose and muscle tissue). For example, despite the fact that anaesthesia is metabolized slowly, the duration of effect is shortened because drug distribution into adipose tissue acts as a storage site or drug reservoir.

Since phenotypic and lifestyle changes of body composition and mass can affect drug distribution and metabolism, the use of imaging modalities to assess the variability and magnitude of the changes early on in the drug development process allows for more efficient clinical trials and more valuable clinical results. The Food and Drug Administration (FDA) has included the use of imaging biomarkers as endpoints for quantifying the size of effect in its *Guidance for Industry Standards for Clinical Trial Imaging Endpoints*. More specifically, the *Guidance for Industry Developing Products for Weight Management* incorporates the use of DXA, CT, or MRI for body composition assessment:

> To ensure that drug or biologic-induced weight loss is caused primarily by a reduction in fat content, not lean-body mass, a representative sample of study subjects should have a baseline and follow-up measurement of body composition by DEXA, or a suitable alternative.
>
> Because the evaluation of investigational weight-management products routinely includes assessment of changes in patients' metabolic profiles, and in some cases may involve measurement of visceral fat content by CT or MRI, waist circumference should not serve as a surrogate for visceral fat content when measured in a clinical trial investigating the efficacy of a product for weight loss.

An additional area of focus for drug development includes the imaging modalities of positron emission tomography (PET), functional MRI (fMRI), and magnetic resonance spectroscopy (MRS) for investigations of mechanisms and in vivo metabolism. These techniques allow for the assessment of tissue and organ quality and composition, fuel utilization, oxygen uptake, blood flow, and other functional properties.

Background

The assessment of body composition for research began in the late 1800s with basic investigations of the human body for fat, protein, salt, and water content [2, 10, 11], while the early 1900s moved into more specific quantifications on the atomic, chemical, and molecular level for the whole body [3, 12–14]. In 1942, Behnke et al. reported on the estimation of lean vs. fat by Archimedes' principle and introduced the two-compartment model and underwater weighing method, which could be implemented by other investigators [4, 15]. With advances in science and technology, the 1960s and 1970s saw development of the three-compartment model by Siri [5, 16] and the introduction of new methods and devices, such as bioimpedance analysis and dual-photon absorptiometry [6, 17, 18]. In 1979, Heymsfield et al. were the first to utilize CT for body composition imaging [7, 19].

Increased clinical adoption of medical imaging in the 1980s allowed body composition assessment to expand from single and multiple slices to whole body imaging, as well as from CT to MRI [8, 20–23]. In the 1990s, continued refinement and cross-validation of the different research methodologies led to the commercial development of bioimpedance analysis (BIA), air displacement plethysmography (BOD POD), and dual-energy X-ray absorptiometry (DXA) systems with widespread clinical, consumer, and research utilization. With the current variety of research techniques available for the assessment of body composition, logistical and scientific considerations play an important role in the selection process. At one end of the spectrum, anthropometric measurements are commonly utilized as surrogates of total body adiposity, where skinfold thickness is a low-cost field measurement, but has a considerable amount of variability in the subcutaneous thickness and compressibility of adipose tissue for a given measurement location. Intermediate techniques, such as the BODPOD or DXA, are more accurate and advanced than the field measures, but still only distinguish between two (fat and fat-free mass) and three (bone, fat, and lean mass) components of body composition, respectively. At the sophisticated end of the spectrum, imaging modalities such as CT and MRI are able to directly quantify adipose tissue in specified regions or the whole body with higher accuracy, but also higher costs and technical requirements.

Key Methods

Body composition imaging has been utilized for over 35 years in scientific research, but has yet to be implemented as a routine clinical measurement. Frequently designated as "non-standard of care", body composition imaging can be classified as a highly technical imaging technique. Since the average imaging technologist does not frequently perform these types of specialized scans in routine clinical practice, there is a need for comprehensive training where emphasis is placed on a number of factors including adherence to a specified acquisition protocol, maximum reproducibility and minimum variability between timepoints, and strict accountability for documentation and transfer of source data. The most accurate and precise use of these imaging techniques in translational research requires an evaluation of the type and maintenance of equipment to be utilized, the experience and training of imaging technologists who will perform the scan, and the protocol to be utilized for acquiring the images and managing the data.

The key methods are organized by imaging modality and typically selected based on the prioritization of logistical concerns versus scientific need. The less complicated methods will be more readily available and can be implemented in a more scalable manner, but only provide a limited number of results. The more advanced techniques require higher end scanners and additional equipment, which are most often located at academic medical centres or large imaging facilities, but are able to produce additional results which are not directly available from other modalities.

Dual-Energy X-Ray Absorptiometry

Methods

DXA is widely accepted for its ability to measure bone mineral density and utilized for the assessment of fracture risk and the diagnosis of osteoporosis from lumbar spine, proximal femur/hip, and distal forearm scans. Broad adoption has lead to the installation of approximately 50,000 whole body DXA scanners worldwide and, because of increased accessibility, the utilization in numerous studies ranging from bone health, exercise and HIV/AIDS to diabetes, muscle wasting/sarcopaenia, and obesity/weight loss. The majority of DXA scanners also include the whole body scan mode for body composition, which emits a low radiation dose between 0.02 and 1.5 mrem, depending on the instrument and the scan speed, and is less exposure than acquired during one transcontinental flight across the USA (4–6 mrems). Since some radiation is involved with all DXA scans, it is contraindicated for women who might be pregnant and requires administration of a pregnancy test prior to scanning in women of childbearing age.

A whole body DXA scan can measure three main body composition compartments (bone mineral content, fat mass, and lean soft tissue mass), divided into separate anatomical sections for arms, legs, and trunk. The typical acquisition time is approximately 15 min for a whole body scan, which is comprised of 5 min for entry of patient biography, 5 min for patient positioning in supine orientation, and 5 min for image acquisition. Patients should be properly screened to ensure that they would be able to fit within the height, weight, and width limitations of the DXA scanner. The weight limit is typically 300 lb (~136 kg) for most DXA scanners, but newer generations have improved table designs to accommodate up to 450 lb (~205 kg). Patients taller than 76 in. (193 cm) or wider than 23–26 in. (58–65 cm) might not fit within the imaging field of view, and some tissue or an entire limb region could be rendered invalid data. Therefore, careful positioning is crucial for the acquisition of reproducible scans to ensure the accuracy and precision of the resulting image analysis.

Standardization of patient preparation should include proper control of hydration status by conducting serial measurements at the same time of day, under fasting conditions, and during the same period of the menstrual cycle for females and wearing a hospital gown after removing jewellery and any undergarments that might contain metal clasps or wires. Positioning should be standardized by ensuring:

1. Patient is resting comfortably in the supine position.
2. Body is centred evenly on the table pad.
3. There is approximately 1–2 in. of space between the top of the head and the topline of the table pad.
4. Hands are placed in a lateral position beside the body.
5. Legs are straight with feet perpendicular to table and toes together.
6. All body parts and tissue are within the field of view (Fig. 6.4).

Some accommodations can be made to wrap a patient's chest, abdomen, and hip regions with a thin sheet in an attempt to keep the tissue within the field or view or to place a small folded pillowcase between arms and hips or between thighs in order to keep separate tissue from overlapping. If a patient is too large to fit within the field of view, even after multiple attempts to reposition and wrap, then scans should be acquired on the right half of the body so that total body composition can be estimated, based on the principle of bilateral symmetry [24] (Fig. 6.5).

For a valid, completed DXA scan, it is an important quality control (QC) step to compare the measured scale weight to the sum of all DXA subregions. The average agreement between measurements should be within a 2.2 lb (1 kg) standard

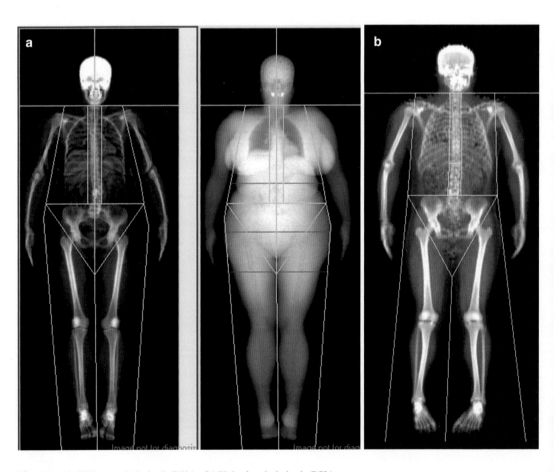

Fig. 6.4 (a) GE lunar whole body DXA. (b) Hologic whole body DXA

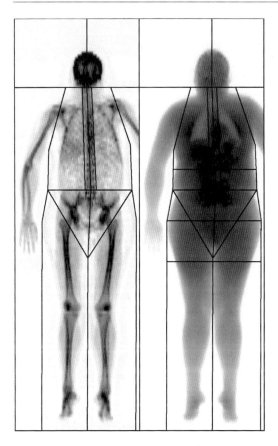

Fig. 6.5 DXA hemi-scan

placed on accuracy, precision, and reproducibility. Therefore, comprehensive training and standard operating procedures for the DXA technologist are essential for the proper instruction and conduct of data management activities, positioning of subjects, and scan acquisition. Additional recommendations for consistent scanning include:

1. Serial measurements should be acquired on the same DXA scanner.
2. All baseline and follow-up timepoints should be acquired by the same DXA technologist and utilizing the same scans mode and settings.
3. Patient positioning should follow a standard operating procedure (SOP) from the scanner manufacturer or a study protocol.
4. Image analysis should follow an SOP for the consistent placement of the regions of interest (ROIs) and the "compare" or "copy" function should always be used when available
5. Auto-analysis features should also be used, but still checked by the DXA technologist, to ensure proper positioning and catch any errors

deviation [25]. Additional calibration and quality assurance (QA) procedures utilize different phantoms and standards depending on the scanner manufacturer, model, and software version. Different forms of calcium hydroxyapatite and aluminium spine phantoms are either included by the scanner manufacturers or available from third parties ("Bona Fide Phantom" from BioClinica or "European Spine Phantom" from QRM GmbH) for daily QC as well as monitoring long-term scanner stability. Phantoms with components to mimic soft tissue include the Hologic "Whole Body Phantom", the BioClinica "Variable Composition Phantom", and the OrthoMetrics "Whole Body Phantom" and are used for body composition measurements and cross-calibrations between similar systems (Fig. 6.6).

While most US states require a licensed radiology technologist to acquire DXA scans, this does not mean they will have experience with clinical trials and understand the importance

Advantages

As a relatively inexpensive imaging modality, compared to CT or MRI, DXA scanners are available for between US $75,000–$100,000, with an annual service contract around US $10,000. Widespread clinical use for osteoporosis means that a large install base of scanners is available for research-focused measurements of body composition. An open table design, minimal patient preparation, and quick scan time all contribute to a user-friendly experience for the patient. A highly automated and guided workflow with a limited number of options/settings creates a user-friendly experience for the technologist. DXA has long been accepted as a precise and reliable measurement of body composition when serial examinations are performed on the same scanner [26]. Reliability and repeatability data from our centre include coefficients of variation (CVs) for total body tissue mass (0.6 %), fat mass (2.1 %), lean mass (1.15 %), and bone mineral content (1.1 %).

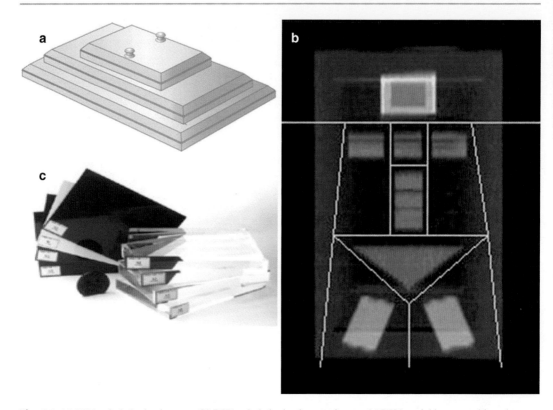

Fig. 6.6 (a) DXA whole body phantom. (b) DXA whole body phantom image. (c) DXA variable composition phantom

Disadvantages

Inherent to DXA is the use of dual-energy X-rays, which exposes the patient to radiation. Although the dose is very low, DXA is contraindicated for women who might be pregnant. While licensed radiology technologists are often required to perform a DXA scan, they are typically responsible for multiple/other imaging modalities and clinical protocols (i.e. bone density scans for osteoporosis), but not always experienced in body composition assessment and clinical trials. As DXA is a mature imaging modality, some legacy systems are often stand-alone computer and scanner systems and not connected to a network. DXA technologists are not always up-to-date on the latest technology developments and quickly become unfamiliar with newer methods to archive and transfer data/scans from their systems.

Although the market is dominated by two main scanner manufacturers, GE Lunar (GE Healthcare, Madison, WI, USA) and Hologic (Hologic, Inc., Bedford, MA, USA), there is still a lack of standardization between the two, as well as a difference in bone mineral content of approximately 20 %. Cross-calibration equations have recently been developed and validated in over 200 individuals ranging in age from 6 to 81 years to allow for the conversion of measurements between specific software versions from the manufacturers [27].

Finally, DXA is only capable of measuring total fat within an individual pixel or specified regions and is therefore unable to differentiate between layers of adipose tissue (intramuscular, subcutaneous, and visceral) occupying the same region. Additionally, in regions with a significant amount of bone surrounding soft tissue (i.e., head, chest, pelvis), DXA is unable to separate the soft tissue into fat or lean components. Because of these limitations, cross-sectional imaging modalities, such as CT and MRI, are utilized for further tissue discrimination.

Fig. 6.7 DXA-VAT region (*Left*, GE; *Right*, Hologic)

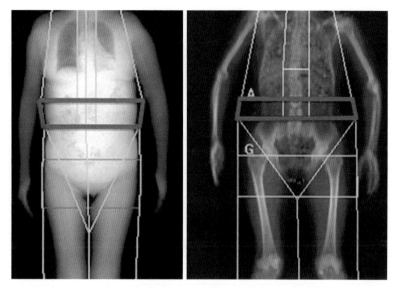

Value in Drug Development

DXA is an imaging modality that is precise and reliable for body composition measurement when serial examinations are performed on the same scanner. It is more objective than manual field methods such as body mass index (BMI), skinfolds, and waist-to-hip ratio and also provides more scientific information with regards to tissue composition and anatomical regions. DXA scanners are widely available and can be incorporated into clinical trials for drug development in a very standardized manner.

Advances in the development of new subregions for the whole body scan have been incorporated in the latest software revisions from both GE and Hologic and include discrimination of the android and gynoid fat regions, as well as the estimation of VAT. Recent publications have reported on the relationship of the android and gynoid regions to metabolic risk factors (hypertension, impaired glucose tolerance, and elevated triglycerides) [28, 29]. Both manufacturers have also developed an estimation of VAT by cross-validation against CT measurement of VAT area for Hologic [30] and VAT volume for GE [31], which demonstrate high correlations and should show increased utilization due to the number of scanners already in place (Fig. 6.7).

Cross-Sectional Imaging

While field measures and intermediate imaging techniques like DXA and ultrasound (US) are widely available, their usefulness becomes limited to correlations and estimates once the research focus turns to the internal components of body composition. In order to perform direct quantitative and qualitative measurements of internal organs (brain, heart, liver, kidneys, spleen, pancreas) and tissues (muscle, SAT, VAT, intermuscular adipose tissue (IMAT)), an advanced imaging modality such as CT or MRI should be utilized [32, 33]. Typically, two-dimensional images are acquired and analysed for area in the axial, coronal, or sagittal planes and then integrated along with their slice thickness and any gaps or spacing to reconstruct a three-dimensional volume. These methods are the gold standard techniques for the measurement of adipose tissue compartments and offer new insights into associations between intra-abdominal adipose tissue and metabolic factors.

Computed Tomography

Methods

CT scanners are widely available (~35,000 worldwide) due to a large install base at hospitals and imaging facilities, as well as utilization for clinical diagnostic imaging. Even though CT does expose individuals to ionizing radiation, it is one of the only available methods (along with MRI) to be able to separate individual organs from VAT, VAT from SAT, as well as muscle from IMAT [3, 34]. The classical CT scan for body composition (SAT/VAT) is a single, axial slice acquired at the anatomic level of the L4–L5 intervertebral space, while for muscle and IMAT it is a single, axial slice acquired at the level of the midthigh, which needs to be determined by measurement and calculation from anatomical landmarks (distance between the anterior superior iliac crest and the inferior margin of the patella) [8, 35]. When these types of scans are acquired with standard settings (120 kVp, 200 mA, and 2 s exposure), the typical radiation dose ranges between 40 and 400 mrem, depending on the total amount of body volume scanned and the spatial resolution required. In comparison, CT scan can be approximately 250 times more radiative than DXA, but provides information and results not available from DXA. Since radiation is involved with all CT scans, it is contraindicated for women who might be pregnant and requires administration of a pregnancy test prior to scanning in women of childbearing age (Fig. 6.8).

A combined abdomen and midthigh CT scan can typically be acquired within a 30 min appointment slot, comprised of 5 min for entry of patient biography, 5 min for patient positioning in supine orientation, 5 min for acquisition of an abdominal localizer image and a single or multiple axial images in the abdomen, 5 min for acquisition of a thigh localizer image, and then 10 min

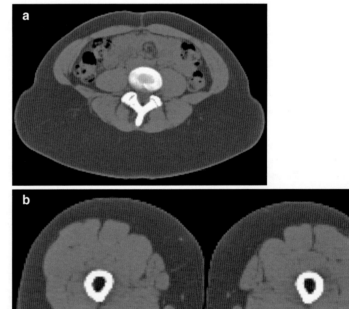

Fig. 6.8 (a) Abdominal CT image. (b) Midthigh CT image

to accurately measure, calculate, and acquire a single or multiple axial images of the midthigh. When acquiring a thigh scan or midthigh slice, approximately 10–15 min should be allocated for the patient to rest in the supine position and ensure an even fluid distribution for the tissue of interest.

Patients should be properly screened to ensure that they would be able to fit within the height, weight, and width limitations of the CT scanner. The typical weight limit is approximately 400–450 lb (~182–204 kg) depending on the make and model of CT scanner, but newer generations with bariatric options or larger bores have improved table designs to accommodate up to 500–650 lb (~226–294 kg). Patients wider than 21–26 in. (55–65 cm) might not fit within the imaging field of view, and some tissues might not be quantified. Therefore, careful positioning is crucial for the acquisition of reproducible scans to ensure the accuracy and precision of the resulting image analysis. Standardization of patient preparation should include wearing a hospital gown after removing jewellery and any undergarments that might contain metal clasps or wires.

While there are no specific CT QC procedures for body composition, each scanner should employ a standard phantom for daily QA activities and follow American College of Radiology (ACR) guidelines or maintain ACR certification. These standard phantom scans will allow for the longitudinal monitoring of scanner performance during the course of a study. Anthropomorphic phantoms are available, with accurate anatomical structures, where synthetic organs and tissues have radiation absorption properties approximate to human tissue and allow for scanning under actual clinical conditions. These advanced phantoms can be used for cross-calibrations between scanners (Fig. 6.9).

Additionally, a standard CT scanner can acquire scans for bone density measurements, quantitative computed tomography (QCT), by utilizing a special calibration phantom (which is scanned with the patient and contains five standards of varying density to be compared against the bone of interest), a quality control phantom to monitor system stability, and separate analysis software (Fig. 6.10).

A licensed radiology technologist is required to operate a CT scanner, but the technologist is often assigned to different locations and/or different scanners throughout an imaging facility, depending on staffing needs. The rapid imaging and throughput capabilities that make CT popular have also lead to shorter appointment times (sometimes as little at 15 min) and less opportunity for the technologist to focus on study documentation. As a result of these time limitations, the CT technologist will have very little flexibility for research scans, and certain activities should be completed either proactively, prior to the scan (case report forms, data transmittal forms, demographic documentation, etc.), or immediately after completion (image data transfer, image analysis).

Since a CT scanner is most often utilized for clinical scans, it is rare that a technologist will have experience with clinical trials; therefore, comprehensive training and standard operating procedures which focus on accuracy, precision, and reproducibility are essential for the proper instruction and conduct of research studies. Additional recommendations for consistent scanning include:

1. Serial measurements should be acquired on the same CT scanner.
2. All baseline and follow-up timepoints should be acquired by the same CT technologist and utilizing the same scan mode and settings.
3. Images from previous timepoints should be reviewed to help maximize reproducibility.
4. Patient positioning should follow a standard operating procedure (SOP) from the scanner manufacturer or a study protocol.

Advantages

A CT scanner is more expensive than field measurements and intermediate imaging methods (DXA and US), but allows more advanced measurements of internal organs and tissues, as well as the separation between similar tissues (IMAT, SAT, and VAT). Compared to MRI, a CT scanner is middle tier based on cost of US $100,000–$300,000, with an annual service

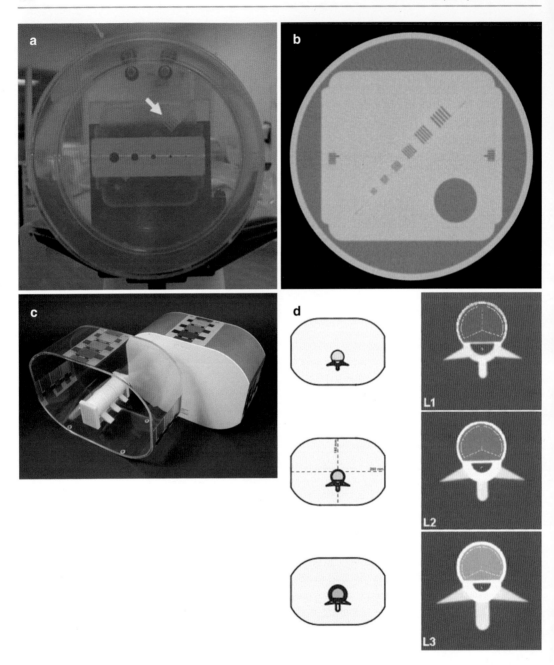

Fig. 6.9 (a) CT phantom. (b) CT phantom image. (c) EU spine phantom from QRM. (d) EU spine phantom image (Images reprinted with permission from ORM GmbH, Moehrendorf, Germany)

contract ranging between US $50,000 and 100,000. CT scanners have a wide bore and short length, which accommodates larger patients while reducing the concern for claustrophobia. Individual images can be acquired in seconds and complete scans can be acquired within 5 min or less. This rapid scanning speed improves image quality, decreases breatholding, and reduces patient discomfort and time. Additionally, patients who have metal in their body (certain types of implants, metallic fragments, cardiac monitors or pacemakers) can often be scanned by

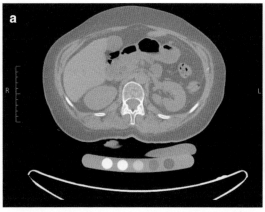 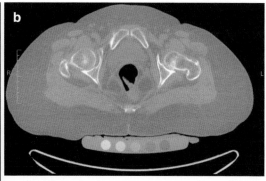

Fig. 6.10 (a) QCT spine scan. (b) QCT hip scan

CT when they would otherwise not be able to be scanned by MRI due to the magnetic field.

Another advantage of CT imaging is the objectivity of the technique, where physical density is the main determinant of X-ray attenuation, called the Hounsfield unit (HU), and each pixel is assigned an HU value on a grey scale that reflects the composition of the tissue (where air = −1,000 and water = 0). The spatial resolution and detail of a CT image allows for separation of adipose from muscle tissue, different regions of adipose tissue, as well as regions within subcutaneous adipose tissue (deep vs. superficial SAT). Simple image analysis can be performed directly on the CT scanner, on a picture archiving and communications system (PACS), or on a personal computing (PC) workstations with commercial off-the-shelf software, by utilizing a histogram or thresholding tool to select pixels within a given HU range (−190 to −30 HU for AT, 0–100 HU for muscle) and then multiplying the area of each pixel by the number of pixels [36].

Disadvantages

Costing approximately US $1,000–2,000, a CT scan is more expensive than a DXA scan (approximately US $300) and several field measures (Bioelectrical Impedance Analysis/Skin Folds) combined. Radiation exposure is a disadvantage for the use of CT, but also becomes increased in obese patients for deeper tissue penetration in order to obtain good image quality. CT scanner table weights are higher than for DXA, but still a limitation for obese patients. A limited field of view up to 70 cm for some new CT scanners can still result in tissue being excluded from imaging and analysis.

CT scanners are primarily utilized for clinical medicine and less frequently available for clinical research. Typically high daily caseloads, due to short scan times, lead to low appoint availability and scheduling difficulties for research cases, which can be intensive and require extra time to complete. CT technologists are more focused on clinical cases, where they utilize their individual knowledge and experience to obtain the best possible diagnostic image from their perspective, which is counter to the reproducible and standardized procedures required for clinical research. Technologists and managers are rarely provided enough time to learn new research techniques that are beyond standard of care imaging, to complete the required study documentation, or to manage data transfer of scans via systems outside of their PACS.

Value in Drug Development

CT is quite valuable in drug development because it is an advanced imaging modality that allows for quantification of internal organs and tissues, as well as a mature technology that is not cost prohibitive. The use of CT is referenced in FDA Draft

Guidance to be used for direct VAT measurement, rather than waist circumference as a surrogate measure, and to utilize a centralized process to better provide verifiable and uniform training, management, and performance. These factors have led to recent use of CT in several large multicentre clinical trials for the evaluation and registration of diabetes and weight loss drugs.

While CT measurements such as the VAT to SAT ratio have been used as an index of abdominal fat distribution, it distinguishes between a more VAT and more SAT profile, which is closely linked to metabolic abnormalities, independent of sex, age, and BMI [37]. Advances in measurement of VAT and SAT with CT and MRI allow investigators to study additional compartments that were previously indistinguishable (e.g. different aspects of VAT), such as intrathoracic and intra-abdominopelvic areas, the latter being composed of intraperitoneal and extraperitoneal compartments and possibly relating differently to metabolic factors [38]. Additional developments have made it possible to measure ectopic fat (fat in non-adipose tissue locations) in the liver and muscle tissue [39].

Imaging biomarkers are important for clinical development as a practical means of demonstrating the activity, safety, and efficacy of a drug in the target population. In this regard, CT has been useful as a clinical endpoint to directly and objectively measure the change in VAT as a pharmacodynamic response to drugs in development for diabetes, weight loss, and even for the reduction of excess abdominal fat in human immunodeficiency virus (HIV)-infected patients with lipodystrophy.

Magnetic Resonance Imaging

Methods

MRI and CT are similar, in that both scanners have the same install base at hospitals and imaging facilities and have primary utilization for clinical diagnostic imaging, but since an MRI scanner is more expensive (US $1–1.5 million) and requires special installation considerations (magnetic shielding), there are fewer scanners (~25,000 worldwide).

MRI is the most advanced imaging modality because of its ability to perform functional, molecular, quantitative, and qualitative/compositional measurements all within the same scanner. The body composition assessment of organs and tissues between MRI and CT is very similar because they are both cross-sectional imaging techniques, but different because of the physics principles used for image acquisition. MRI does not use ionizing radiation, but instead, is based on the magnetic interaction between protons. Since there is no X-ray exposure by MRI, it is an accepted modality for use in infants, children, normal volunteers, and women of childbearing age. MRI is especially suitable for comparisons between individuals and can be used for body composition assessment in longitudinal studies without concern for accumulated radiation exposure over time. MRI can also function as a reference method for quantification of organ and tissue volumes, as the estimates will be reliable independent of age. MRI is the only in vivo method that has been used to study foetal body composition [40] and may help provide an understanding of physiological and pathological conditions in both pregnant women and newborns.

The main body composition protocols of interest for MRI include abdominal scans (for VAT and SAT), limb scans (for IMAT, SAT, and Muscle), whole body scans (for IMAT, SAT, VAT, and muscle), and organ-specific scans (brain, heart, liver, kidney, spleen, and pancreas). These types of scans typically involve the acquisition of axial images throughout the whole body or anatomical region of interest, although coronal and sagittal images are also possible. Depending on the spatial resolution required, and thus the number of slices acquired, a complete scan can take between 30 and 60 min. The most convenient acquisition protocol utilizes 10 mm thick axial slices with 40 mm spacing between slices, which are organized into a 7-slice series that can be acquired in under 30 s to accommodate a single breath hold and minimize motion artefacts [41–43]. Individual series are stacked together to create a continuous set of images (typically between 40 and 60 images) to cover the entire body with a total examination duration of 30 min.

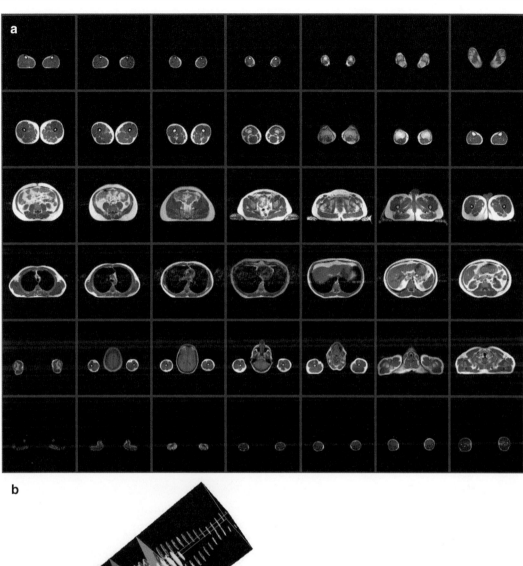

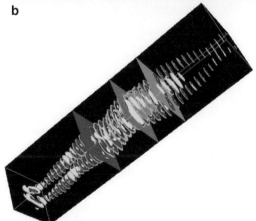

Fig. 6.11 (a) Whole body MRI protocol images. (b) Whole body MRI analysis

The whole body scan is often broken down into an upper body half and a lower body half, with the L4–L5 anatomical landmark as the origin (Fig. 6.11).

Patient preparation begins with appropriate screening and education to ensure that everyone involved correctly understands the amount of compliance and effort required to complete the MRI scan. The initial concern and question should be whether or not the patient is claustrophobic and would be able to remain calm and still during the length of the MRI scan. A patient's physical characteristics should be reviewed and screened to ensure that they are below the limits of 350 lb (~160 kg) for the table, within 60–70 cm to fit within the opening of the MRI scanner, and ideally within 65 cm to fit all tissue within the field of view. Therefore, careful positioning is crucial for the acquisition of reproducible scans to ensure the accuracy and precision of the resulting image analysis. Standardization of patient preparation should include wearing a hospital gown after special attention is paid to removing jewellery and any undergarments that might contain metal clasps or wires, due to the high magnetic field produced by the MRI scanner.

Similar to CT, there are no specific quality control (QC) procedures for body composition; therefore, each scanner should employ a standard phantom for daily quality assurance (QA) activities and follow American College of Radiology (ACR) guidelines or maintain ACR certification. These standard phantom scans will allow for the longitudinal monitoring of scanner performance (homogeneity and linearity of images) during the course of a study. Anthropomorphic phantoms are available, with accurate anatomical structures, where synthetic organs and tissues have radiation absorption properties approximate to human tissue and allow for scanning under actual clinical conditions. These advanced phantoms can be used for cross-calibrations between scanners, and some can even be used for both CT and MRI scanners (Fig. 6.12).

A licensed radiology technologist is required to operate an MRI scanner and is often assigned to

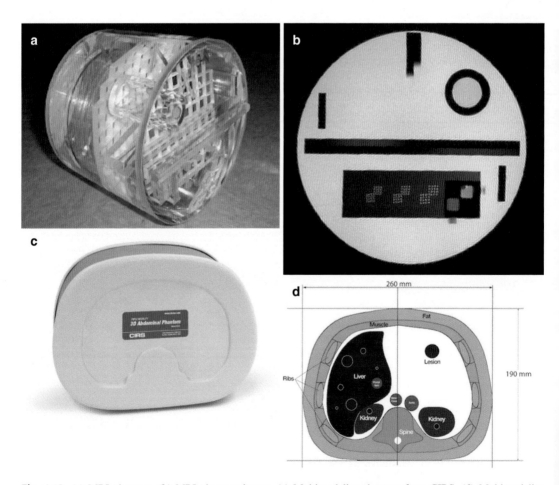

Fig. 6.12 (a) MRI phantom. (b) MRI phantom image. (c) Multimodality phantom from CIRS. (d) Multimodality phantom specifications from CIRS (Images reprinted with permission from CIRS, Norfolk, VA, USA)

a single machine, or at least a single location, during a shift, unlike a CT technologist. Clinical MRI scans often take between 30 and 60 min, which is similar to research MRI scans, and appointment slots are often prearranged in 30 min increments. Due to the lengthier appointment times and acquisition times for individual series, the MRI environment is slightly more relaxed and allows the opportunity for the technologist to complete study documentation or reviewing images. Even with greater flexibility, certain activities should be completed either proactively, prior to the scan (case report forms, data transmittal forms, demographic documentation, etc.), or immediately after completion (image data transfer, image analysis).

Since MRI technology is younger than CT technology, and new applications are continuously being developed, the technologist is more likely to have some experience with clinical trials. Comprehensive training and standard operating procedures are still necessary, with a focus on accuracy, precision, and reproducibility for the proper instruction and conduct of research studies. Additional recommendations for consistent scanning include:

1. Serial measurements should be acquired on the same MRI scanner.
2. All baseline and follow-up timepoints should be acquired by the same MRI technologist and utilizing the same scans mode and settings.
3. Images from previous timepoints should be reviewed to help maximize reproducibility.
4. Patient positioning should follow a standard operating procedure (SOP) from the scanner manufacturer or a study protocol.

Additionally, a wide range of radio frequency (RF) coils are available that cover the entire anatomy: body, head, knee, shoulder, spine, and surface coils, which are used for transmitting energy and receiving signals in order to boost the signal-to-noise ratio (SNR) and offer the option of parallel imaging. These coils are frequently used for magnetic resonance spectroscopy (MRS), a method to obtain metabolic composition and information from tissues in vivo.

Advantages

MRI poses minimal risk to patients, because it does not utilize ionizing radiation, and can be used in utero, in infants and children, and in normal healthy adults. In general, MRI is able to provide higher detail in soft tissue than CT and is actually able to change the contrast of images through various settings, in order to highlight different types of tissues. Another advantage of MRI is the ability to change the image acquisition plane without having to reposition the patient. Contrast agents for MRI have paramagnetic properties and are not made from iodine; thus, they are considered to be safer than X-ray dyes.

Disadvantages

MRI scanners are very expensive (US $1–1.5 million) and require significant service contracts and special considerations, like the use of helium (currently in limited supply) to keep the MRI magnets cooled. An individual MRI scan can cost between US $1,000 and $5,000. Since the MRI scanners produce very high magnetic fields, special considerations and precautions must be taken to ensure that no metal is brought into or near the entry of the MRI scanner's magnetically shielded room. Additionally, the physical dimensions of the MRI scanner are limited to 350 lb (~159 kg) for the table and 60–70 cm for the opening of the bore, which does not accommodate very large patients.

Value in Drug Development

MRI is valuable for drug development because of the ability to quantify internal organs and tissues and surpasses CT scanning with MRS and additional applications to identify the composition and metabolic information of tissues in vivo. As with CT, MRI is referenced in FDA Draft Guidance to be used for direct VAT measurement, but there is a need for standardization both in the acquisition and the analysis in order to extend its benefit to multicentre clinical trials.

Single or multiple slice measurements of muscle, SAT, and VAT by CT or MRI are a good start, but it is the acquisition and analysis of whole body MRI data that offers the most distinct advantages and value for assessing changes in body composition. Whether during weight loss or other

Fig. 6.13 (a) MRS voxel placement. (b) MRS spectrum

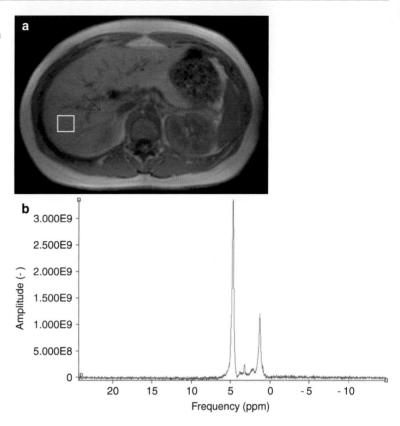

interventions that might induce regional changes in body composition, MRI would be the only technique to accurately quantify a muscle or SAT decrease in one region that is countered by a muscle or SAT increase in another region. Whole body MRI protocols have been implemented in trials on age-related muscle loss or sarcopaenia, cancer cachexia, diet and exercise changes, effects of space travel, and pharmaceutical interventions for obesity and diabetes, which has provided novel insights into the pattern of body compositions changes and can be utilized for the development or refinement of optimal intervention strategies.

Magnetic resonance spectroscopy (MRS) is most commonly used for neurological studies, but has also been used to quantify the lipid content of non-adipose tissues [39, 44]. MRS can be utilized to reliably quantify intramyocellular lipid (IMCL) and extramyocellular lipid (EMCL) in the tibialis anterior and soleus of the lower leg, in vivo [45], and associations have been reported between intramyocellular lipid and metabolic variables such as insulin resistance [46]. Lipid content of the liver can also be quantified with MRS [47], further demonstrating this is a non-invasive methodology to quantify the content and metabolism of ectopic fat in tissue and organs of the human body (Fig. 6.13).

New Imaging Methods

MRI technology is undergoing continuous development leading to new applications and techniques that allow for quantitative mapping of body composition. Quantitative mapping techniques include magnetic resonance (MR) relaxometry for fat fraction imaging (Dixon method) and iron concentration mapping, sodium MRI, magnetic resonance elastography (MRE), dynamic contrast-enhanced (DCE)-MRI, and diffusion MRI. An important focus for all of the techniques will be the interaction between organ and tissue structure, composition, and function.

Magnetic Resonance Relaxometry

Quantitative relaxometry enables measurement and mapping of various pathophysiological properties that is not feasible from conventional MR images [48]. The contrast in conventional images is dependent on the density of H1 nuclei and various relaxation mechanisms such as T1, T2, and T2*, in addition to scanner dependencies such as coil configuration and sensitivity. Consequently, the signal intensity in conventional images can only be measured in arbitrary units. Assessment of pathophysiology from conventional MR images thus remains qualitative and subjective and is mostly limited to comparative assessment of adjacent anatomical structures.

In quantitative relaxometry, the underlying contrast mechanisms are extracted from the MR signal free of scanner dependencies, providing absolute maps of tissue relaxation characteristics that directly relate to tissue microstructure. Relaxometry maps can thus be used to assess body composition serially and across multiple sites in a reliable and consistent manner, enabling large-scale multicentre studies to be performed with differing hardware. Adherence to specified imaging protocols is however required, to ensure that the MR signal behaviour is adequately sampled for extraction of the underlying tissue contrast mechanisms.

To accurately extract relaxometry maps, an appropriate time course of images must be measured that adequately capture the range of relaxation values that occur in both normal and abnormal tissue. Relaxation component models of the MR signal decay are then fit to the image signal intensities as a function of measurement time. The fitting is performed voxel by voxel to generate relaxation rate (or relaxation time) maps. The fitting process however can be perturbed by a number of confounds, including the degree of noise in the images, whether the signal model is sufficiently representative of the behaviour induced by the tissue microstructure, as well as on the numerical fitting routines used [48].

The accuracy and precision of the fitting routines is particularly important when multicomponent relaxometry (MCR) is used [49]. Relaxation in any given voxel is typically contributed to by more than one dominant hydrogen proton pool, where each pool is characterized by its own relaxation behaviour. Consequently, the derivation of "characteristic" relaxation rate maps assuming only one hydrogen proton pool can be misleading, resulting in measurements that suffer from reduced dynamic range and bias, limiting accuracy. Such results have been observed for both fat and iron measurement in phantoms and humans [50, 51].

A limitation on the use of relaxometry in clinical practice has been the time required to collect an appropriate span of MR images. Multi-echo sequences are thus favourable to repeated single echo acquisitions, but are not always feasible. However, new techniques are emerging based on compressed sensing and sparsity principles to achieve acceptable scan times [52].

In all cases of relaxometry, it is important to verify the accuracy and precision of the derived relaxation maps through phantom studies, where contributions of the biophysical property of interest can be accurately isolated and measured. The generation of synthetic image data sets also assists to define the theoretical range over which relaxation values can be reliably determined, in addition to enabling the simulation of noise and other confounds. In addition, where separate image acquisitions are performed to collect the image series, it is important to fix receiver gain settings between acquisitions or include an external reference object of known relaxation characteristics to correct for absolute intensity differences between images [53].

Fat Fraction Imaging (Dixon Method)

Numerous chemical shift methods have been developed to separate water and fat images from a combination of source images acquired at different echo times [54–56]. These techniques are based on the differences in physical properties of the hydrogen nuclei in water and fat and have been further developed to create fat fraction maps from the composite images. Gradient echo sequences used to measure fat fraction are widely available on numerous makes of scanner and can collect the required data within a single breath hold.

There are a number of confounders that affect the accuracy of fat fraction maps, which impact the choice of scanning parameters and the signal analysis technique. Key factors to consider include T1 bias, T2* relaxation effects, and the multi-peak spectral nature of fat [57]. T1 bias can be adequately compensated for by choosing a sufficiently low flip angle and long TR [58], but T2* relaxation and multi-peak spectral behaviour are best accounted for by incorporation into signal models that are fitted to the measured signal decay through MCR approaches. Commercial applications that account for such factors are available for the latest MRI scanners (IDEAL-IQ, GE Healthcare, Waukesha, WI and mDIXON-Quant, Philips Healthcare, Best, The Netherlands) to further non-invasive assessment of diffuse liver disease. Recent applications of fat fraction imaging have also focused on the ability to detect brown adipose tissue (BAT) [59], which metabolizes fat to generate heat, and whole body imaging [60–62].

An advantage of MCR approaches employing multi-peak spectral modelling of fat is that it enables resolution of the fat-water ambiguity problem that has previously limited the use of magnitude only images to discrimination of fat percentages below 50 % [63]. Complex-based measurement techniques such as IDEAL-IQ have successfully resolved the fat-water ambiguity problem through the use of phase information and field mapping, but can be sensitive to phase errors and require the additional data [64]. FatMap™ is a new magnitude-based MCR approach for mapping percentage fat that accounts for the aforementioned confounds and can be readily adopted in routine imaging across various makes and models of scanner (Fig. 6.14).

FatMap® - Putting Fat in the Picture

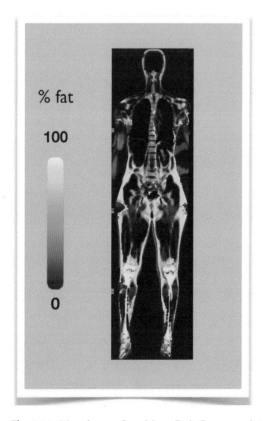
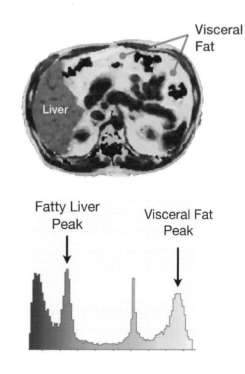

Fig. 6.14 Liver fat map from MagnePath (Image reprinted with permission from MagnePath)

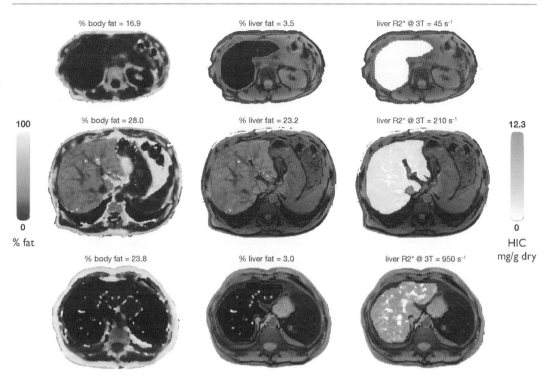

Fig. 6.15 Liver iron map from MagnePath (Image reprinted with permission from MagnePath)

Iron Magnetic Resonance Imaging

MR relaxometry methods also provide for cardiac or liver iron concentration measurement, where the rate of signal decay (R2 or R2*) has been calibrated against biopsy-derived hepatic iron concentration (HIC) measurements [65, 66]. Given the dominant effect of hemosiderin iron on MR signal relaxation, these techniques are robust in the presence of inflammation or fibrosis. No contrast agents are required, nor additional software or hardware for the standard MRI scanner. The resulting map of liver iron concentration and calculated mean value is used to report on distribution throughout the liver and guide chelation therapy.

For R2*-based measurement of iron concentration, increasing levels of fat above 30 % have been shown to result in progressive underestimation of R2* where a common relaxation rate is attributed to water and fat [50]. MCR techniques that model separate relaxation rates for water and fat can overcome this bias to provide R2* maps of the water component linearly related to iron concentration, in addition to fat fraction maps, as demonstrated by FatMap™ (Fig. 6.15).

Sodium Magnetic Resonance Imaging

Sodium content in the body can also be measured non-invasively by MRI, but requires specialized coils and pulse sequences to enhance the signal-to-noise ratio and allow acceptable spatial resolution for tissue sodium concentration [67–69]. The resulting images allow for the direct visualization and quantification of sodium in the skin and muscle tissue, as opposed to estimates of extracellular water content, 24-h urine collections, and serum sodium concentrations [70, 71]. Future application will support utilization of MRI to obtain additional insight into the composition of tissues, the role of sodium storage, and the evaluation of medication-induced fluid retention. As with H1-MRI, sodium relaxometry offers the potential to objectively quantify sodium between intracellular and extracellular compartments, which cannot be achieved by the qualitative assessment of sodium MR images alone [72].

Magnetic Resonance Elastography

Magnetic resonance elastography is a recent development which enables quantitative assessment of the mechanical properties of soft tissue and has been applied to liver and skeletal muscle, as well as brain, heart, kidneys, lungs, and other organs [73, 74]. The technique can be implemented on a standard MRI scanner and involves three steps: installed device for generation of mechanical vibrations in the tissue of interest, a special image acquisition sequence to capture the minute tissues changes, and image post processing to create quantitative maps of tissue stiffness. This method has been used to assess skeletal muscle stiffness and the physiological response of diseased and damaged muscles [75–77] and has been established as an accurate method for diagnosing hepatic fibrosis [78–82].

Dynamic Contrast-Enhanced-Magnetic Resonance Imaging

DCE-MRI is an established method for assessing tumour biology and treatment response by utilizing an intravenous contrast agent and repeated imaging to quantify tumour perfusion and capillary vessel leakage [83]. New investigations are applying DCE-MRI techniques for the quantification of fibrosis and cirrhosis before morphologic changes can be detected [84, 85]. Specialized acquisition sequences and post processing analysis software are under evaluation and have shown the ability to accurately assess liver fibrosis and cirrhosis for patients with chronic liver disease [86, 87].

Diffusion Magnetic Resonance Imaging

Diffusion-weighted imaging (DWI) by MRI has become a mature and reliable technique for the characterization of tissue properties, originally applied in the brain for the evaluation of neurological conditions. DWI is increasingly utilized in other body regions such as the abdomen, breast, liver, musculoskeletal, pelvis, and prostate. The DWI methodology enables the quantification and qualitative assessment of the random motion of water through specific tissues under investigation without the need for contrast agents. Recent technical advances have improved image quality and acquisition times, which are increasing adoption and incorporation into clinical protocols. For investigating liver fibrosis, DWI has compared well against other non-invasive methods (DCE-MRI, MRE, and ultrasound), can quantify the degree of liver fibrosis, and can be used for early diagnosis and following the response to treatment [88, 89]. On a similar basis to MCR, the quantification of separate diffusion and perfusion compartments through intra-voxel incoherent motion (IVIM) analysis [90] may provide greater sensitivity and specificity in the assessment of fibrosis than a single representative apparent diffusion coefficient (ADC) in the liver [91].

Diffusion tensor imaging (DTI) incorporates information from several DWI images in different gradient directions, to measure diffusion in multiple directions to create parametric maps. Recent investigations focusing on muscle tissue have found that elongated muscle fibres exhibit similar water diffusion properties to nerve fibres and can be studied with DTI [92]. Additional findings suggest that DTI measurements of ADC, eigenvalues, and fractional anisotropy (FA) from skeletal muscle can be utilized to estimate physiologic cross-sectional area, fibre length, fibre type, and pennation angle [93].

This synopsis of new imaging methods is intended to highlight some of the scientific and technical advances in imaging, which is rapidly progressing from simple descriptive and structural measurements to more advanced functional techniques and understanding of the imaging modalities and the organs/tissues of interest. Functional studies of body composition in obesity and type 2 diabetes will greatly improve with novel methods which combine the quantitative and qualitative aspects of anatomical volumes and metabolic functions.

Translating Results into Clinical Practice

It is well established that excess adiposity is associated with cardiovascular disease and type 2 diabetes, yet obesity has maintained at epidemic status despite a continued increase in the number of approved treatments. Investigations of diet, exercise, lifestyle, pharmacological, and surgical interventions are producing new results every day, but there is limited translation from research into clinical practice of accurately assessing body composition even in its simplest form, by BMI. In clinical practice, these technically advanced and highly sensitive methods are not currently being utilized.

By utilizing in vivo imaging, scientists are able to directly quantify tissue changes earlier and more accurately, as opposed to physical measurements or field techniques which can only estimate IMAT, SAT, and VAT. With increased accuracy, precision, and sensitivity of detection, imaging has enabled faster "go/no go" decisions in early phase drug development, by allowing for more measurement timepoints at closer intervals in addition to reducing the number of subjects required to assess a statistically significant difference. Decisions based on imaging biomarkers have been utilized for trials in support of recently approved type 2 diabetes and weight loss drugs, as well as for trials where imaging confirmed a lack of efficacy and resulted in decisions to terminate further development. Examples include lorcaserin [94] and phentermine/topiramate [95] for weight management.

While these imaging techniques are primarily utilized in a research capacity, they are based on clinical imaging modalities, which are increasingly accessible and available for clinicians via referral to academic medical centres, independent hospitals, and private radiology facilities. The barrier to clinical adoption of body composition assessment remains the current determination as "non-standard of care". While clinicians could incorporate body composition imaging into their treatment plans, this would remain non-diagnostic because of a lack of current procedural terminology (CPT) codes and a lack of coverage/reimbursement from insurance companies. Scale weight is the only widely accepted measurement for a determination of overweight or obese, eventhough CT or MRI imaging is the only way to directly quantify IMAT, SAT, and VAT.

EGRIFTA® (tesamorelin for injection) has been approved by the FDA based on imaging biomarkers and is the first and only treatment indicated to reduce excess abdominal fat in HIV-infected patients with lipodystrophy. Other similar pharmaceutical compounds are under investigation for cosmetic spot reduction of adipose tissue, so continued development should lead to more specific targeting of adipose tissue for obesity and type 2 diabetes. The FDA has also recently approved FerriScan™, previously cleared for measuring liver iron concentration (LIC) non-invasively using MRI, as an imaging companion diagnostic to select patients and to manage therapy for Exjade (deferasirox) treatment for the removal of excess iron in patients with non-transfusion-dependent thalassaemia. It is promising that continued publication and dissemination of research findings, along with patients' direct dialogue with their physicians and organized public advocacy, will increase the emphasis on the issue and eventually lead to a shift in acceptance, policy, and reimbursement.

Conclusions

Body composition imaging is more technical than general clinical imaging and should be constrained to a rigorous protocol in order to provide reproducibility and scalability for translational research. Since image acquisition and processing technologies are rapidly evolving, researchers and scientists should thoroughly evaluate logistical concerns and scientific needs before selecting an imaging modality. As with any scientific methodology, the quality and validity of results are only as good as the source data; therefore, engineers, physicists, and technologists should be included in discussions with clinical researchers in order to address technical issues that must be resolved for use in translational research. Body composition imaging has long been utilized for obesity/diabetes research and drug development and is expanding into other disease and therapeutic areas. Broader implementation will increase the familiarity and quality of these techniques while building a solid foundation for new investigations.

Despite the widespread availability of field measures for assessing body composition, there remains a growing need to utilize more advanced methods and technologies which are more accurate, objective, and reliable for the estimation of total and regional adipose tissue accumulation. The current imaging modalities of CT and MRI are able to more discretely quantify and separate internal depots of adipose tissue that are not possible with the more basic techniques. The ability to separately quantify and further subdivide SAT, VAT, and IMAT allows for more advanced investigations and enables stronger associations with physiological and pathological processes compared to overall total body fatness. More advanced methods, modalities, and technologies are being developed on a continuous basis and will require more intricate collaboration for translational research between the clinical researchers leading the investigations and the engineers, physicists, and technologists required to appropriately validate and implement the protocols for widespread adoption and utilization.

References

1. Wajchenberg BL. Subcutaneous and visceral adipose tissue: their relation to the metabolic syndrome. Endocr Rev. 2000;21(6):697–738.
2. Bermudez OI, Tucker KL. Total and central obesity among elderly Hispanics and the association with type 2 diabetes. Obesity (Silver Spring). 2001;9(8): 443–51.
3. Shen W, Wang Z, Punyanita M, Lei J, Sinav A, Kral JG, et al. Adipose tissue quantification by imaging methods: a proposed classification. Obes Res. 2003;11(1):5–16.
4. Després J-P. The insulin resistance-dyslipidemic syndrome of visceral obesity: effect on patients' risk. Obes Res. 1998;6(S1):8S–17.
5. Kelley DE, Williams KV, Price JC, McKolanis TM, Goodpaster BH, Thaete FL. Plasma fatty acids, adiposity, and variance of skeletal muscle insulin resistance in type 2 diabetes mellitus. J Clin Endocrinol Metab. 2001;86(11):5412–9.
6. Kelley DE, Thaete FL, Troost F, Huwe T, Goodpaster BH. Subdivisions of subcutaneous abdominal adipose tissue and insulin resistance. Am J Physiol Endocrinol Metab. 2000;278(5):E941–8.
7. Goodpaster BH, He J, Watkins S, Kelley DE. Skeletal muscle lipid content and insulin resistance: evidence for a paradox in endurance-trained athletes. J Clin Endocrinol Metab. 2001;86(12):5755–61.
8. Goodpaster BH, Thaete FL, Kelley DE. Thigh adipose tissue distribution is associated with insulin resistance in obesity and in type 2 diabetes mellitus. Am J Clin Nutr. 2000;71:885–92.
9. Goodpaster BH, Krishnaswami S, Resnick H, Kelley DE, Haggerty C, Harris TB, et al. Association between regional adipose tissue distribution and both type 2 diabetes and impaired glucose tolerance in elderly men and women. Diabetes Care. 2003;26(2):372–9.
10. Moleschott J. Physiologie der Nahrungsmittel: Ein Handbuch der Diätetik, Ferber, Giessen, 2nd Edition, 1859, p 224 (https://archive.org/details/physiologiedern00molegoog).
11. Bischoff E. Einzelne Gewichts- und Trocken-Bestimmungen der Organe des menschlichen Korpers. Fresenius, Zeitschrift f anal Chemie. 1864;3(1):250–4.
12. Camerer W Jr, Sölder, Camerer Jr. Die chemische Zusammensetzung des Neugeborenen – Google Scholar. Z Biol. 1900;39:173–92.
13. Mitchell HH, Hamilton TS, Steggerda FR, Bean HW. The chemical composition of the adult human body and its bearing on the biochemistry of growth. J Biol Chem. 1945;158:625–37.
14. Widdowson EM, McCance RA, Spray CM. The chemical composition of the human body. Clin Sci. 1951;10(1):113–25.
15. Behnke AR, Feen BG, Welham WC. The specific gravity of healthy men. JAMA. 1942;118(7): 495–8.
16. Siri WE. Techniques for measuring body composition: proceedings of a conference, quartermaster research and engineering center, Natick, 22–23 Jan 1959. National Academies, 1961.
17. Thomasset A. Bio-electric properties of tissues. Estimation by measurement of impedance of extracellular ionic strength and intracellular ionic strength in the clinic. Lyon Med. 1963;209:1325–50.
18. Mazess RB, Cameron JR, Sorenson JA. Determining body composition by radiation absorption spectrometry. Nature. 1970;228(5273):771–2.
19. Heymsfield SB, Olafson RP, Kutner MH, Nixon DW. A radiographic method of quantifying protein-calorie undernutrition. Am J Clin Nutr. 1979;32: 693–702.
20. Borkan GA, Hults DE, Gerzof SG, Burrows BA, Robbins AH. Relationships between computed tomography tissue areas, thicknesses and total body composition. Ann Hum Biol. 1983;10(6):537–45.
21. Tokunaga K, Matsuzawa Y, Ishikawa K, Tarui S. A novel technique for the determination of body fat by

computed tomography. Int J Obes (Lond). 1983; 7(5):437–45.
22. Foster MA, Hutchison JMS, Mallard JR, Fuller M. Nuclear magnetic resonance pulse sequence and discrimination of high- and low-fat tissues. Magn Reson Imaging. 1984;2(3):187–92.
23. Sjöström L, Kvist H, Cederblad A, Tylén U. Determination of total adipose tissue and body fat in women by computed tomography, 40K, and tritium. Am J Physiol. 1986;250(6 Pt 1):E736–45.
24. Tataranni PA, Ravussin E. Use of dual-energy X-ray absorptiometry in obese individuals. Am J Clin Nutr. 1995;62(4):730–4.
25. Houtkooper LB, Going SB, Sproul J, Blew RM, Lohman TG. Comparison of methods for assessing body-composition changes over 1 y in postmenopausal women. Am J Clin Nutr. 2000;72(2):401–6.
26. Russell-Aulet M, Wang J, Thornton J, Pierson RN. Comparison of dual-photon absorptiometry systems for total-body bone and soft tissue measurements: dual-energy X-rays versus gadolinium 153. J Bone Miner Res. 1991;6(4):411–5.
27. Shepherd JA, Fan B, Lu Y, Wu XP, Wacker WK, Ergun DL, et al. A multinational study to develop universal standardization of whole-body bone density and composition using GE Healthcare Lunar and Hologic DXA systems. J Bone Miner Res. 2012;27(10):2208–16.
28. Lee K, Lee S, Kim Y-J, Kim Y-J. Waist circumference, dual-energy X-ray absortiometrically measured abdominal adiposity, and computed tomographically derived intra-abdominal fat area on detecting metabolic risk factors in obese women. Nutrition. 2008;24(7–8):625–31.
29. Wiklund P, Toss F, Weinehall L, Hallmans G, Franks PW, Nordström A, et al. Abdominal and gynoid fat mass are associated with cardiovascular risk factors in men and women. J Clin Endocrinol Metab. 2008;93(11):4360–6.
30. Micklesfield LK, Goedecke JH, Punyanitya M, Wilson KE, Kelly TL. Dual-energy X-ray performs as well as clinical computed tomography for the measurement of visceral fat. Obesity (Silver Spring). 2012;20(5):1109–14.
31. Kaul S, Rothney MP, Peters DM, Wacker WK, Davis CE, Shapiro MD, et al. Dual-energy X-ray absorptiometry for quantification of visceral fat. Obesity (Silver Spring). 2012;20(6):1313–8.
32. Heymsfield S. Human body composition. 2nd ed. Champaign: Human Kinetics; 2005. 1 p.
33. Sjöström L. A computer-tomography based multicompartment body composition technique and anthropometric predictions of lean body mass, total and subcutaneous adipose tissue. Int J Obes (Lond). 1991;15 Suppl 2:19–30.
34. Gallagher D, Belmonte D, Deurenberg P, Wang Z, Krasnow N, Pi Sunyer FX, et al. Organ-tissue mass measurement allows modeling of REE and metabolically active tissue mass. Am J Physiol. 1998;275(2 Pt 1):E249–58.
35. Kelley DE, McKolanis TM, Hegazi RAF, Kuller LH, Kalhan SC. Fatty liver in type 2 diabetes mellitus: relation to regional adiposity, fatty acids, and insulin resistance. Am J Physiol Endocrinol Metab Am Physiol Soc. 2003;285(4):E90–16.
36. Kvist H, Sjöström L, Tylén U. Adipose tissue volume determinations in women by computed tomography: technical considerations. Int J Obes (Lond). 1986;10(1):53–67.
37. Fujioka S, Matsuzawa Y, Tokunaga K, Tarui S. Contribution of intra-abdominal fat accumulation to the impairment of glucose and lipid metabolism in human obesity. Metab Clin Exp. 1987;36(1):54–9.
38. Mårin P, Andersson B, Ottosson M, Olbe L, Chowdhury B, Kvist H, et al. The morphology and metabolism of intraabdominal adipose tissue in men. Metab Clin Exp. 1992;41(11):1242–8.
39. Goodpaster BH. Measuring body fat distribution and content in humans. Curr Opin Clin Nutr Metab Care. 2002;5(5):481–7.
40. Deans HE, Smith FW, Lloyd DJ, Law AN, Sutherland HW. Fetal fat measurement by magnetic resonance imaging. Br J Radiol. 1989;62(739):603–7.
41. Shen W, Wang Z, Tang H, Heshka S, Punyanitya M, Zhu S, et al. Volume estimates by imaging methods: model comparisons with visible woman as the reference. Obes Res. 2003;11(2):217–25.
42. Shen W, Punyanitya M, Wang Z, Gallagher D, St-Onge M-P, Albu J, et al. Visceral adipose tissue: relations between single-slice areas and total volume. Am J Clin Nutr. 2004;80(2):271–8.
43. Shen W, Punyanitya M, Wang Z, Gallagher D, St-Onge M-P, Albu J, et al. Total body skeletal muscle and adipose tissue volumes: estimation from a single abdominal cross-sectional image. J Appl Physiol. 2004;97(6):2333–8.
44. Szczepaniak LS, Babcock EE, Schick F, Dobbins RL, Garg A, Burns DK, et al. Measurement of intracellular triglyceride stores by H spectroscopy: validation in vivo. Am J Physiol. 1999;276(5 Pt 1): E977–89.
45. Boesch C, Slotboom J, Hoppeler H, Kreis R. In vivo determination of intra-myocellular lipids in human muscle by means of localized 1H-MR-spectroscopy. Magn Reson Med. 1997;37(4):484–93.
46. Jacob S, Machann J, Rett K, Brechtel K, Volk A, Renn W, et al. Association of increased intramyocellular lipid content with insulin resistance in lean nondiabetic offspring of type 2 diabetic subjects. Diabetes. 1999;48(5):1113–9.
47. Petersen KF, West AB, Reuben A, Rothman DL, Shulman GI. Noninvasive assessment of hepatic triglyceride content in humans with 13C nuclear magnetic resonance spectroscopy. Hepatology. 1996; 24(1):114–7.
48. Cheng H-LM, Stikov N, Ghugre NR, Wright GA. Practical medical applications of quantitative MR relaxometry. J Magn Reson Imaging. 2012;36(4):805–24.

49. MacKay A, Whittall K, Adler J, Li D, Paty D, Graeb D. In vivo visualization of myelin water in brain by magnetic resonance. Magn Reson Med. 1994;31(6): 673–7.
50. Chebrolu VV, Hines CDG, Yu H, Pineda AR, Shimakawa A, McKenzie CA, et al. Independent estimation of T*2 for water and fat for improved accuracy of fat quantification. Magn Reson Med. 2010; 63(4):849–57.
51. Clark PR, Chua-anusorn W, St Pierre TG. Bi-exponential proton transverse relaxation rate (R2) image analysis using RF field intensity-weighted spin density projection: potential for R2 measurement of iron-loaded liver. Magn Reson Imaging. 2003;21(5):519–30.
52. Huang C, Graff C, Bilgin A, Altbach MI. Fast MR Parameter Mapping from Highly Undersampled Data by Direct Reconstruction of Principal Component Coefficient Maps Using Compressed Sensing. ISMRM Stockholm; 2010.
53. Clark PR, St Pierre TG. Quantitative mapping of transverse relaxivity (1/T(2)) in hepatic iron overload: a single spin-echo imaging methodology. Magn Reson Imaging. 2000;18(4):431–8.
54. Dixon WT. Simple proton spectroscopic imaging. Radiology. 1984;153(1):189–94.
55. Reeder SB, Wen Z, Yu H, Pineda AR, Gold GE, Markl M, et al. Multicoil Dixon chemical species separation with an iterative least-squares estimation method. Magn Reson Med. 2004;51(1):35–45.
56. Berglund J, Johansson L, Ahlström H, Kullberg J. Three-point Dixon method enables whole-body water and fat imaging of obese subjects. Magn Reson Med. 2010;63(6):1659–68.
57. Reeder SB, Robson PM, Yu H, Shimakawa A, Hines CDG, McKenzie CA, et al. Quantification of hepatic steatosis with MRI: the effects of accurate fat spectral modeling. J Magn Reson Imaging. 2009;29(6):1332–9.
58. Hines CDG, Yokoo T, Bydder M, Sirlin CB, Reeder SB. Optimization of flip angle to allow tradeoffs in T1 bias and SNR performance for fat quantification. Proc Intl Soc Mag Reson Med. 18th Annual Meeting, Stockholm; 2010.
59. Hu HH, Yin L, Aggabao PC, Perkins TG, Chia JM, Gilsanz V. Comparison of brown and white adipose tissues in infants and children with chemical-shift-encoded water-fat MRI. J Magn Reson Imaging. 2013;38(4):885–96.
60. Ma J, Costelloe CM, Madewell JE, Hortobagyi GN, Green MC, Cao G, et al. Fast dixon-based multi-sequence and multiplanar MRI for whole-body detection of cancer metastases. J Magn Reson Imaging. 2009;29(5):1154–62.
61. Costelloe CM, Madewell JE, Kundra V, Harrell RK, Bassett RL, Ma J. Conspicuity of bone metastases on fast Dixon-based multisequence whole-body MRI: clinical utility per sequence. Magn Reson Imaging. 2013;31(5):669–75.
62. Hu HH, Börnert P, Hernando D, Kellman P, Ma J, Reeder S, et al. ISMRM workshop on fat-water separation: insights, applications and progress in MRI. Magnetic Resonance in Medicine. 2012;68(2): 378–88.
63. Hu HH, Nayak KS, Goran MI. Assessment of abdominal adipose tissue and organ fat content by magnetic resonance imaging. Obes Rev Off J Int Assoc Study Obes. 2011;12(5):e504–15.
64. Reeder SB, Hu HH, Sirlin CB. Proton density fat-fraction: a standardized MR-based biomarker of tissue fat concentration. J Magn Reson Imaging. 2012;36(5):1011–4.
65. St Pierre TG, Clark PR, Chua-anusorn W, Fleming AJ, Jeffrey GP, Olynyk JK, et al. Noninvasive measurement and imaging of liver iron concentrations using proton magnetic resonance. Blood. 2005;105(2):855–61.
66. Hernando D, Levin YS, Sirlin CB, Reeder SB. Quantification of liver iron with MRI: state of the art and remaining challenges. J Magn Reson Imaging. 2014. DOI: 10.1002/jmri.24584.
67. Ouwerkerk R, Sodium MRI. Methods Mol Biol. 2011;711:175–201.
68. Wetterling F, Corteville DM, Kalayciyan R, Rennings A, Konstandin S, Nagel AM, et al. Whole body sodium MRI at 3T using an asymmetric birdcage resonator and short echo time sequence: first images of a male volunteer. Phys Med Biol. 2012;57(14):4555–67.
69. Kopp C, Linz P, Wachsmuth L, Dahlmann A, Horbach T, Schöfl C, et al. Na magnetic resonance imaging of tissue sodium. Hypertension. 2012;59(1):167–72.
70. Zuo CS, Villafuerte RA, Henry ME, Dobbins RL, Lee C, Sung Y, et al. MRI assessment of drug-induced fluid accumulation in humans: validation of the technology. Magn Reson Imaging. 2008;26(5):629–37.
71. Kopp C, Linz P, Dahlmann A, Hammon M, Jantsch J, Müller DN, et al. 23Na magnetic resonance imaging-determined tissue sodium in healthy subjects and hypertensive patients. Hypertension. 2013;61(3):635–40.
72. Madelin G, Regatte RR. Biomedical applications of sodium MRI in vivo. J Magn Reson Imaging. 2013;38(3):511–29.
73. Mariappan YK, Glaser KJ, Ehman RL. Magnetic resonance elastography: a review. Clin Anat. 2010;23(5):497–511.
74. Glaser KJ, Manduca A, Ehman RL. Review of MR elastography applications and recent developments. J Magn Reson Imaging. 2012;36(4):757–74.
75. Dresner MA, Rose GH, Rossman PJ, Muthupillai R, Manduca A, Ehman RL. Magnetic resonance elastography of skeletal muscle. J Magn Reson Imaging. 2001;13(2):269–76.
76. Ringleb SI, Bensamoun SF, Chen Q, Manduca A, An K-N, Ehman RL. Applications of magnetic resonance elastography to healthy and pathologic skeletal muscle. J Magn Reson Imaging. 2007;25(2):301–9.
77. Basford JR, Jenkyn TR, An K-N, Ehman RL, Heers G, Kaufman KR. Evaluation of healthy and diseased

muscle with magnetic resonance elastography. Arch Phys Med Rehabil. 2002;83(11):1530–6.
78. Huwart L, Peeters F, Sinkus R, Annet L, Salameh N, ter Beek LC, et al. Liver fibrosis: non-invasive assessment with MR elastography. NMR Biomed. 2006;19(2):173–9.
79. Rouvière O, Yin M, Dresner MA, Rossman PJ, Burgart LJ, Fidler JL, et al. MR elastography of the liver: preliminary results. Radiology. 2006;240(2):440–8.
80. Yin M, Talwalkar JA, Glaser KJ, Manduca A, Grimm RC, Rossman PJ, et al. Assessment of hepatic fibrosis with magnetic resonance elastography. Clin Gastroenterol Hepatol. 2007;5(10):1207–13.e2.
81. Huwart L, Salameh N, ter Beek L, Vicaut E, Peeters F, Sinkus R, et al. MR elastography of liver fibrosis: preliminary results comparing spin-echo and echoplanar imaging. Eur Radiol. 2008;18(11):2535–41.
82. Huwart L, Sempoux C, Vicaut E, Salameh N, Annet L, Danse E, et al. Magnetic resonance elastography for the noninvasive staging of liver fibrosis. Gastroenterology. 2008;135(1):32–40.
83. Do RKG, Rusinek H, Taouli B. Dynamic contrast-enhanced MR imaging of the liver: current status and future directions. Magn Reson Imaging Clin N Am. 2009;17(2):339–49.
84. Patel J, Sigmund EE, Rusinek H, Oei M, Babb JS, Taouli B. Diagnosis of cirrhosis with intravoxel incoherent motion diffusion MRI and dynamic contrast-enhanced MRI alone and in combination: preliminary experience. J Magn Reson Imaging. 2010;31(3):589–600.
85. Shim JH, Yu J-S, Chung J-J, Kim JH, Kim KW. Segmental difference of the hepatic fibrosis from chronic viral hepatitis due to hepatitis B versus C virus infection: comparison using dual contrast material-enhanced MRI. Korean J Radiol. 2011;12(4):431–8.
86. Leporq B, Dumortier J, Pilleul F, Beuf O. 3D-liver perfusion MRI with the MS-325 blood pool agent: a noninvasive protocol to asses liver fibrosis. J Magn Reson Imaging. 2012;35(6):1380–7.
87. Chen B-B, Hsu C-Y, Yu C-W, Wei S-Y, Kao J-H, Lee H-S, et al. Dynamic contrast-enhanced magnetic resonance imaging with Gd-EOB-DTPA for the evaluation of liver fibrosis in chronic hepatitis patients. Eur Radiol. 2012;22(1):171–80.
88. Lewin M, Poujol-Robert A, Boëlle P-Y, Wendum D, Lasnier E, Viallon M, et al. Diffusion-weighted magnetic resonance imaging for the assessment of fibrosis in chronic hepatitis C. Hepatology. 2007;46(3):658–65.
89. Zhou M-L, Yan F-H, Xu P-J, Chen C-Z, Shen J-Z, Li R-C, et al. Comparative study on clinical and pathological changes of liver fibrosis with diffusion-weighted imaging. Zhonghua Yi Xue Za Zhi. 2009;89(25):1757–61.
90. Le Bihan D, Breton E, Lallemand D, Aubin ML, Vignaud J, Laval-Jeantet M. Separation of diffusion and perfusion in intravoxel incoherent motion MR imaging. Radiology. 1988;168(2):497–505.
91. Dyvorne HA, Nevers T, Galea N, Fiel MI, Carpenter D, Wong E, et al. Intravoxel incoherent motion diffusion-weighted imaging for detection of liver fibrosis in HCV: comparison of four sequences. Proc Intl Soc Mag Reson Med. 20th Annual Meeting, Melbourne; 2012.
92. Longwei X. Clinical application of diffusion tensor magnetic resonance imaging in skeletal muscle. Muscles Ligaments Tendons J. 2012;2(1):19–24.
93. Scheel M, von Roth P, Winkler T, Arampatzis A, Prokscha T, Hamm B, et al. Fiber type characterization in skeletal muscle by diffusion tensor imaging. NMR Biomed. 2013;26(10):1220–4.
94. Hoy SM. Lorcaserin: a review of its use in chronic weight management. Drugs. 2013;73(5):463–73.
95. Rueda-Clausen CF, Padwal RS, Sharma AM. New pharmacological approaches for obesity management. Nat Rev Endocrinol. 2013;9(8):467–78.

Measurement of Energy Expenditure

Klaas R. Westerterp

Keywords

Indirect calorimetry • Doubly labelled water • Basal metabolic rate • Diet-induced energy expenditure • Physical activity • Food intake

Summary

Background

At the present state of the art, energy expenditure is measured with indirect calorimetry, where energy production is calculated from oxygen consumption, carbon dioxide production and urine-nitrogen loss. Daily energy expenditure consists of three components, i.e. maintenance expenditure, diet-induced energy expenditure and activity-induced energy expenditure.

Key Methods

Indirect calorimetry methods for the assessment of gaseous exchange as presented in this chapter include a mouthpiece or facemask, ventilated hood, respiration chamber and doubly labelled water.

Method	Measurement	Advantages	Disadvantages	Value in drug development decisions
Mouthpiece or facemask	O_2 consumption and CO_2 production from breathing	Minimal response time; no dilution of respiratory gases	Mouthpiece and facemask are tolerated for limited time interval	Limited; measurement of energy expenditure for defined activities including VO_2 max
Ventilated hood	O_2 consumption and CO_2 production from breathing	Standardised measurement conditions	Mainly applicable under resting conditions	Limited; measurement of basal metabolic rate and diet-induced energy expenditure

K.R. Westerterp, PhD
Department of Human Biology, Maastricht University, Maastricht, The Netherlands
e-mail: k.westerterp@maastrichtuniversity.nl

Method	Measurement	Advantages	Disadvantages	Value in drug development decisions
Respiration chamber	O_2 consumption and CO_2 production from breathing	Definition of living environment including diet and physical activity	High dilution of respiratory gases; confined environment	High; evaluation of effects of diet, physical activity and sleep on energy expenditure
Doubly labelled water	CO_2 production from isotope elimination as measured in urine, saliva or blood	Assessment of total energy expenditure without any interference	Minimal observation time several days or weeks, depending on the physical activity level of the subject	Moderate; evaluation of daily energy requirement and validation of reported food intake and physical activity assessment

Conclusions

Designing studies to evaluate intervention effects on energy expenditure, including drugs, should be based on the energy expenditure component as targeted. The indicated method for the measurement of maintenance expenditure is a ventilated hood. Diet-induced energy expenditure can be measured with a ventilated hood or in a respiration chamber. Activity-induced energy expenditure is measured under standardised conditions with a mouthpiece, facemask or in a respiration chamber and under free-living conditions with doubly labelled water. Energy expenditure can be estimated and evaluated with alternative methods including prediction equations for maintenance expenditure, based on height, weight, age and gender; doubly labelled water validated accelerometers to assess activity-induced energy expenditure; and measurements of food intake as evaluated with the doubly labelled water technique.

Introduction

Energy expenditure is measured primarily to assess energy requirement. Measured energy expenditure is the basis for food intake recommendations including nutritional advice and for enteral and parenteral nutrition in a clinical setting. The level of resting energy expenditure, as affected by maintenance metabolism, is a reflection of the health status of a subject. Activity-induced energy expenditure is a measure for the physical activity level. Maximal energy expenditure is a measure for physical fitness.

The design of weight-maintenance diets, as applicable in clinical settings, is based on energy requirement as derived from measured energy expenditure. Alternatively, energy requirement can be based on reported food intake. However, reported intake is often lower than habitual energy intake, resulting in weight loss when subjects are fed according to what they report they normally eat.

Measured energy expenditure is a criterion method for the evaluation of methods for the assessment of food intake and physical activity. Nowadays, the validity of reported food intake, with questionnaires, interviews or dietary records, can be evaluated with a measurement or estimate of energy expenditure under daily living conditions. The validity of methods to assess the physical activity level of a subject like questionnaires, interviews, activity records, heart rate monitoring, pedometers or accelerometers can be evaluated by measurement of daily energy expenditure in combination with a measurement or estimate of resting energy expenditure.

Studies on energy expenditure in large numbers of subjects have resulted in prediction equations based on subject characteristics, for situations preventing real measurements or usage as a reference. A well-known example is the Harris and Benedict equation for the prediction of resting energy expenditure, based on height, weight, age and gender [1]. Body weight and habitual physical activity are the main determinants of energy requirements for subjects with different lifestyles. Total energy expenditure, expressed as a multiple of resting or maintenance expenditure, is an expression of the physical activity level (PAL) of a subject. The Food and Agriculture Organization of the United Nations (FAO), World Health Organization (WHO) and United Nations University (UNU) classified lifestyles in relation to the intensity of habitual physical activity or PAL. A sedentary or light activity lifestyle has a PAL value of 1.40–1.69, an active or moderately activity lifestyle has a PAL value of 1.70–1.99 and a vigorous or vigorously activity lifestyle has a PAL value of 2.00–2.40 [2].

Nutrition and pharmacological research uses human energetics for the study of the efficacy of nutrients and drugs for body weight regulation. Then, effects are studied in relation to energy expenditure as well as substrate utilisation. Substrate utilisation, i.e. the oxidation of protein, carbohydrate and fat, can be calculated from the simultaneous measurement of oxygen consumption, carbon dioxide production and urine-nitrogen loss. Thus, it can be evaluated whether a nutrient or drug is thermogenic or affects, for instance, fat oxidation in subjects with overweight and obesity.

Background

Sanctorius (Italy, 1561–1636) started to assess energy expenditure from weight measurements. He observed that the weight of what he ate and drank was larger than the weight loss in faeces and urine. The difference was ascribed to insensible perspiration. We now know insensible perspiration is more a measure for water loss through evaporation than for energy expenditure [3]. The next step was a calorimeter, measuring the heat given off by the body. Lavoisier (Paris, 1780) placed a guinea pig in a cage surrounded by ice. As the ice melted from the animal's body heat, the water was collected in a container. The amount of melted water was a measure for heat production. Heat exchange with the environment was prevented with an outer jacket around the inner jacket surrounding the cage, packed with ice as well. The method of measuring energy expenditure by heat loss is named direct calorimetry. Around 1900, the first direct calorimeter for humans was developed. In between, indirect calorimetry was developed, measuring energy expenditure by measuring oxygen consumption and/or carbon dioxide production. The present state of the art is assessing energy expenditure with indirect calorimetry. Measurement of gas exchange discloses more about metabolic processes.

In indirect calorimetry, energy expenditure is calculated from oxygen consumption, carbon dioxide production and urine-nitrogen loss. The method is based on the relationship between the amount of energy produced in oxidation of the energy substrates carbohydrate, fat and protein and the amount of carbon dioxide produced by this process. Protein oxidation results in carbon dioxide, water and nitrogen, where the latter is excreted in the urine. The resulting three equations with three unknowns can be solved for energy expenditure. Examples of equations for the calculation of energy expenditure derived from these figures are the Weir equation [4]:

$$\text{Energy expenditure}(kJ) = 16.32\,\text{oxygen consumption}(l) + 4.60\,\text{carbon dioxide production}(l) - 2.17\,\text{urine} - \text{nitrogen}(g);$$

and the Brouwer equation [5]:

$$\text{Energy expenditure}(kJ) = 16.20\,\text{oxygen consumption}(l) + 5.00\,\text{carbon dioxide production}(l) - 0.15\,\text{urine} - \text{nitrogen}(g).$$

Differences in the coefficients are caused by differences in assumptions on gaseous exchange and energy release from the metabolised carbohydrate, fat and protein. The contribution of measured urine-nitrogen loss to calculated energy expenditure, the so-called protein correction, is only small. In the case of a normal protein oxidation of 10–15 % of daily energy production, the protein correction for the calculation of energy expenditure is smaller than 1 %. Usually, urine-nitrogen is only measured when information on the contribution of carbohydrate, fat and protein to energy expenditure is required. For calculating the energy expenditure, the protein correction is often neglected.

Comparing indirect calorimetry with direct calorimetry provides information on work efficiency, the fraction of energy expenditure for external work. Webb et al. [6] simultaneously measured energy production and heat loss in subjects at rest, walking on a treadmill and cycling on an ergometer. Subjects stayed in a respiration chamber for measuring energy production from gaseous exchange while wearing a suit calorimeter to quantify heat loss. At rest, indirect calorimetry-assessed energy expenditure matched heat loss as measured with direct calorimetry. Resting energy expenditure was on average 100 Watt, typical for a young adult. During physical activity, heat loss was systematically lower than indirect calorimetry-assessed energy expenditure. The difference increased with walking speed and cycling load. During cycling, indirect calorimetry-assessed energy expenditure matched the sum of heat loss and power output. The work efficiency during cycling, power output divided by energy expenditure, was in the range of 15–25 %. Thus, heat loss matches total energy expenditure at rest but can be up to 25 % lower than total energy expenditure during endurance exercise.

Key Techniques

Current techniques utilising indirect calorimetry for the measurement of energy expenditure in man are a mouthpiece or facemask, ventilated hood, respiration chamber and doubly labelled water.

Mouthpiece or Facemask

Metabolic gas analysis systems with a mouthpiece or facemask are typically used to determine physical fitness in patients and athletes. Oxygen consumption and carbon dioxide production are measured on a breath-by-breath basis. The oxygen and carbon dioxide concentrations are commonly measured with a paramagnetic oxygen analyser and an infrared carbon dioxide analyser, respectively. Flow is measured with a variety of mass flow detectors. Generally, results are based on mathematical integration after reconstructing the waveforms of gas concentrations and matching the curves with the flow signal. Then, the critical aspect is the reconstruction procedure and the temporal alignment of the gas flow with the gas analysis. Alternatively, the system has a mixing chamber, providing mean values for a specified number of breaths or a specified time interval. Measurement systems have evolved from metabolic carts to portable systems for field-based studies. Before and after usage, the system is calibrated with gases of known concentration including ~16 % oxygen, 4–5 % carbon dioxide and room air, and the flow detector is checked by passing a fixed air volume with a syringe. Mouthpiece and facemask systems supply the most direct information on gaseous exchange with minimal response time. Expiration gases can be measured without dilution. Disadvantages are interference with the measurement of breathing through a mouthpiece with nose clip or facemask, also limiting the time interval of measurements.

Ventilated Hood

A ventilated hood is typically used to measure resting energy expenditure and energy expenditure for food processing or diet-induced energy expenditure. The subject lies with his head enclosed in a plastic canopy, sealed off by plastic straps around the neck. Air is sucked through the canopy with a pump and blown into a mixing chamber where a sample is taken for analysis. Measurements taken are those of the airflow and of the oxygen and carbon dioxide concentrations of the air flowing in and out. The airflow is adjusted to keep differences in oxygen and carbon dioxide concentrations between inlet and outlet within a range of 0.5–1.0 %. For adults this means airflow rates around 50 l/min. A ventilated hood allows the subject to relax completely. Discarding the first minutes of an observation interval can eliminate effects of habituation. Calibration with gases of known concentration can be performed before and after as well as during observations, by automated switching. Flow metres usually do not require frequent calibration, showing little or no drift in time. Subjects getting restless limit observation time.

Respiration Chamber

A respiration chamber is an airtight room, which is ventilated with fresh air. Basically the difference between a respiration chamber and a ventilated hood system is size. In a respiration chamber the subject is fully enclosed instead of enclosing the head only, allowing physical activity depending on the size of the chamber. With both methods, the airflow rate and the oxygen and carbon dioxide concentration difference between inlet and outlet air are measured in the same way. The flow rate to keep differences for oxygen and carbon dioxide concentrations between inlet- and outlet air in the range of 0.5–1.0 % is slightly higher in the respiration chamber than in the ventilated hood system as in the chamber subjects never lie down over the full length of an observation interval. In a sedentary adult a typical flow rate is 50–100 l/min, while in exercising subjects the flow has to be increased to over 100 l/min. In the latter situation one has to choose a compromise for the flow rate when measurements are to be continued over 24 h including active and inactive intervals. During exercise bouts the 1 % carbon dioxide level should not be surpassed for long periods. During resting bouts, like an overnight sleep, the level should not fall too far below the optimal measuring range of 0.5–1.0 %. Changing the flow rate during an observation interval reduces the accuracy of the measurements due to the response time of the system. A normal size respiration chamber has a volume of 10–30 m^3 and is equipped with a bed, toilet, washbasin and communication facilities like telephone, radio, television and Internet. Basically it is a hotel room. The experimenter sets the room temperature. Food and drink is delivered through an air lock according to the experimental design. Physical activity is often monitored with a radar system to know when and how often subjects are physically active. A respiration chamber can be equipped with a cycle-ergometer or a treadmill to perform standardised workloads. A respiration chamber has a much longer response time than a ventilated hood. Though the flow rate in both systems is comparable, the volume of a respiration chamber is more than 20 times the volume of a ventilated hood. Consequently, the minimum length of an observation period in a respiration chamber is in the order of 5–10 h.

Doubly Labelled Water

The doubly labelled water technique is the most recent variant of indirect calorimetry. The doubly labelled water technique for the measurement of energy expenditure is based on the discovery that oxygen in the respiratory carbon dioxide is in isotopic equilibrium with the oxygen in body water. The technique involves enriching the body water with an isotope of oxygen and an isotope of hydrogen and then determining the washout kinetics of both isotopes. Most of the oxygen isotope is lost as water, but some is also lost as carbon dioxide because CO_2 in body fluids is in isotopic equilibrium with body water due to exchange in the bicarbonate pools. The hydrogen isotope is lost as water only. Thus, the washout for the oxygen isotope is faster than for the hydrogen isotope, and the difference represents the CO_2 production. The isotopes of choice are the stable, heavy, isotopes of oxygen and hydrogen, oxygen-18 (^{18}O) and deuterium (^2H), since these avoid the need to use radioactivity and can be used safely. Both isotopes naturally occur in drinking water and thus in body water. Oxygen-18 (^{18}O) has eight protons and ten neutrons instead of the eight protons and eight neutrons found in normal oxygen (^{16}O). Deuterium (^2H) has one proton and one neutron instead of one neutron for normal hydrogen (^1H). 'Normal' water consists largely of the lighter isotopes ^1H and ^{16}O, the natural abundance for ^2H is about 150 parts per million or 150 ppm and for ^{18}O 2,000 ppm. Enriching the body water with doubly labelled water ($^2H_2^{18}O$) for the measurement of energy expenditure implies an increase of the background levels as mentioned with 200–300 ppm for ^{18}O and with 100–150 ppm for ^2H. The CO_2 production, calculated from the subsequent difference in elimination between the two isotopes, is a measure of energy expenditure (Fig. 7.1). In practice, the observation duration is set by the biological half-life of the isotopes as a function of the level of the energy expenditure. The minimum observation duration is about 3 days in subjects with a high energy turnover like premature infants or endurance athletes. The maximum duration is 30 days or about 4 weeks in elderly (sedentary) subjects. An observation starts by collecting a baseline sample. Then, a weighed isotope dose is administered, usually a mixture of 10 % ^{18}O and 5 % ^2H in water. For a 70 kg adult, between 100 and 150 cc water would be used. Subsequently the isotopes equilibrate with the body water and the initial sample is collected. The equilibration time is dependent on body size and energy expenditure. For an adult the equilibration time would take between 4 and 8 h. During equilibration the subject usually does not consume any food or drink. After collecting the initial sample, the subject performs routines according to the instructions of the experimenter. Body water samples (blood, saliva or urine) are collected at regular intervals until the end of the observation period. There are different sampling protocols, i.e. multi-point versus two-point method. The ideal protocol is a combination of both, taking two independent samples: at the start, the midpoint and at the end of the observation period. Thus, an independent comparison can be made within one run, calculating CO_2 production from the first samples and the second samples over the first half and the second half of the observation interval. Validation studies, comparing the method with respirometry, have shown that results based on the doubly labelled water method elicit an accuracy of 1–3 % and a precision of 2–8 %. The method requires high-precision isotope ratio mass spectrometry, in order to utilise low amounts of the very expensive ^{18}O isotope. The doubly labelled water technique gives precise and accurate information on carbon dioxide production. Converting CO_2 production to energy expenditure needs information on the energy equivalent of CO_2, which can be calculated with additional information on the substrate mixture being oxidised. One option is the calculation of the energy equivalent from the macronutrient composition of the diet. In energy balance, substrate intake and substrate utilisation are assumed to be identical. Doubly labelled water provides an excellent method to measure energy expenditure in unrestrained humans in their normal surroundings over a time period of 1–4 weeks.

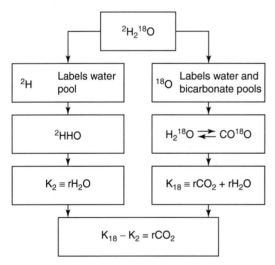

Fig. 7.1 The principle of the doubly labelled water method. The two isotopes, ^{18}O and ^2H as administered as doubly labelled water ($^2H_2^{18}O$), mix with the body water, where ^{18}O exchanges with CO_2 in the bicarbonate pools as well. Thus, the elimination rate of ^2H (K_2) is a measure for water loss (rH_2O) and the elimination rate of ^{18}O (K_{18}) is a measure for rH_2O plus carbon dioxide production (rCO_2), and $rCO_2 = K_{18} - K_2$

Validation of Methods

Calibration of indirect calorimetry methods is usually performed by calibrating the analytic procedures involved, i.e. flow detector and gas analysers or isotope ratio mass spectrometry. Independent validation of the final result should

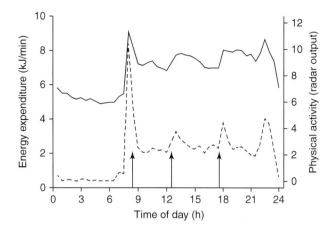

Fig. 7.2 Variation of energy expenditure (*left axis, continuous line*) and physical activity (*right axis, broken line*) throughout a day, as measured in a respiration chamber [11]. *Arrows* denote meal times

be performed as well. Indirect calorimetry systems require regular validation [7]. Mouthpiece and facemask systems are usually validated against the Douglas bag method as a gold standard [8]. For a ventilated hood and respiration chamber, alcohol combustion is a valid and easy-to-use procedure [9]. The result of the doubly labelled method has been evaluated with simultaneous respiratory gas exchange measurements in a respiration chamber [10].

The easiest and reliable method for validating indirect calorimetry is alcohol combustion. Alcohol (99.8 % methanol GR for analysis) is combusted by using a gas burner. The burner is placed on a calibrated balance connected to a computer to measure the rate of combustion during the experiment. The rate of combustion and the time interval for validation are set to mimic the oxygen consumption and carbon dioxide (CO_2) production of subjects to be measured and the experimental design of the study. Mouthpiece and facemask systems can be validated indirectly by performing the test with a subject in a respiration chamber, allowing simultaneous measurement of oxygen consumption and carbon dioxide production with both systems and adopting the validated respiration chamber outcome as the criterion.

Technique Application

Indirect calorimetry methods are used to assess physical performance from energy expenditure for defined activities including VO_2 max and for assessment of daily energy expenditure and its components. Here the focus is on the application for assessment of daily energy expenditure and its components. The components of daily energy expenditure are sleeping metabolic rate (SMR), energy cost of arousal, thermic effect of food or diet-induced energy expenditure (DEE) and energy cost of physical activity or activity-induced energy expenditure (AEE). Sometimes daily energy expenditure is divided into three components, taking sleeping metabolic rate and the energy cost of arousal together as energy expenditure for maintenance or basal metabolic rate (BMR). BMR usually is the main component of daily energy expenditure.

Variation of energy expenditure throughout a day, as measured in a respiration chamber, is presented in Fig. 7.2. Overnight, there generally is no food intake and, when one sleeps quietly, there is little or no physical activity. Energy expenditure gradually decreases to a daily minimum before increasing again at awakening and getting up. Then, the increase is primarily caused by activity-induced energy expenditure and subsequently by diet-induced energy expenditure as soon as one has breakfast. Thus, variation in energy expenditure throughout a day is a function of body size and body composition as determinants of SMR and BMR, physical activity as determinant of AEE and food intake as determinant of DEE.

The indicated method for the measurement of SMR is a respiration chamber and for BMR a ventilated hood, and DEE can be measured in a respiration chamber or with a ventilated hood, as explained in the subsequent sections. Activity-induced energy expenditure can be measured under standardised conditions, as in a respiration chamber, or under free-living conditions with the doubly labelled water method. For the latter, the measurement of total energy with doubly labelled water is combined with a measurement of BMR under a ventilated hood, or alternatively, BMR is estimated with a prediction equation based on height, weight, age and gender of the subject.

Sleeping Metabolic Rate and Basal Metabolic Rate

Basal metabolic rate is defined as the daily rate of energy expenditure to maintain and preserve the integrity of vital functions. The measurement of basal metabolic rate must meet four conditions: the subject is awake, is in a thermoneutral environment to avoid heat production for the maintenance of body temperature, is fasted long enough to eliminate DEE and is at rest to eliminate AEE. For the measurement of sleeping metabolic rate, subjects must be asleep and meet the remaining three conditions for the measurement of BMR.

To perform accurate measurement of BMR, one usually adopts an inpatient protocol. A subject stays overnight in the facility, where food intake and physical activity are strictly controlled, and BMR is measured directly after waking up in the morning. A 10–12-h fast before BMR measurement is the accepted procedure to eliminate DEE. Thus, when BMR is measured at 7.00 AM, subjects should be fasted from about 8.00 PM the day before. High-intensity exercise should be prevented on the day before BMR measurement. An outpatient protocol, where subjects are transported by car or public transport to the facility after spending the night at home, produces sufficiently reproducible results when subjects are carefully instructed and behave accordingly [12].

A protocol for a BMR measurement with a ventilated hood system takes about 30 min. To eliminate effects of subject habituation to the testing procedure, the respiratory measurements

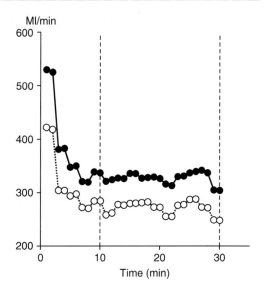

Fig. 7.3 A typical example of a basal metabolic rate measurement with a ventilated hood system, where oxygen consumption (closed dots) and carbon dioxide production (open dots) are plotted in time. To eliminate effects of subject habituation to the testing procedure, the respiratory measurements over the first 10 min are discarded and the following 20 min are used to calculate basal metabolic rate

over the first 10 min are discarded and the following 20 min are used to calculate BMR (Fig. 7.3). The criterion for the chosen time interval is the reproducibility of the calculated BMR value. Longer measurements tend to result in higher values because subjects become restless. It is discouraged to use a mouthpiece or facemask for collection of respiratory gases, introducing stress during breathing and resulting in an overestimate of the BMR value. Similarly, values are generally higher for subjects observed in a sitting position than for subjects in a more relaxed supine position.

Sleeping metabolic rate is based on a number of subsequent data points, as measured in a respiration chamber. The minimum interval for the measurement of energy expenditure in a respiration chamber, set by chamber volume and ventilation rate, is around 30 min. Then, sleeping metabolic rate is defined as the average value of six subsequent 30-min intervals with the lowest value or the lowest residual of the individual relationship between energy expenditure and physical activity over 24 h [13]. Both procedures generally result in the last 3 h of the night before waking up between 3.00 and 7.00 AM (Fig. 7.2). It is advised to measure SMR during a night following free-living conditions. Sleeping metabolic rate tends to be higher during a subsequent night of a longer stay in a respiration chamber due to increased overnight restlessness [14].

Basal metabolic rate and SMR are usually compared between subjects by standardising BMR and SMR to an estimate of metabolic body size, where fat-free mass is the main predictor. The reliable way of comparing BMR or SMR data is by regression analysis. BMR or SMR should never be divided by the absolute fat-free mass value, since the relationship between energy expenditure and fat-free mass has an axis intercept that is significantly different from zero. Comparing SMR per kg fat-free mass between women and men results in significantly higher values for women than for men. The smaller the fat-free mass, the higher the SMR/kg, and thus, the SMR per kg fat-free mass is on average higher in women with a lower fat-free mass compared to men. When fat-free mass and gender are included as covariates in a regression analysis, gender does not come out as a significant contributor to the explained variation.

In conclusion, basal metabolic rate or sleeping metabolic rate measurements should meet the conditions of being awake or asleep, respectively, being post absorptive, at rest and in the thermoneutral zone. Measured values can be compared between subjects in a regression analysis with fat-free mass and fat mass as covariates.

Diet-Induced Energy Expenditure

Diet-induced energy expenditure (DEE) is the energy expenditure for intestinal absorption of nutrients, the initial steps of their metabolism and the storage of the absorbed but not immediately oxidised nutrients. It is measured as the increase in energy expenditure above the basal fasting level after consumption of a meal, defined as the increase in energy expenditure above the basal fasting level divided by the energy content of the food ingested and commonly expressed as a percentage.

The experimental design of most studies on DEE is a measurement of resting energy expenditure before and after a test meal, with a ventilated hood system. The observation is started after an overnight fast, where subjects are refrained from eating after the last meal at 8.00 PM at the latest. Thus, with observations starting between 8.00 and 9.00 h AM the next morning, the fasting interval is at least 12 h. Postprandial measurements are made for several hours while subjects have to remain stationery, most often in a supine position, for the duration of the measurements. In some studies, measurements are 30 min with 15-min intervals allowing, e.g. for sanitary activities. A study in 131 different subjects, measured for 6 h after a breakfast covering 25 % of usual intake, indicated that DEE lasted beyond 6 h for the majority of subjects [15].

The use of a respiration chamber to measure DEE has the advantage of reproducing more physiological conditions over a longer period of time while regular meals are consumed throughout the day. The DEE, as observed in a respiration chamber over 24 h has been evaluated in different ways: (1) as the difference in 24-h energy expenditure between a day in the fed state and a day in the fasted state, (2) as the difference in daytime energy expenditure adjusted for the variability of spontaneous activity and basal metabolic rate and (3) as the difference in 24-h energy expenditure adjusted for the variability of spontaneous activity and basal metabolic rate [16]. Method 1 tends to overestimate DEE as fasting excludes DEE but might reduce AEE as well. Method 2 results in an underestimate of DEE, as DEE does not stop at bedtime [17]. Thus, method 3 is the indicated approach for the measurement of DEE in a respiration chamber.

The pattern of DEE throughout the day, calculated by plotting the residual of the individual relationship between energy expenditure and physical activity, as measured over 30-min intervals from a 24-h observation in a respiration chamber, in time is presented in Fig. 7.4. The level of resting metabolic rate after waking up in the morning, and directly before the first meal, was defined as basal metabolic rate. Resting metabolic rate did not return to basal metabolic rate

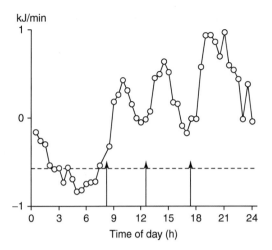

Fig. 7.4 The mean pattern of diet-induced energy expenditure throughout the day, calculated by plotting the residual of the individual relationship between energy expenditure and physical activity, as measured over 30-min intervals from a 24-h observation in a respiration chamber, in time [18]. *Arrows* denote meal times

before lunch at 4 h after breakfast or before dinner at 5 h after lunch. Overnight, basal metabolic rate was reached at 8–9 h after dinner consumption. It confirms DEE lasts beyond 6 h and a 10–12-h fast before BMR measurement is the accepted procedure to eliminate DEE.

Reported intra-individual variability in DEE, determined with ventilated hood systems, is 5–30 % [19]. Reported within-subject variability in DIT, determined with a respiration chamber, is 40–50 % [16]. The figures for the respiration chamber measurements are for the 24-h DEE calculation as described above under method 3, 24-h energy expenditure adjusted for the variability of spontaneous activity and basal metabolic rate. Method 2, daytime energy expenditure adjusted for the variability of spontaneous activity and basal metabolic rate, resulted in an intra-individual variability of 125 %.

Based on the amount of ATP required for the initial steps of metabolism and storage, the DEE is different for each nutrient. Reported DEE values for separate nutrients are 0–3 % for fat, 5–10 % for carbohydrate, 20–30 % for protein [20] and 10–30 % for alcohol [21]. In healthy subjects with a mixed diet, DEE represents about 10 % of the total amount of energy ingested over 24 h. Thus, when a subject is in energy balance, where intake equals expenditure, DEE is 10 % of daily energy expenditure.

Activity-Induced Energy Expenditure

Activity-induced energy expenditure (AEE) is the most variable component of daily energy expenditure. The indicated method for the measurement of AEE is the doubly labelled water method for the measurement of total energy expenditure (TEE) in combination with a measurement of basal metabolic rate under a ventilated hood as described above. Then, AEE is calculated as TEE − (DEE + BMR) or $0.9 \times$ TEE − BMR, where DEE is 10 % of daily energy expenditure when intake equals expenditure as described above as well.

The observation interval for the measurement of TEE with doubly labelled water ideally covers a representative interval of daily life activity, i.e. 1 or more weeks. The number of weeks is a function of the biological half-life of the isotopes as determined by the level of physical activity. One week is the optimal observation interval for extremely active subjects like professional endurance athletes. Adults with a light or moderately active lifestyle are usually observed for 2 weeks. Subjects with a sedentary lifestyle like elderly and nursing home residents can be observed for 3 or 4 weeks. Thus, the doubly labelled water method provides a weekly average for AEE.

There are several methods to compare the physical activity level between subjects. The most common method, as adopted by the Food and Agricultural Organization of the United Nations, the World Health Organization and the United Nations University, is to express TEE as a multiple of BMR: physical activity level (PAL) = TEE/BMR [2]. It assumes that variation in TEE is due to body size and physical activity, where the effect of body size is corrected for by expressing TEE as a multiple of BMR. Additionally, it assumes the relationship between TEE and BMR has no significant intercept. The most sophisticated way to compare the physical activity level between subjects is a linear regression analysis.

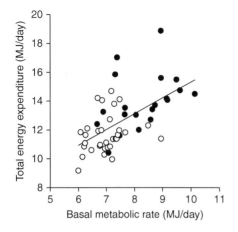

Fig. 7.5 Total energy expenditure plotted as a function of basal metabolic rate with the calculated linear regression line. Subjects were 31 women (*open dots*) and 20 men (*closed dots*) from a study in obese subjects observed before weight loss [22]

Then, the activity measure is the residual of the regression of TEE on BMR. Subjects with a positive residual have a higher physical activity than the group average and subjects with a negative residual have a lower physical activity than the group average. An example is presented in Fig. 7.5. Data are from a study in obese subjects, 20 men and 31 women before weight loss [22]. There was a close correlation between the individual values of the residual of the regression of TEE on BMR and the PAL ($r=0.94$, $p<0.0001$). The three men with the highest residual had the highest PAL value as well, 2.2, 2.3 and 2.1, respectively.

The common method to adjust AEE for differences in body size is by expressing AEE per kg body mass. It assumes that subjects weighing 100 kg spend twice as much energy for the same activities as subjects weighing 50 kg. However, not all daily activities are mass dependent. Normalising AEE by dividing by body mass to the exponent 1.0 might overcorrect for body size in heavier subjects, making them appear less active. Thus, caution must be exercised when interpreting AEE data from individuals of markedly different body size. So far, physical activity level calculated as TEE divided by BMR, where BMR scales to metabolic body mass or body mass to the exponent 0.66–0.75, seems to be the best compromise. The majority of the population has a physical activity level ranging from 1.5 to 2.0. The World Health Organization defined an activity factor below 1.7 as sedentary or light activity lifestyle, between 1.7 and 2.0 moderately active to active and above 2.0 as vigorously active [2].

Validation of Alternative Methods

Energy requirement is ideally based on measured energy expenditure. When individual energy requirements cannot be measured by indirect calorimetry, there are alternative methods to estimate energy expenditure. Here, methods are presented for the estimation of resting energy expenditure, activity-induced energy expenditure and total energy expenditure. Resting metabolic rate or BMR is often estimated with prediction equations, based on weight, sex, age and height of a subject or on body composition. Activity-induced energy expenditure can be estimated from observation, self-report and physiological measures like heart rate or body movement. Total energy expenditure can be estimated from a combination of estimated BMR and AEE and from reported food intake. All estimation procedures should be validated with indirect calorimetry.

Basal Metabolic Rate

The oldest prediction equations for BMR, still in use, are the Harris and Benedict equations [1]. The equations are based on measurements of BMR in one laboratory over a 10-year interval. Subject characteristics covered a wide range for age, weight and height and included similar numbers of both genders (Table 7.1). The equations were developed to predict BMR from age, weight and height, separately for women and men. Prediction equations from later years sometimes include body composition, i.e. fat-free mass (FFM) and fat mass (FM), instead of age, weight and height. Then, data from women and men are often combined in the same equation. Here, an example is the Westerterp equation [23]:

Table 7.1 Characteristics of the subjects of the Harris and Benedict prediction equation for basal metabolic rate [1]

	Women n=103			Men n=136		
	Mean	SD	Range	Mean	SD	Range
Age (years)	31	14	15–74	27	9	16–63
Height (m)	1.62	0.05	1.51–1.76	1.73	0.08	1.48–1.98
Body mass (kg)	56	11	36–94	64	10	33–109
BMR (MJ/day)	5.6	0.7	4.1–7.4	6.8	0.9	4.2–10.7

BMR basal metabolic rate

Table 7.2 Characteristics of the subjects of the Westerterp et al. prediction equation for basal metabolic rate [23]

	Women n=105			Men n=85		
	Mean	SD	Range	Mean	SD	Range
Age (years)	42	20	20–95	42	19	19–80
Height (m)	1.63	0.08	1.38–1.81	1.77	0.08	1.60–2.05
Body mass (kg)	62	16	38–130	80	24	55–215
Fat-free mass (kg)	42	6	29–60	61	10	44–93
Fat mass (kg)	19	12	3–76	19	17	2–128
BMR (MJ/day)	5.6	0.9	3.4–8.2	7.6	1.4	4.7–12.7

BMR basal metabolic rate

$$\text{BMR} \, (\text{MJ}/\text{day}) = 0.102 \, \text{FFM} \, (\text{kg}) + 0.024 \, \text{FM} \, (\text{kg}) + 0.85$$

The database for the Westerterp equation covers a slightly wider range of subjects (Table 7.2) than the Harris and Benedict equation, especially with regard to age and weight. Applying the Harris and Benedict equation to predict the BMR of the subjects in the database for the Westerterp equation results in a mean difference of only 1.5 % with the measured value, showing the applicability of equations to predict BMR.

Nowadays, the most widely used prediction equations for BMR are the Schofield equations [24] and the FAO/WHO/UNU equations [25], based on hundreds of data from many laboratories. Surprisingly, more data does not necessarily imply better equations. Heterogeneity between publications is greater than might be expected by chance, probably due to undocumented technique differences between laboratories [26]. Based on a review of more extended data sets generated between 1985 and 2000, the FAO decided to continue to use the Schofield prediction equations as mentioned in the last report [2]. The validity of the equations has been shown for patients, including outpatients and inpatients [27].

Most prediction equations, like the ones mentioned above, are based on measurements in white subjects. Application in non-white subjects might lead to systematic errors. Wouters-Adriaens and Westerterp [28] showed measured BMR in Asian subjects was significantly lower than predicted with the Schofield equations based on height, weight, age and gender. Basal metabolic rate predicted with the Westerterp equation, based on fat-free mass and fat mass, was not different from measured values. Thus, racial differences in body composition should be taken into account by using a body composition based equation for predicting BMR in non-white subjects. Comparing measured BMR between subjects by adjusting for differences in body composition should be performed in a regression analysis, with fat-free mass and fat mass as covariates, as mentioned in the section on sleeping metabolic rate and basal metabolic rate.

Activity-Induced Energy Expenditure

Activity-induced energy expenditure can be estimated from behavioural observation, self-report and physiological measures like heart rate or body movement. The method of choice is

Table 7.3 Ranking of methods for the estimation of activity-induced energy expenditure on four different parameters where 1 denotes the highest and 4 the lowest rank

	Subject interference	Subject effort	Observer effort	Data quality
Behavioural observation	4	1	4	3
Self-report	3	4	2	4
Heart rate monitoring	2	3	3	2
Motion sensors	1	2	1	1

a function of input parameters including subject interference and subject effort and output parameters including observer effort and data validity. Methods can be ranked, based on the four parameters mentioned (Table 7.3). Motion sensors minimally interfere with the activity behaviour of a subject, the application takes little effort for the subject as well as the observer and the data quality is potentially high, depending on the choice of a properly validated sensor. For behavioural observation, the subject effort is minimal though the risk of interference with the activity behaviour of the subject is maximal. Direct observation of subjects is very time consuming and the translation of activity behaviour to activity-induced energy expenditure is subjective with regard to the estimation of activity intensity. Self-report, where the subject does the classification, is even more subjective with regard to the estimation of activity intensity. On the other hand, short questionnaires can have surprisingly good results as shown by a doubly labelled water validation of the assessment of the physical activity level with two questions [29]. Heart rate monitoring was one of the first objective methods for the assessment of physical activity. However, heart rate requires individual calibration with indirect calorimetry for the translation to activity-induced energy expenditure, and heart rate is affected by more factors than physical activity.

Motion sensors are the most promising for the assessment of activity-induced energy expenditure. Sensors can be applied in free-living subjects over prolonged periods of time. When equipped with a data memory to store information on body movement, they can also be used to study patterns of physical activity in time. Various sensors have been developed from mechanical devices to electronic accelerometers. Accelerometers can provide information about the total amount, the frequency, the intensity and the duration of physical activity. The validity is generally based on a comparison between accelerometer output and doubly labelled water-assessed energy expenditure in a multiple regression analysis with subject characteristics as additional covariates. The separate contribution of accelerometer counts to the explained variation in activity-induced energy expenditure is often not presented and standard errors or limits of agreement are large or not presented [30]. So far, the best results were found for the Tracmor, a device with the first published doubly labelled water validation [31]. A recent version (DirectLife, Philips New Wellness Solutions, the Netherlands) allows determining outcome parameters of physical activity such as total energy expenditure, physical activity level and activity-induced energy expenditure [32]. Validity of energy expenditure prediction equations developed in lean subjects was extended to overweight and obese subjects [33].

Total Energy Expenditure

Total energy expenditure is a function of body size and physical activity. Body size and body composition determine maintenance expenditure or basal metabolic rate. Body movement or physical activity determines activity-induced energy expenditure. The remaining component, diet-induced energy expenditure, is a fixed fraction of total energy expenditure, i.e. about 10 % when intake equals energy expenditure.

The first step in the estimation of total energy expenditure is the calculation of maintenance expenditure or basal metabolic rate with a prediction equation based on gender, age, weight and height or on fat-free mass and fat mass of the subject. Subsequently, maintenance expenditure or basal metabolic rate is multiplied with a value for the physical activity level to get at total energy expenditure. The physical activity level is ideally based on a measurement with a doubly labelled water-validated accelerometer.

In the absence of an accelerometer-based estimate of the physical activity level, one can make a reasonable estimate with questions on physical activity at home, at work and during leisure time. The physical activity level is around 1.4 for somebody staying home and not performing specific physical exercise. A value of 2.3 is for someone doing heavy industrial or construction work or farming and performing strenuous activities several times a week during leisure time. The values in between are a weighed average of what one does at work and during leisure time. Somebody who is very inactive at work and very active during leisure time reaches an activity factor of 1.9. One who has a lot of free time with very little physical activity only reaches this value when very active at work. The average value for an adult aged 20–50 years is around 1.7.

The value of accelerometer-based estimations of total energy expenditure should be interpreted with care. Estimations are usually based on proprietary formulas, where one has to put in gender, height, age and weight of the subject. The algorithm for the calculation of resting energy expenditure and the contribution of accelerometer counts to the explained variation in total energy expenditure is an unknown. Then, validation studies, ideally with simultaneously doubly labelled water-measured total energy expenditure, only apply for the hardware and software as applied and cannot be extrapolated to other devices or subject populations.

Food Intake as Measure for Energy Expenditure

Food intake in humans in their own environment is one of the most difficult parameters to measure. Still, until the application of the doubly labelled water method for the measurement of daily energy expenditure, energy requirement was based on energy intake as calculated from food intake. Additionally, measured food intake is often related to health and disease.

Food intake can be measured on national, household or individual level. Here, the focus is on the measurement of individual food intake. Then, all methods rely on self-report. Typical methods for the measurement of individual food intake are diet history and diet record methods. Diet history methods involve an estimation by recall of food consumed over the last day, week or longer. Diet record methods involve measurement and recording of food intake as it is eaten in daily life for 1, 3, 7 or more days. Measured food intake is converted to intake of energy, macronutrients and micronutrients using food composition tables.

Assessment of food intake is subject to different types of error, depending on the method used. Errors in food composition tables and coding errors are for all methods the same and are relatively small. Larger errors in the assessment of food intake are due to the phenomenon that subjects tell the interviewer or record their perception of what they eat instead of their real consumption. Thus, the information can be qualitatively and quantitatively wrong. Weighing all foods consumed in a weighed dietary record can solve the latter. However, weighing all foods might interfere more with habitual consumption than other methods do.

The length of the observation period depends on the day-to-day variability in intake. Humans do not balance intake and expenditure on a daily basis, as smaller animals do. Of course, humans maintain a perfect energy balance in the long term as shown by a constant body weight in adult life. Energy intake strongly correlates with energy expenditure on a weekly basis. Discrepancies on a daily basis between intake and expenditure are especially large when days with a high energy expenditure are alternated with quieter intervals. Military cadets did not show an increase in energy intake on days with higher energy expenditure when they joined a drill competition. The corresponding increase in energy intake came about 2 days afterwards

[34]. Generally, weekdays are different from weekend days with respect to energy intake or energy expenditure or both. Ideally, the observation period covers a full week, like a 7-day dietary record.

Validation of intake methods must be independent of the dietary assessment method used. Validating a diet history method with a diet record method is useless, where both methods are similarly biased by the phenomenon that subjects tell the interviewer or record their perception of what they eat instead of their real consumption. The indicated reference method is measured or estimated total energy expenditure. The doubly labelled water method is the most accurate method for the validation of reported intake by subjects in their own environment. However, costs make it less practical for validation in a large number of subjects. Then, a combination of measured or estimated basal metabolic rate and physical activity is an alternative. A further simplification is the identification of invalid reporting with defined cut-off limits for the ratio between reported energy intake and estimated basal metabolic rate. Values of energy intake/BMR lower than 1.35 are recognised as under-reporting, assuming that values below 1.35 are not very likely unless someone has a very inactive lifestyle [35]. However, a value higher than 1.35 does not guarantee a higher agreement of reported intake with energy requirement. Individual energy requirement has a wide range with a minimum value of 1.35 times BMR for very inactive subjects to a maximum value of 2.0–2.5 times BMR for extremely active individuals.

Validation studies of food intake reporting show over-reporting and under-reporting. Over-reporting often happens when caregivers and nurses report what they feed children or patients. Under-reporting usually occurs when subjects report intake their selves. A clear example of the first, over-reporting, is a study in children and adolescents with cerebral palsy [36]. Most subjects had severe feeding problems and were fed by the caregivers, recording intake as well. Recorded intake was 45 % higher than doubly labelled water-measured energy expenditure, reflecting perceived instead of actual intake. Under-reporting of habitual intake can be explained by under-recording and undereating. Comparing reported food intake and water intake with energy expenditure and water loss could separate the two errors. Since most foodstuffs contain water, when subjects record food intake, they are also recording water intake. In healthy individuals, water balance is preserved and is therefore an independent indicator for under-recording. The recording precision of water intake is assumed to be representative for total food recording, as most foodstuffs contain water. Undereating during food recording was monitored by measurement of body mass. Body mass changes over a food-recording period are compared with normal body mass fluctuations. Figure 7.6 shows the percentage under-reporting, divided into undereating and under-recording (open bar) as observed in lean women [37],

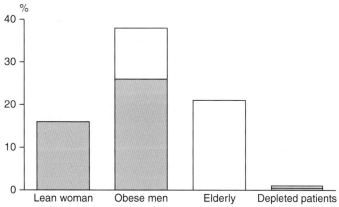

Fig. 7.6 The percentage under-reporting of habitual food intake, divided into undereating (*stippled bar*) and under-recording (*open bar*), as observed in lean women [37], obese men [38], elderly men and women [39] and depleted patients [40]

obese men [38], elderly men and women [39] and depleted patients [40]. Both the obese men and lean women ate less while recording food intake, but probably for different reasons. The lean women ate less because weighing and recording food intake was perceived as a great burden, which might also count for the obese men. However, the obese men used the recording period also as an opportunity to start dieting. The recording error observed in the obese men and in the elderly men and women was probably due to underestimation of self-determined food portion sizes and to not recording of all foods consumed. Only the depleted patients reported their food intake accurately and they did not change their diet while recording food intake.

Under-reporting has consequences for interventions where subjects are fed according to energy requirement based on reported intake. In a controlled intervention study, a control group was planned to receive a weight-maintenance diet, while the experimental group was planned to receive a diet containing 20 % less than the energy of their habitual diet, estimated by means of a 7-day dietary record [41]. Reported energy intake appeared to be 82.5 % of daily energy expenditure as measured with doubly labelled water. Thus, the control group lost weight and the actual level of energy restriction of the experimental group was 33 % rather than 20 %. Under-reporting increases with successive measurements, complicating the evaluation of interventions on food intake. In a study on the effect of exercise training on food intake, reported energy intake was unchanged, whereas energy expenditure increased more than 20 % and body weight did not change much over a 40-week interval [42]. Measurement of energy intake, with a 7-day dietary record, was performed before the start of the training and at 8, 20 and 40 weeks after the start of the training. At the start, the difference between reported energy intake and simultaneously measured energy expenditure (with doubly labelled water) was -4 ± 16 %. The difference between reported energy intake and measured energy expenditure at week 40 was -19 ± 17 %, which was approximately equivalent to the increase in energy requirements. The misreporting prevented the detection of intervention effects on food intake and on the nutrient composition of the diet.

Under-reporting of food intake seems to be selective. In a study in obese men, the reported percentage of energy from fat was negatively correlated with the amount of under-reporting [38]. In subjects with the highest level of under-reporting, the reported fraction of energy from fat was only 25–30 %. In subjects with the lowest level of under-reporting, the reported fraction of energy from fat was as much as 45–50 %. In case of no under-reporting, the percentage of energy from fat would be 46 ± 5 %, much higher than the reference intake value of up to 30 %. Thus, campaigns aimed at changing food intake might not be as successful as concluded from the results of national food consumption methods. Subjects might be reporting according to expected instead of real intake.

There is not yet a method for the accurate determination of dietary intake. A potential solution is to confront subjects with earlier results of food reporting [43]. The use of a combination of basal metabolic rate, measured or estimated, and physical activity assessed with a triaxial accelerometer is a good method for validating reported intake [44].

Applications in the Clinical Setting

Energy expenditure measurements in the clinical setting are the basis for the prevention of disease-induced weight loss – here, the example of chronic obstructive pulmonary disease (COPD). Patients with COPD often suffer from weight loss due to an inadequate dietary intake combined with increased energy expenditure. Physical activity, as the main determinant of variation in energy requirement, plays an important role. Interestingly, there was no difference in total energy expenditure between COPD patients with normal resting energy expenditure and those with increased resting energy expenditure [45]. Patients with normal resting energy expenditure appeared to have higher energy expenditure for activities than those patients with COPD who had increased resting energy expenditure. The activity factor was significantly higher in the former group (1.78) than in the latter group (1.58). Physical activity affects the energy need of the COPD patient and determines energy balance. In depleted ambulatory outpatients with COPD, energy balance could be reached with oral nutritional supplements as a function of physical activity. Weight change was negatively associated with the energy requirement for physical activity. Patients with an activity factor above 1.55 lost weight and with an activity factor below 1.55 gained weight [40]. The disease appears to be an important limitation for an active lifestyle.

Energy expenditure measurements are the basis for the opposite as well, induction of weight loss in obese subjects. Weight loss results in a disproportionate reduction of energy expenditure as a persistent risk factor of weight regain. A smaller body has a lower maintenance requirement and resting energy expenditure of a postobese subject is even lower than resting energy expenditure of a 'normal' subject with the same body composition [46]. Measurements in subjects at more than 3 years after surgical weight loss showed similar results [47]. Weight loss induced by energy restriction leads to a decrease in physical activity as well [22]. However, physical activity returns to baseline levels when weight loss is maintained. Physical activity and sustained intakes of dietary protein may be the best strategies available to prevent the decline in resting energy expenditure [48]. Antiobesity drugs often show effects on both sides of the energy balance equation, where measurable effects on energy expenditure are generally small and the main effect must be ascribed to a reduction of appetite and an increase in satiety [49–51].

Conclusions

To ensure maintenance of body weight, subjects should be fed according to measured or estimated energy expenditure rather than reported intake. Evaluations of interventions to affect energy balance are preferably based on measured energy expenditure as well. The indicated method, including facemask, ventilated hood, respiration chamber or doubly labelled water, depends on the energy expenditure component as targeted. Alternative methods are subject characteristic-based prediction equations for maintenance expenditure and doubly labelled water validated-accelerometers for activity-induced energy expenditure. Applications show intervention effects on energy expenditure to be generally small, where larger effects on energy balance must be ascribed to effects on energy intake.

References

1. Harris JA, Benedict FG. A biometric study of the basal metabolism in man. Washington: Carnegie Institution; 1919, publ 279.
2. FAO/WHO/UNU. Human energy requirement. Rome 2004.
3. Westerterp KR. Body weight change during over- and underfeeding as an indicator of adaptive thermogenesis. Br J Nutr. 2004;92:541–4.
4. de V Weir JB. New methods for calculating metabolic rate with special reference for protein metabolism. J Physiol. 1949;109:1–9.
5. Brouwer E. On simple formulae for calculating the heat expenditure and the quantities of carbohydrate and fat oxidized in metabolism of men and animals, from gaseous exchange (oxygen intake and carbonic acid output) and urine-N. Acta Physiol Pharmacol Neerl. 1957;6:795–802.
6. Webb P, Saris WHM, Schoffelen PFM, Van Ingen Schenau GJ, Ten Hoor F. The work of walking: a calorimetric study. Med Sci Sports Exerc. 1988;20:331–7.
7. Schadewaldt P, Nowotny B, Straßburger K, Kotzka J, Roden M. Indirect calorimetry in humans: a postcalorimetric evaluation procedure for correction of metabolic monitor variability. Am J Clin Nutr. 2013;97:763–73.
8. Rietjens GJWM, Kuipers H, Kester ADM, Keizer HA. Validation of a computerized metabolic measurement system (Oxycon-Pro®) during low and high intensity exercise. Int J Sports Med. 2001;22:291–4.
9. Schoffelen PFM, Westerterp KR, Saris WHM, Ten Hoor F. A dual-respiration chamber system with automated calibration. J Appl Physiol. 1997;83:2064–72.
10. Schoeller DA. Measurement of energy expenditure in free-living humans by using doubly labeled water. J Nutr. 1988;118:1278–89.
11. Verboeket-van de Venne WPHG, Westerterp KR, Hermans-Limpens TJFMB, De Graaf C, Van het Hof KH, Weststrate JA. Long-term effects of consumption of full-fat or reduced-fat products in healthy non-obese

volunteers; assessment of energy expenditure and substrate oxidation. Metabolism. 1996;45:1004–10.
12. Adriaens MPE, Schoffelen PFM, Westerterp KR. Intra-individual variation of basal metabolic rate and the influence of physical activity before testing. Br J Nutr. 2003;90:419–23.
13. Westerterp KR, Wilson SAJ, Rolland A. Diet-induced thermogenesis measured over 24h in a respiration chamber: effect of diet composition. Int J Obes. 1999;23:287–92.
14. Schoffelen PFM, Westerterp KR. Intra-individual variability and adaptation of overnight- and sleeping metabolic rate. Physiol Beh. 2008;94:158–63.
15. Reed GW, Hill JO. Measuring the thermic effect of food. Am J Clin Nutr. 1996;63:164–9.
16. Tataranni PA, Larson DE, Snitker S, Ravussin E. Thermic effect of food in humans: methods and results from use of a respiratory chamber. Am J Clin Nutr. 1995;61:1013–9.
17. Goldberg GR, Prentice AM, Davies HL, Murgatroyd PR. Overnight and basal metabolic rates in men and women. Eur J Clin Nutr. 1988;42:137–44.
18. Westerterp KR. Diet induced thermogenesis. Nutr Metab. 2004;1:5.
19. Weststrate JA. Resting metabolic rate and diet-induced thermogenesis: a methodological reappraisal Am J Clin Nutr. 1993;58:592–601.
20. Tappy L. Thermic effect of food and sympathetic nervous system activity in humans. Reprod Nutr Dev. 1996;36:391–7.
21. Suter PM, Jequier E, Schutz Y. Effect of ethanol on energy expenditure. Am J Physiol. 1994;266:R1204–12.
22. Camps SG, Verhoef SP, Westerterp KR. Weight loss-induced reduction in physical activity recovers during weight maintenance. Am J Clin Nutr. 2013;98:917–23.
23. Westerterp KR, Donkers J, Fredrix EWHM, Boekhoudt P. Energy intake, physical activity and body weight; a simulation model. Br J Nutr. 1995;73:337–47.
24. Schofield WN. Predicting basal metabolic rate, new standards and review of previous work. Hum Nutr Clin Nutr. 1985;39C:5–41.
25. FAO/WHO/UNU. Energy and protein requirements. WHO technical report series. Geneva 1985.
26. Cole TJ, Henry CJK. The Oxford Brookes basal metabolic rate database – a reanalysis. Publ Health Nutr. 2005;8:1202–12.
27. Weijs PJM, Kruizinga HM, Van Dijk AE, Van der Meij BS, Langius JAE, Knol DL, et al. Validation of predictive equations for resting energy expenditure in adult outpatients and inpatients. Clin Nutr. 2008;27:150–7.
28. Wouters-Adriaens MP, Westerterp KR. Low resting energy expenditure in Asians can be attributed to body composition. Obesity. 2008;16:2212–6.
29. Johansson G, Westerterp KR. Assessment of the physical activity level with two questions: validation with doubly labeled water. Int J Obes. 2008;32:1031–3.
30. Plasqui G, Westerterp KR. Physical activity assessment with accelerometers: an evaluation against doubly labeled water. Obesity. 2007;15:2371–9.
31. Bouten CVC, Verboeket-van de Venne WPHG, Westerterp KR, Verduin M, Janssen JD. Physical activity assessment: comparison between movement registration and doubly labeled water. J Appl Physiol. 1996;81:1019–26.
32. Bonomi AG, Plasqui G, Goris AH, Westerterp KR. Estimation of free-living energy expenditure using a novel activity monitor designed to minimize obtrusiveness. Obesity. 2010;18:1845–51.
33. Valenti G, Camps S, Verhoef S, Bonomi AG, Westerterp KR. Validating measures of free-living physical activity in overweight and obese subjects using an accelerometer. Int J Obes. 2014;38(7):1011–4.
34. Edholm OG, Fletcher JG, Widdowson EW, McCance RA. The energy expenditure and food intake of individual men. Br J Nutr. 1955;9:286–300.
35. Goldberg GR, Black AE, Jebb SA, Cole TJ, Murgatroyd PR, Coward WA, Prentice AM. Critical evaluation of energy intake data using fundamental principles of energy physiology: 1. Derivation of cut-off limits to identify under-recording. Eur J Clin Nutr. 1991;45:569–81.
36. Stallings VA, Zemel BS, Davies JC, Cronk CE, Charney EB. Energy expenditure of children and adolescents with severe disabilities: a cerebral palsy model. Am J Clin Nutr. 1996;64:627–34.
37. Goris AHC, Westerterp KR. Underreporting of habitual food intake is explained by undereating in highly motivated lean women. J Nutr. 1999;129:878–82.
38. Goris AHC, Westerterp-Plantenga MS, Westerterp KR. Undereating and underrecording of habitual food intake in obese men: selective underreporting of fat intake. Am J Clin Nutr. 2000;71:130–4.
39. Goris AHC, Meijer EP, Westerterp. Repeated measurement of habitual food intake increases under-reporting and induces selective under-reporting. Br J Nutr. 2001;85:629–34.
40. Goris AHC, Vermeeren MAP, Wouters EFM, Schols AMWJ, Westerterp KR. Energy balance in depleted ambulatory patients with chronic obstructive pulmonary disease; the effect of physical activity and oral nutritional supplementation. Br J Nutr. 2003;89:725–9.
41. Velthuis-te Wierik EJM, Westerterp KR, Van den Berg H. Impact of a moderately energy-restricted diet on energy metabolism and body composition in non-obese men. Int J Obes. 1995;19:318–24.
42. Westerterp KR, Meijer GAL, Janssen EME, Saris WHM, Ten Hoor F. Long term effect of physical activity on energy balance and body composition. Br J Nutr. 1992;68:21–30.
43. Goris AHC, Westerterp KR. Improved reporting of habitual food intake after confrontation with earlier results on food reporting. Br J Nutr. 2000;83:363–9.
44. Goris AHC, Meijer EP, Kester A, Westerterp KR. The use of a tri-axial accelerometer for the validity of reported food intake. Am J Clin Nutr. 2001;73:549–53.

45. Baarends EM, Schols AMWJ, Westerterp KR, Wouters EFM. Total daily energy expenditure relative to resting energy expenditure in clinically stable patients with COPD. Thorax. 1997;52:780–5.
46. Camps SG, Verhoef SP, Westerterp KR. Weight loss, weight maintenance and adaptive thermogenesis. Am J Clin Nutr. 2013;97:990–4.
47. Van Gemert WG, Westerterp KR, Greve JWM, Soeters PB. Reduction of sleeping metabolic rate after vertical banded gastroplasty. Int J Obes. 1998;22:343–8.
48. Thivel D, Brakonieki K, Duche P, Morio B, Boirie Y, Laferrère B. Surgical weight loss: impact on energy expenditure. Obes Surg. 2013;23:255–66.
49. Hansen DL, Toubro S, Stock MJ, Macdonald IA, Astrup A. Thermogenic effects of sibutramine in humans. Am J Clin Nutr. 1998;68:1180–6.
50. Wyne K, Park AJ, Small CJ, Meeran K, Ghatei MA, Frost GS, Bloom SR. Oxyntomodulin increases energy expenditure in addition to decreasing energy intake in overweight and obese humans: a randomised controlled trial. Int J Obes. 2006;30:1729–36.
51. Sjödin A, Gasteyger C, Nielsen A-LH, Raben A, Mikkelsen JD, Jensen JKS, Meier D, Astrup A. The effect of the triple monoamine reuptake inhibitor tesofensine on energy metabolism and appetite in overweight and moderately obese men. Int J Obes. 2010;34:1634–43.

Omics: Potential Role in Early-Phase Drug Development

Harald Grallert, Carola S. Marzi, Stefanie M. Hauck, and Christian Gieger

Keywords

Genomics • Epigenomics • Transcriptomics • Proteomics • Metabolomics • Microarray • Sequencing • Disease prediction • Pharmacogenomics • Personalized medicine

Summary

Background

The development of high-throughput omics technologies has nourished the hope to improve our understanding and treatment of the pathophysiology of globally increasing diseases such as type 2 diabetes and obesity. These technologies provide innovative tools that have the potential to truly revolutionize patient care.

H. Grallert, PhD (✉) • C.S. Marzi, PhD
Research Unit of Molecular Epidemiology,
Institute of Epidemiology II, Helmholtz Zentrum
München, German Research Center for Evironmental
Health (GmbH), Neuherberg, Germany
e-mail: harald.grallert@helmholtz-muenchen.de

S.M. Hauck, PhD
Research Unit Protein Science,
Helmholtz Zentrum München – German Research
Center for Environmental Health (GmbH),
Ingolstädter Landstr. 1, Neuherberg, Germany

C. Gieger, PhD
Research Unit of Molecular Epidemiology, Institute
of Genetic Epidemiology, Helmholtz Zentrum
München, German Research Center
for Environmental Health (GmbH),
Neuherberg, Germany

Key Methods

Genomics, Epigenomics, Transcriptomics

	Methodology/ platforms	Measurement	Advantages	Disadvantages	Value in drug development decisions
Single locus (<100) determination	PCR-based assays on different platforms	PCR products depending on allele by fluorescence, gel electrophoresis, or matrix-assisted laser desorption/ionization- time of flight (MALDI-TOF)	Provides data for single to few targets of interest; relatively inexpensive; customizable	Only applicable for sites of known value, i.e., requires a priori knowledge	Screening for known loci influencing drug efficiency, customizable for pharmacogenomic testing
Genomewide arrays	Microarray platforms from Illumina and Affymetrix	Hybridization and or extension products measured by fluorescence	Simple; relatively fast (high throughput) and inexpensive; applicable for many subjects	Predesigned sets different genome coverage, restricted to common variants; limited addition of customized sites	Hypothesis-free testing/potential of identification of unknown loci/pathways; screening for loci influencing drug efficiency/pharmacogenomic testing; customizable for large scales
Sequencing	Wide range of classical and NGS technologies for both whole genome or locus-specific analysis	Full sequence of bases of small fragments of DNA that are sequentially identified from fluorescence signals emitted as each fragment is resynthesized from a DNA template strand	Determination of DNA sequences without prior knowledge of genome or specific regions	Very cost intensive, high requirements for data handling	Determines full information on genome, epigenome, or transcriptome for decisions on treatment or disease prediction

Proteomics

	Method	Measurement	Advantages	Disadvantages	Value in drug development decisions
2DE and MALDI-MS	Two-dimensional protein separation coupled to peptide mass fingerprinting mass spectrometry	Stained separated protein spots; relative quantification based on differential intensity; after tryptic proteolysis a set of peptide masses indicative for the protein is measured	Protein isoforms and modifications can be detected	Restricted proteome coverage, very low throughput, technically challenging, low reproducibility	Identification of relevant targets
Shotgun proteomics	High-resolution peptide liquid chromatography mass spectrometry (LC-MSMS)	Peptide masses; relative abundance of peptide based on intensity of extracted ion chromatogram; peptide fragment spectra translating into peptide sequence information	High coverage of proteomes, robust quantification methods available	Complex sample preparation for complete proteome coverage, low to medium throughput	Identification of relevant targets

8 Omics: Potential Role in Early-Phase Drug Development

	Method	Measurement	Advantages	Disadvantages	Value in drug development decisions
Interaction proteomics	Isolation of intact functional protein-protein complexes with specific affinity binders and identification of constituents by LC-MSMS	Peptide masses; relative abundance of peptide based on intensity of extracted ion chromatogram; peptide fragment spectra translating into peptide sequence information	Very sensitive discovery of novel functionalities of relevant proteins	Complex sample preparation, long development times including molecular engineering, low to medium throughput	Discovery of novel functional entities within disease relevant pathways
Targeted proteomics	Selected reaction monitoring coupled with LC-MSMS	Transitions from peptide mass to peptide fragment mass; area under curve used for relative and absolute quantifications	Selected and specific coverage of proteomes, robust absolute quantification methods available	Long assay development times, high throughput once assay is set	Validation of targets detected in discovery approaches

Metabolomics

	Method	Measurement	Advantages	Disadvantages	Value in drug development decisions
Nontargeted profiling	Mass spectrometry (MS) based: e.g., Metabolon applies tandem MS combining gas- (GC) and liquid-phase (LC) chromatography Nuclear magnetic resonance (NMR): e.g., Chenomx uses a compound database that matches NMR acquisition capabilities with support for field strengths of 400, 500, 600, 700, and 800 MHz	MS based: ion peaks organized by mass, retention time, peak areas NMR: Resonance frequency spectra, chemical shift compared to a reference is used to detect metabolites	The methods cover a wide nontargeted panel of known and unknown metabolites A combination of LC-MS and GC-MS assures a maximum coverage of a wide metabolite spectrum NMR has the advantage of leaving the sample intact but requires much larger (10–100×) sample volumes	Nontargeted methods often only provide semiquantitative traits, such as ion counts per sampling time, which may vary extensively between experiments	Allows the discovery of novel metabolites in disease relevant pathways and in reactions on drug treatment
Targeted profiling	Mass spectrometry based (MS): e.g., Biocrates AbsoluteIDQ Kits are based on tandem MS and apply targeted metabolomics	Ion peaks organized by mass; detection is based on isotope-labeled internal standards	The metabolites are in advance known and thereby provide more precise measurements and are easy to replicate The methods provide absolute quantification by comparison to isotope-labeled external standards	The methods are limited to analyzing only a subset of preselected compounds The targeted panel comes at the cost of missing potentially interesting metabolites	Validation of targets detected in discovery

Conclusions

Technologies continue to propel the omics fields forward. However, translating research discovery into routine clinical applications use is a complex process not only from scientific prospective but also from ethical, political, and logistic points of view. Particularly the implementation of omics based tests requires changes in fundamental processes of regulation, reimbursement, and clinical practice. Altogether, developments in the field of omics technologies hold great promise to optimize patient care and improve outcomes and eventually lead to new tests and treatments that are well integrated in routine medical care.

Introduction

During the past few decades, there have been dramatic increases in type 2 diabetes and obesity worldwide with prevalence estimates expected to rise even further in the future [1]. Classic epidemiological studies have already successfully identified multiple key risk factors for many metabolic diseases including both, obesity and type 2 diabetes, by typically relating lifestyle and environmental exposures to disease end points. However, often molecular mechanisms that underlie the observed associations remain unclear.

Recent developments in the field of high-throughput omics technologies have nourished the hope of incorporating novel biomarkers at multiple levels ranging from genetic predisposition (genome) and epigenetic changes (epigenome) to the expression of genes (transcriptome), proteins (proteome), and metabolites (metabolome) into epidemiological studies with the potential of obtaining a more holistic picture of disease pathophysiology [2, 3]. Thus, being at the intersection of classical epidemiology and systems biology, this "systems epidemiology" approach combines traditional research with modern high-throughput technologies to understand complex phenotypes [3]. The major advantage of systems epidemiology is its hypothesis-free approach which does not require a priori knowledge about possible mechanistic pathways or associations. By potentially improving our understanding of biological mechanisms that underlie disease pathophysiology in humans, this approach might also spur translational innovation and provide opportunities for personalized medicine through stratification according to an individual person's risk and more precise classification of disease subtypes [4]. Examples for successful integration of omics data into epidemiology is provided by two recent studies in the field of metabolomics. In these studies several metabolites were identified to play a role in the pathogenesis of type 2 diabetes. The identified set of metabolite biomarkers may successfully be used to help to predict the future risk for type 2 diabetes long before any clinical manifestations [5, 6]. Another example derives from the field of genomics where a number of type 2 diabetes susceptibility loci such as adipokines, *TCF7L2*, *IRS1*, *NOS1AP*, and *SLC30A8* have been shown to be associated with a distinct response to pharmacological and/or lifestyle intervention [7]. However, in general the results of most omics studies to date have shown that although an improved understanding of some pathogenic mechanisms is already emerging, the majority of identified omics-based biomarkers and signatures typically cannot be translated into clinical practice in a fast and straightforward process [3, 4]. To take genomics as an example, the recent development of high-throughput technology has led to large genome-wide association studies (GWAS) in which to date about 12,000 genetic susceptibility loci for common diseases, and in the case of type 2 diabetes, more than 70 genetic susceptibility loci have been identified [4, 8, 9]. Yet, these loci typically display rather modest effect sizes as exemplified by *TCF7L2*. Genetic variants of this gene display the strongest replicated effect in European populations on type 2 diabetes so far but confer odds ratios (OR) of only 1.3–1.6 [10]. Likewise, in spite of these large numbers of identified genetic susceptibility loci, the proportion of explained genetic heritability is still only marginal for the quantitative obesity traits body mass index (BMI) (2.7 % estimated [11]) and waist-to-hip ratio (WHR) (1.4 % estimated [12]) as well as for type 2 diabetes for which a proportion of only up to 10 % explained heritability is assumed [10]. Furthermore, the identified susceptibility loci so far do not add to the clinical prediction of type 2 diabetes beyond that of traditional risk factors, such as obesity, physical inactivity, family history of diabetes, and certain clinical parameters. These examples show that in spite of some early success, most of the omics fields are still in the discovery phase. This has been attributed to the time-consuming, expensive, and uncertain development process from disease biomarker discovery to clinical test, the underdeveloped and inconsistent standards to assess biomarker validity, the heterogeneity of patients with a given diagnosis, and the lack of appropriate study designs and analytical methods for these analyses [13]. Some critics have already questioned the excitement afforded omics-based discoveries, suggesting that advancements will have primarily modest effects in patient care [14]. It is generally agreed that methods used in systems epidemiology provide potential tools for future clinical application using omics-based tests. However, the discoveries of omics analyses as yet are insufficient to support clinical decisions. Altogether, it can be assumed that further developments in omics research together with the integration of omics data into risk interaction with relevant environmental exposures and lifestyle factors might yield the potential of a holistic understanding of molecular pathways underlying epidemiologic observations. Yet, the extent to which systems epidemiology can be translated into clinical practice will only become evident in a few years' time.

Background

Several omics technologies can be used to identify genetic susceptibility loci or biomarkers which are associated with a certain disease of interest and could potentially be used to better understand the disease mechanisms or to develop an omics-based test for clinical application. In this chapter we aim to give an overview of the most important omics research fields along with their potential clinical value to date.

Genomics

The genome is the complete sequence of DNA in a cell or organism. This genetic material may be found in the cell nucleus or in other organelles, such as mitochondria. A major advantage of genomic research is that except for mutations and chromosomal rearrangements, the genome of an organism remains essentially constant over time and is consistent in distinct cell types and tissues. Thus, the genome can easily be assessed in appropriate blood samples at any time. With the introduction of the first sequencing technologies allowing the readout of short deoxyribonucleic acid (DNA) fragments, the year 1977 heralded a new era of genomics research [15, 16]. However, due to the enormous costs of sequencing, researchers focused on candidate approaches to assess genetic variation, involving a number of polymerase chain reaction (PCR)-based methods to determine few single nucleotide polymorphisms (SNPs). In 2005, the first successful GWAS identified a major susceptibility gene for a complex trait, the factor H gene as a genetic cause of age-related macular degeneration [17]. Since then, rapid technological development has been an enabling force, providing transformative tools for genomic research including GWAS and next-generation sequencing (NGS) to assess complete genetic variation of the genome or specific genetic regions [18]. GWAS are performed using arrays of thousands of oligonucleotide probes that hybridize to specific DNA sequences in which SNPs are known to occur. Despite of its restriction to common variants, incomplete genome coverage, and inherent challenge of discerning the actual causal genetic variant, GWAS have been a transformative technology, representing a major advance over the candidate gene approach previously used for decades. By assessing variation across the entire human genome in an unbiased hypothesis-free fashion, this approach offers an unprecedented opportunity to uncover new genetic susceptibility loci for certain diseases with a potential clinical utility [18]. Apart from SNPs, genomic analyses can detect insertions, deletions, and copy number variations, referring to loss or amplification of the expected two copies of each gene. Personal genome sequencing is a more recent and powerful technology, which allows for direct and complete sequencing of genomes. Initially not affordable for large-scale studies, the costs of sequencing a human genome has now dropped to about $1,000 US to date; these costs continue to decline. Current sequencing machines can read about 250 billion bases in a week compared to only about 5 million in 2000 [19]. This massively parallel sequencing applied in NGS technology now allows for direct measurement of all variation in a genome [20], which is estimated to be about three million variants by the data from the 1,000 Genomes Project [21]. Effects of genetic variants in the ~1 % coding regions are more or less predictable. However, the biological implications of variants that occur in the vast remaining noncoding regions of the genome remain largely unknown. This challenge is addressed by the National Human Genome Research Institute initiated project ENCODE, the Encyclopedia of DNA Elements, which aims to functionally annotate noncoding regions of the genome (7). Waiting for those results, researchers have focused on exome sequencing, examining rare and potentially deleterious coding region variants. Today, GWAS and NGS are integral tools in basic genomic research but are increasingly being explored for clinical applications. Because of its high complexity, the elucidation of the genetic basis of common diseases has been challenging. However, research in this area has already broadened our understanding of underlying disease mechanisms and has revealed new therapeutic approaches through repurposing of existing drugs for treating diseases they were not originally intended to treat [22–24].

Epigenomics

Epigenetic regulation of gene expression is mediated through diverse mechanisms such as several kinds of reversible chemical modifications of the DNA or histones that bind DNA as well as non-histone proteins and noncoding ribonucleic acid (RNA) forming the structural matrix of the chromosomes [25]. Epigenomic modifications can occur in a tissue-specific manner, in response to environmental factors or in the development of disease states, and can persist across generations. The epigenome can vary substantially over time and across different cell types within the same organism. Since epigenetic mechanisms may function as an interface between genome and environment, epigenetic deregulation is likely to be involved in the etiology of human diseases associated with environmental exposures [26, 27]. As of today, biochemically epigenetic changes that are measured at high throughput belong to two categories: methylation of DNA cytosine residues (at CpG sites) and multiple kinds of modifications of specific histone proteins in the chromosomes. Human studies to date concentrate particularly on DNA methylation which is why this chapter focuses mainly on methods for DNA methylation profiling. Analogous to early genomics studies, DNA methylation studies were initially confined to a candidate gene approach to identify alterations occurring in disease states. New powerful technologies, such as comprehensive DNA methylation microarrays [28, 29] and genome-wide bisulphite sequencing [30] reinforce the notion of epigenetic disruption at least as a signature of human diseases [31]. As DNA methylation patterns are affected by genetic variation and due to their variability over time, it is one of the major challenges today to distinguish whether the methylation profile is a result of the disease or whether it is a contributing cause of it. First results from candidate regions as well as epigenome-wide association studies (EWASs) indicate that epigenetic profiles will be useful in practical clinical situations, providing a promising tool for the diagnosis and prognosis of disease and for the prediction of drug response. The pioneering efforts at generating a whole-genome single-base-pair resolution methylome map of eukaryotic organisms were made by two independent groups in 2008. Using two different shotgun bisulphite high-throughput sequencing protocols named BS-seq [32] and MethylC-seq [33], both groups generated comprehensive cytosine methylation maps of the *Arabidopsis thaliana* genome. MethylC-seq was also later applied to generate the first ever single-base resolution map of human methylome in embryonic stem cells and fetal fibroblasts [34]. Remarkably, this study identified that nearly one quarter of cytosine methylation in embryonic stem cells is in non-CG context, which emphasizes the need of an unbiased, genome-wide approach.

Transcriptomics

The transcriptome is the complete set of transcripts in a cell, and their quantity, at a specific developmental stage or physiological condition. Understanding the transcriptome is essential not only for the interpretation of functional elements of the genome but also for understanding of the pathogenic mechanisms and disease manifestation. The key aims of transcriptomics comprise indexing of all species of transcript, including mRNAs, noncoding RNAs, and small RNAs; determination of transcriptional structure of genes, in terms of their start sites, 5′ and 3′ ends, splicing patterns, and other posttranscriptional modifications; as well as quantification of changing expression levels of each transcript during development and under different conditions. Various technologies such as hybridization or sequence-based approaches have been developed to deduce and quantify the transcriptome. Hybridization-based approaches typically involve incubating fluorescently labeled cDNA with custom-made microarrays or commercial high-density oligo microarrays. Furthermore, specialized microarrays have been designed, for example, with probes spanning exon junctions that can be used to detect and quantify distinct spliced isoforms [35]. Genomic tiling microarrays that represent the genome at high density have been constructed and allow the mapping of transcribed regions to a very high resolution, from several base pairs to ~100 bp [36–39]. Hybridization-based approaches are high throughput and relatively inexpensive, except for high-resolution tiling arrays that interrogate large genomes. However, these methods have several limitations, which include: reliance upon existing knowledge about genome sequence; high background levels owing to cross-hybridization [40, 41]; and a limited dynamic range of detection owing to both background and saturation of signals. Moreover, comparing expression levels across different experiments is often difficult and can require complicated normalization methods.

Proteomics

The proteome is the complete set of proteins expressed by a cell, tissue, or organism. The proteome is inherently quite complex because proteins can undergo posttranslational modifications (glycosylation, phosphorylation, acetylation, ubiquitylation, and many other modifications to the amino acids comprising proteins), have different spatial configurations and intracellular localizations, and interact with other proteins as well as other molecules. This complexity may be substantially challenging for the development of a proteomics-based test that might be used in clinical practice. The proteome can be assayed using mass spectrometry and protein microarrays [42, 43]. Unlike RNA transcripts, proteins do not have obvious complementary binding partners, so the identification and characterization of capture agents is critical to the success of protein arrays. The field of proteomics has benefited from a number of recent advances. One example is the development of selected reaction monitoring (SRM) proteomics based on automated techniques [44]. During the past 2 years, multiple peptides which are specific for distinct proteins derived from each of the 20,300 human protein-coding genes known today have been synthesized and their mass spectra determined. The resulting SRMAtlas is publicly available for the entire scientific community to use in choosing targets and purchasing peptides for quantitative analyses [45]. In addition, data from untargeted "shotgun" mass spectrometry-based proteomics have been collected and uniformly analyzed to generate peptide atlases which are specific for plasma, liver, and other organs and biofluids [46]. Furthermore, antibody-based protein identification and tissue expression studies have progressed considerably [47, 48]. The

Human Protein Atlas has antibody findings for more than 12,000 of the 20,300 gene-encoded proteins. Already now the Protein Atlas is a useful resource for planning experiments and will be further enhanced by linkage with mass spectrometry findings through the emerging Human Proteome Project [49]. In addition, recently developed protein capture-agent aptamer chips also can be used to make quantitative measurements of approximately 1,000 proteins from the blood or other sources [50]. A major bottleneck in the successful deployment of large-scale proteomic approaches is the lack of high-affinity capture agents with high sensitivity and specificity for particular proteins. This challenge is exacerbated in highly complex mixtures such as whole blood, where concentrations of different proteins vary by more than ten orders of magnitude. One technology that holds great promise in this regard is "click chemistry" [51], which uses a highly specific chemical linkage to "click" together low-affinity capture agents to create a single capture agent with much higher affinity.

Metabolomics

The metabolome is the complete set of small molecule metabolites found within a biological sample (including metabolic intermediates in carbohydrate, lipid, amino acid, nucleic acid, and other biochemical pathways, along with hormones and other signaling molecules, as well as exogenous substances such as drugs and their metabolites). The metabolome is dynamic and can vary within a single organism and among organisms of the same species because of many factors such as changes in diet, stress, physical activity, pharmacological effects, and disease. The components of the metabolome can be measured with mass spectrometry [52] as well as by nuclear magnetic resonance spectroscopy [53]. This method also can be used to study the lipidome [54], which is the complete set of lipids in a biological sample and a rich source of additional potential biomarkers [55]. Improved technologies for measurements of small molecules [56] also enable the use of metabolomics for the

development of candidate omics-based tests with potential clinical utility [57]. Promising early examples include a metabolomic and proteomic approach to diagnosis, prediction, and therapy selection for heart failure [58].

Key Methods

Various emerging omics technologies are likely to influence the development of omics-based tests in the future, as both the types and numbers of molecular measurements continue to increase. Furthermore, advancing bioinformatics and computational approaches and a larger integration of different data types steadily improve evaluation and assessment of omics data. Given the rapid pace of development in these fields, it is not possible to give detailed description of all current and emerging technologies or data analytic techniques. Instead the following section focuses on key methods and techniques which are most relevant in today's practical research.

Genomics

When designing a study to assess genetic variation, the selection of an appropriate genotyping or sequencing platform for particular types of experiments is an important consideration. The decision depends on various factors, including speed, cost, error rate, and coverage of different genotyping arrays.

In spite of immense technological advance since the introduction of the first sequencing technologies, a number of early genotyping technologies which are capable of genotyping small numbers of previously selected SNPs and which were thus originally used in candidate gene studies are still in use to replicate susceptibility loci identified in discovery GWAS. For example, the iPLEX Assay developed by Sequenom provides the possibility to custom design a set of assays for up to 36 SNPs using single nucleotide extensions with mass modified nucleotides that are distinguished in MALDI-TOF MS [59]. Also the TaqMan System allows a high flexibility through customizability. This technology uses hybridization of allele-specific oligonucleotides with discriminative fluorescent labeling and a quencher suppressing fluorescence while the oligonucleotide is intact. Applying PCR the hybridized oligonucleotides are destroyed and the label is released to distinguish alleles by different fluorescence. These technologies have the potential to design specific low-scale arrays for clinical use. One example for a small custom array used successfully in pharmacogenomics is a genotyping array that was designed based on TaqMan chemistry providing a broad panel of SNPs chosen from PharmGKB to cover 120 genes of pharmacogenetic relevance including 25 drug metabolism genes and 12 drug transporter genes [60]. Together with the sequencing methods mentioned below, up to now, customized SNP chips are the most cost-efficient methods available to assess genetic variation in specific regions with a moderate number of variants.

Current genotyping arrays used in GWAS can detect up to five Mio SNPs with different designs in terms of genome coverage. These genotyping chips are widely used for the discovery of new loci associated with a certain disease as they are relatively cheap for the amount of information generated. Based on information from the 1,000 genomes project [21], DNA array data can be enhanced by estimating SNPs that are not covered by the chip. This so-called imputing of SNPs gives reasonably good information on the genotypes for all known common SNPs throughout the whole genome with some limitations regarding some problems to estimate rarer variants. The two most prominent genotyping platforms are provided by the companies Illumina and Affymetrix. While the genome-wide bead arrays (Illumina) were mainly designed to cover coding regions, chip arrays (Affymetrix) focused on the more or less evenly coverage of the whole genome. Both technologies are based on hybridization, but while chip arrays bind labeled fragments of the targets genomic DNA to multiple probes for the specific alleles, bead arrays bind genomic DNA using single-base elongation with labeled nucleotide to detect the specific alleles. Furthermore, the different length of probes between chip arrays (25 nucleotides) and bead arrays (50 nucleotides) influences selectivity [61]. The latest generation of SNP chips provides the possibility to include custom SNPs, mutations, and CNVs to increase flexibility. One example for a complete custom genome-wide bead array is the Illumina Cardio-Metabochip, which was designed by a number of GWAS consortia (viz., DIAGRAM, MAGIC, CARDIoGRAM, GIANT, ICBP GWAS + QT-IGC, Global Lipid Consortium) investigating different but related disease and quantitative phenotypes. All participating consortia selected SNPs of interest either to replicate previous findings or for finemapping of previously identified candidate loci. Because costs for the Illumina Cardio-Metabochip were below those of the genotyping chips used in discovery, this customized chip could be applied for a much larger number of cohorts. The approach turned out to lead to the successful identification of new loci for all traits and clinical endpoints being in the focus of the participating consortia.

Not quite a quarter of a century after the implementation of classical DNA sequencing technologies, the advance of sequencing technologies named "next-generation sequencing" (NGS) succeeded in decoding of (almost) the whole human genome (2.7 billion bp). The advance was to some extent an extension of readout lengths but was mainly based on a massive parallelization of the sequencing process. In the currently used advanced Sanger capillary sequencing systems, for example, millions of copies of the sequence are determined in parallel using an enzymatic primer extension and a mixture of deoxynucleotides (the "natural" building blocks of DNA) and base-specific labeled dideoxynucleotides which cause a nonreversible termination of the extension reaction and thereby DNA products of different lengths and molecular weight. Eventually, this can be used to sort the distinct DNA products and readout sequences with a high validity (error rates between 10^{-4} and 10^{-5}) [62, 63]. After the introduction of genotyping array platforms, GWA studies conducted in large samples sizes boosted the knowledge of the influence of common genetic variants on type 2 diabetes as well as on measures of adiposity. Meanwhile, sequencing technologies were mainly used for finemapping or replication of previously identified susceptibility regions. Because of its high validity, besides the MALDITOF-Sequenom technology, particularly Sanger sequencing has been as yet the most frequently used technology for a valid sequencing of a limited number of previously identified InDels or SNPs and the finemapping of low-complex regions of interest in small sample sizes [63]. The lately developed NGS technologies all allowed an even higher parallelization and throughput of data mainly by usage of beads or well plates and the development of new methodologies like bridge amplification. Some of these technologies are like the Sanger sequencing principally based on an allele-specific primer elongation of DNA polymerases such as the 454/Roche pyrosequencing in which the enzymatic extension of the DNA strand together with a sulphurylase and luciferase is translated into a light reaction, the Illumina GA sequencing which uses reversible terminator chemistry with blocked and labeled nucleotides [64] and the allele-specific primer extension Sequenom iPLEX techonolgy while others incorporate distinct methodologies such as Applied Biosystem's SOLiD which uses oligonucleotide ligation or HeliScope which sequences single molecules using asynchronous virtual terminator chemistry [63].

As a cost-saving and efficient alternative to whole genome sequencing, innovative study designs refine to whole exome sequencing. Exomes are the part of the genome which is eventually translated into a protein and may therefore have direct clinical importance. For patients with extreme phenotypes, this approach has already yielded some successes, as was shown exemplarily by the identification of *DCTN4* in the case of clinical sequelae in cystic fibrosis patients infected with Pseudomonas aeruginosa [65]. In the case of type 2 diabetes and obesity, large-scale associations by huge consortia are currently under way. However, the success of whole-exome sequencing is not quite guaranteed as GWA studies have revealed that a lot of genetic susceptibility loci are not located within an exome or can even not be clearly assigned to a protein coding region in the genome. Traditional Sanger sequencing delivers highly valid DNA sequences but has a slow throughput and is rather cost intensive compared to next-generation methods. Recent advances in sequence-based technology permit massive parallel sequencing. Real-time sequencing has replaced natural nucleotides or reversible terminators by detection of continuously added fluorescence-labeled nucleotides to the growing DNA strand thereby enhancing the speed and output length of nucleotides (18). Established sequencing libraries and post-sequencing bioinformatics algorithms have further facilitated the generation, reconstruction, and analysis of sequence reads, while the optimization of the sequencing accuracy together with redundant sequencing has constantly reduced sequencing errors. Bioinformatics tools are continuously being refined to store and process the massive amount of sequence data. In spite of all these advances, there are several challenges which remain with next-generation sequencing. Firstly, platforms differ by template preparation, sequencing chemistry, imaging, read length, and quantity per run. And although quality measures are provided by the respective manufacturers, a uniform quality assessment protocol has not been implemented so far. Secondly, statistical analyses need to account for a possible type I error (i.e., false-positive findings) in the resulting huge data sets and thus need to develop methods to dissect phenotypically relevant variants from commonly shared alleles. Finally, the identification of disease-specific genetic variants from bystanders remains a challenge. Despite these limitations, next-generation sequencing has already been applied, for example, to follow up GWAS loci for CVD phenotypes, to identify rare forms of CVD traits by exome sequencing, and to identify structural variation in the genome [66]. Altogether, next-generation sequencing has already shown great success and the methods for sequencing have evolved to the point that sequencing of an entire genome has become considerably less expensive and straightforward.

Epigenomics

A wide range of methods and approaches for the identification, quantification, and mapping of DNA methylation within the genome are available [67]. While the earliest approaches were nonspecific and were at best useful for the quantification of total methylated cytosines in the chunk of DNA, there has been a considerable progress and development over the past decades. Methods for DNA methylation analysis differ in their coverage and sensitivity, and the method of choice depends on the intended application and desired level of information. Potential results include global methyl cytosine content, degree of methylation at specific loci, or genome-wide methylation maps.

Numerous methods have been reported for locus-specific analysis. While the earlier ones relied exclusively on restriction enzymes (RE), application of bisulphite conversion has revolutionized the field. Methylation at one or more CpG sites within a particular locus can be determined either qualitatively (presence or absence) or quantitatively. DNA samples are usually derived from a heterogeneous population of cells, in which individual cells may vary vastly in their DNA methylation patterns. Hence, most of the methods aimed at quantitative measurement of DNA methylation determine the average methylation level across many DNA molecules.

Methylation-specific PCR (MSP) is one of the most widely used methods in DNA methylation studies. Using primers that can discriminate between methylated (M primer pair) or unmethylated (U primer pair) target region after bisulphite treatment, DNA is amplified using PCR. One primer in both M and U primer pairs necessarily contains a CpG site near its 3′ end. This CpG site is the one under investigation, and both M and U primers contain the same site. A forward primer in M pair having the C nucleotide in its sequence for the CpG position under investigation will fail to amplify the region if that particular cytosine is unmethylated (hence, converted to uracil during bisulphite reaction) and vice versa. Success or failure in amplification can qualitatively determine the methylation status of the target site [68]. Although rapid and easy to use, MSP suffers from various disadvantages such as reliance on gel electrophoresis and the fact that only a very few CpG sites can be analyzed using a given primer pair. Using TaqMan technology in a method, named as MethyLight, bisulphite-converted DNA is amplified and detected by methylation-state-specific primers and TaqMan probes in a real-time PCR [69]. As the two strands of DNA no longer remain complementary after bisulphite conversion, primers and probes are targeted for either of the resulting strands. Initial template quantity can be measured by traditional real-time PCR calculations. Incorporation of various quality controls for bisulphite conversion and recovery of DNA after bisulphite treatment have improved the quantitative reliability of this method. MethyLight has many advantages over MSP and other locus-specific DNA methylation analysis methods. It avoids gel electrophoresis, restriction enzyme digestion, radiolabeled dNTPs, and hybridization probes, yet there are a few shortcomings above all PCR bias a phenomenon owing to the investigation of cell mixtures. Caused by a potentially distinct cytosine content of heterogeneous cell populations and a resulting distinct amplification with varying efficiencies, PCR bias can potentially affect the accurate quantitative estimation of DNA methylation [70].

In addition, pyrosequencing, a sequencing by synthesis approach, has been widely used for locus-specific DNA methylation analyses. Pyrosequencing offers a highly reliable, quantitative, and high-throughput method for analysis of DNA methylation at multiple CpG sites with built-in internal control for completeness of bisulphite treatment. As bisulphite treatment converts unmethylated cytosines into uracils (which will be converted to thymine upon subsequent PCR amplification) leaving methylated ones unchanged, the methylation difference between cytosines is converted into a C/T genetic polymorphism [71]. Although bisulphite pyrosequencing is one of the most widely used methods for quantitative determination of methylation, it is limited by a few drawbacks. Thermal instability of enzymes used in pyrosequencing reactions, particularly luciferase, requires the reaction to be carried out at 28 °C. Therefore, optimal amplicon size to be subsequently used for pyrosequencing reaction is around 300 bp or less to avoid secondary structures [72]. As bisulphite conversion results in low-complexity DNA molecules (A, T, and G nucleotides, except very few methylated cytosines), designing optimal primer sets for every region of interest is a difficult task [73].

In yet another high-throughput quantitative approach, Sequenom's EpiTYPER assay, bisulphite-treated DNA is first amplified with specific primers. The reverse primer is tagged at the 5′ end with a T7 promoter sequence to facilitate in vitro transcription by phage RNA polymerase in the next step. Endonuclease RNase A, which cuts after every C and U in an RNA molecule, is used to generate short fragments. However, for only C-specific or U-specific cleavage, two separate in vitro transcription reactions are run. In a U-specific cleavage reaction, dCTP is used instead of CTP. This blocks cleavage after C and RNaseA only cut after U. Similarly, a separate C-specific cleavage reaction is set up. That way, a complex mixture of short oligonucleotides of varying lengths is generated. Methylation-dependent C/T polymorphism in bisulphite-converted DNA is reflected as G/A in transcribed RNA molecules and results in a 16-Da mass difference for each CpGsite in cleavage products, which is then analyzed by MALDI-TOF spectrometry [74].

The introduction of microarray technologies opened unprecedented horizons in methylome research. In contrast to methods discussed above, thousands of regions of interest can be analyzed simultaneously. Various platforms differing in their resolution and targeted regions have been used to study the DNA methylome. Ranging from CGI or promoter region-specific platforms to oligonucleotide-tiling arrays virtually covering the whole genome with high resolution, various arrays have been custom designed or are commercially available [67]. As only a very small portion of the methylome can be studied using restriction enzyme-based approaches, affinity enrichment of DNA has emerged as an effective alternative. As a general approach, DNA is first sheared randomly, and a portion of DNA is set aside to be used later as reference. The resulting enriched fraction and input control are differentially labeled and hybridized to a custom-made or commercially available array platform [75, 76].

Bisulphite treatment of DNA results in reduced sequence complexity and increased redundancy, thus reducing hybridization specificity [77]. Therefore, coupling bisulphite treatment with array hybridization has not been much successful. However, the Illumina GoldenGate BeadArray and the Infinium platform are well suited for this purpose and have been widely used.

On the Illumina GoldenGate platform, two pairs of oligos, allele-specific oligo (ASO) and locus-specific oligo (LSO), each ASO-LSO pair specific for methylated or unmethylated target CpG, are used. Each ASO has two parts: a sequence complementary to target and a priming site (P1 or P2). LSO consists of three parts: a stretch of sequence complementary to target, a priming site (P3), and an address sequence which identifies its genomic location and is complementary to capture probes on the BeadArray. The hybridization of pooled oligos to bisulphite converted fragmented immobilized DNA results in specific hybridization. ASO is then extended and ligated to corresponding LSO. During the following PCR amplification, methylated and unmethylated fractions are differentially labeled with fluorescent dyes using differentially labeled P1 and P2 primers. The hybridization to the bead array results in annealing of address sequence in LSO with a unique capture probe on the array. Resulting fluorescence intensities can be compared to quantitatively measure the methylation status at a particular locus [78]. The Infinium platform which is a modification of the genotyping array is based on a similar principle but uses slightly distinct design. On an Illumina methylation assay chip, two types of beads are present, one for methylated (M) and one for unmethylated (U) template. Each bead is covered with hundreds of thousands of copies of a specific 50-mer oligonucleotide. Bisulphite-converted DNA is subjected to whole-genome amplification, fragmented, and hybridized to the chip. Only in case the specific bases match, this is followed by a single-base extension using hapten-labeled ddNTPs. Complex immunohistochemical assays differentiate the two bead types and produce type-specific signals, of which relative intensities are used for quantitative estimation of methylation status of the corresponding CpG site [79]. While the GoldenGate assay can be used to assess up to 1,536 CpG sites, which are completely customizable [78], the actual version of the Infinium platform, the HumanMethylation450 BeadChip, covers >485,000 CpG sites per sample including more than 99 % of RefSeq genes with multiple CpG sites per gene spread across the promoter, 5′ untranslated region (UTR), first exon, gene body, and 3′ UTR. In addition to 96 % CGIs, the Infinium chip also includes various CpG sites corresponding to CGI shores and flanking regions [29].

Whole-genome bisulphite sequencing (WGBS) allows for an unbiased assessment of the profile of complete DNA methylomes. Using bisulphite-treated DNA converting unmethylated cytosines into thymidines [80], next-generation sequencing (NGS) technology is used to obtain a complete overview of CpG methylation level at base-pair resolution. Massively parallel revolution in sequencing has shifted the paradigm of genome-wide DNA methylation analysis. A whole methylome map of a particular cell type can now be generated in a matter of 3–5 days [81]. As for genomics compared to array hybridization, sequencing-based analysis provides more detailed information with less DNA input. Restriction enzyme treatment and affinity enrichment methods have been adapted to downstream massive sequencing, with additional advantage of reduction in target DNA complexity and amount of sequencing. Improving the original HpaII tiny-fragment enrichment by ligation-mediated PCR (HELP) assay by using two sets of adaptors to amplify <200-bp fragments during the LM-PCR step and coupling HELP output with NGS, Oda et al. analyzed 98.5 % of CGIs in the human genome. In this study, methylated spots were identified by their absence in the HpaII-cut fraction's sequence reads using MspI digestion as control [82]. Using a similar approach named Methyl-seq [83] revealed important differences in methylation patterns between hESCs, their in vitro differentiated derivatives, and human tissues. Another widely used method, so-called reduced representation bisulphite sequencing (RRBS), couples restriction enzyme representation followed by bisulphite sequencing on a massively parallel platform [84]. MspI digestion before bisulphite conversion allows reducing redundancy by selecting a CpG-rich genomic subset [84]. The affinity-enrichment-based methods MIRA-seq [85], MeDIP-seq [86], MethylCap-seq [87], and MBD-isolated genome sequencing [88], which have been adapted to downstream analysis by massive parallel sequencing, follow more or less similar protocols. However, enrichment methods target different compartments of the genome. For example, while MeDIP captures methylated regions with low CpG density, MBD favors high-CpG-density regions.

Raw sequencing reads from each type of high-throughput platform need to undergo dedicated and complex bioinformatics analysis pipelines, which differ from each other according to the platform used and the particular type of experiment and protocol. As a general approach, enzyme- and affinity-based sequencing methods determine the relative abundance of different genomic regions in enriched fraction by counting the number of reads that uniquely map to the reference genome as compared to input control. On the other hand, bisulphite sequencing extracts information directly from the sequence [77]. All sequencing approaches discussed above have their own advantages and shortcomings. Shotgun bisulphite sequencing, though still a gold standard because of its genome coverage, is cost and effort intensive which makes this approach unfeasible for studies involving large numbers of samples. Sequence selection strategies though useful are invariably prone to particular biases. While RE-based strategies are limited by the number and distribution of enzyme recognition sites, affinity enrichment methods cannot yield information on individual CpG dinucleotides [77]. Therefore, while the whole-genome approach is useful to generate reference methylome maps, sequence selection strategies can yield useful information about most relevant regions. Relative merits and demerits of each method have been excellently reviewed elsewhere [77].

DNA methylation is a dynamic modification that is put in place and removed by a range of enzymes that may be targeted for disease treatment [89]. Given their dynamic nature, epigenetic disease biomarker genes have to be determined by considering interindividual and intraindividual variations. In this respect, the definition of reference DNA methylation data sets will be of a high value, facilitating biomarker selection by initially defining sites that show consistent levels of DNA methylation in healthy individuals. The comprehensive study of profiles in different healthy individuals and across different types of tissue allows a reasonable estimate of the variance of specific CpG sites or regions such as promoters. Reference data sets are now being created in consortia such as Blueprint, the International Human Epigenome Consortium (IHEC), and Roadmap using high-resolution technologies [90, 91]. Focusing on healthy tissue types, these joint efforts aim to release reference data sets of integrated epigenomic profiles of stem cells, as well as developmental and somatic tissue types allowing for free access by the research community. As a paradigm, the estimation of genetic variance in the human population and the identification of SNPs improved mutational analyses by excluding false-positive hits for disease-linked mutations before screening. Concordantly, filtering out loci that are unstable in DNA methylation between individuals excludes unsuitable CpG sites before selection of appropriate biomarker candidates. Systematic screening of reference data sets will allow us to identify and to exclude variable CpG sites and regions, highly facilitating future biomarker selections.

Transcriptomics

Like the field of genomics and epigenomics, also the field of transcriptomics profits from the rapid development in microarray as well as sequencing technologies. Various microarray systems have been developed. While some platforms of high quality and low cost are commercially available, others are produced primarily in research laboratories. Microarrays used for transcriptomics differ according to type of solid support used, the surface modifications containing various substrates, the type of DNA fragments used on the array, as well as whether the transcripts are synthesized in situ or presynthesized and spotted onto the array, and how DNA fragments are placed on the array [92]. Widely used probes on array platforms are complementary DNA (cDNA) or oligonucleotides. Ideal probes should be sequence validated, unique, and representative of a significant portion of the genome, and they should have minimal cross-hybridization to related sequences. Probes for cDNA arrays are composed of cDNAs from cDNA libraries or clone collections that are "spotted" onto glass slides or nylon membranes at precise locations. Spotted arrays composed of a collection of cDNAs allow for a larger choice of sequences incorporated in the array and may thus enhance the discovery of genes in case unselected clones from cDNA libraries are used [93]. Oligonucleotide arrays consist of probes composed of short nucleotides (15–25 nt) or long oligonucleotides (50–120 nt) that are directly synthesized onto glass slides or silicon wafers, using either photolithography or ink-jet technology. The usage of longer oligonucleotides (50–100 mers) may increase the specificity of hybridization and increase sensitivity of detection [94]. Arrays fabricated by direct synthesis offer the advantage of using reproducible, high-density probe arrays containing more than 300,000 individual elements, with probes specifically designed to contain the most unique part of a transcript. This method allows for increased detection of closely related genes or splice variants.

In contrast to microarray methods, sequence-based approaches determine the cDNA sequence directly. Apart from being expensive and generally not quantitative, Sanger sequencing of cDNA or EST libraries is relatively low throughput [95, 96]. To overcome these limitations tag-based methods were developed, including serial analysis of gene expression (SAGE) [97, 98], cap analysis of gene expression (CAGE) [99, 100], and massively parallel signature sequencing (MPSS) [101–103]. These tag-based sequencing approaches have a high throughput and can provide precise, "digital" gene expression levels. However, most of these approaches are based on the rather cost-intensive Sanger sequencing technology. Furthermore, a significant proportion of the short tags cannot be uniquely mapped to the reference genome, only few transcripts can be analyzed, and isoforms are generally indistinguishable from each other. These disadvantages restrict the application of traditional sequencing technology in transcriptomics research. Like in all omics fields also for transcriptomics, development of novel high-throughput DNA sequencing methods has opened new possibilities for both mapping and quantifying of whole transcriptomes. This method, termed RNA-seq (RNA sequencing), has clear advantages over existing approaches and is expected to revolutionize the manner in which transcriptomes are analyzed. It has already been applied in several species like *Saccharomyces cerevisiae, Schizosaccharomyces pombe, Arabidopsis thaliana*, and mouse but also human cells [104–109].

RNA-seq uses deep-sequencing technologies. In general, a population of RNA is converted to a library of cDNA fragments with adaptors attached to one or both ends. Each molecule, with or without amplification, is then sequenced in a high-throughput manner to obtain short sequences derived from one end (single-end sequencing) or both ends (paired-end sequencing). The reads are typically 30–400 bp, depending on the DNA sequencing technology used. In principle, any high-throughput sequencing technology can be used for RNA-seq [110]. For example, Illumina IG [104–108], Applied Biosystems SOLiD [109], and Roche 454 Life Science [111, 112] systems have already been applied for this purpose. Following sequencing, the resulting reads are either aligned to a reference genome or reference transcripts or assembled de novo without the genomic sequence to produce a genome-scale transcription map that consists of both the transcriptional structure and/or level of expression for each gene. Although RNA-seq is still a technology under active development, it offers several key advantages over existing technologies. First, unlike hybridization-based approaches, RNA-seq is not limited to detecting transcripts that correspond to existing genomic sequence. RNA-seq can reveal the precise location of transcription boundaries, to a single-base resolution. Furthermore, 30-bp short reads from RNA-seq give information about how two exons are connected, whereas longer reads or paired-end short reads should reveal connectivity between multiple exons. These factors make RNA-seq useful for studying complex transcriptomes. In addition, RNA-seq can also reveal sequence variations (e.g., SNPs) in the transcribed regions [107, 109]. A second advantage of RNA-seq relative to DNA microarrays is that RNA-seq has very low background noise and DNA sequences can be unambiguously mapped to unique regions of the genome. There is no upper limit for quantification, which correlates with the number of sequences obtained. Consequently, RNA-seq has a large dynamic range of expression levels over which transcripts can be detected. For example, one study analyzed 16 million mapped reads corresponding to more than 9,000-fold, the estimated number in *Saccharomyces cerevisiae* analyzed [105], another study analyzing assessed 40 million mouse sequence reads making up a range spanning five orders of magnitude of what was estimated [106]. By contrast, DNA microarrays lack sensitivity for genes expressed either at low or very high levels. Determined by usage of quantitative PCR (qPCR), RNA-seq has been shown to be highly accurate for quantifying expression levels [105] and spike-in RNA controls of known concentrations [106]. The reproducibility is rather high, for both technical and biological replicates [105, 109]. Finally, because there are no cloning steps, and with the Helicos technology, there is also no amplification step, RNA-seq requires only small amounts of biomaterial. Taking all of these advantages into account, RNA-seq is the first sequencing-based method that allows for assessment of the entire transcriptome in a high-throughput and quantitative manner. This method offers both single-base resolution for annotation and "digital" gene expression levels at the genome scale, often at a much more cost efficient than either tiling arrays or large-scale Sanger EST sequencing.

The ideal method for transcriptomics should be able to directly identify and quantify all

RNAs, small or large. Although there are only a few steps in RNA-seq, it does involve several manipulation stages during the production of cDNA libraries, which can complicate its use in profiling all types of transcript. Unlike miRNAs, piRNAs, and siRNAs, which can be directly sequenced after adaptor ligation, larger RNA molecules must be fragmented into smaller pieces (200–500 bp) to be compatible with most deep-sequencing technologies. Common fragmentation methods include RNA fragmentation by RNA hydrolysis or nebulization and cDNA fragmentation by DNase I treatment or sonication. Each of these methods creates a different bias in the outcome. For example, RNA fragmentation has little bias over the transcript body [106] but is depleted for transcript ends compared to other methods. Conversely, cDNA fragmentation is usually strongly biased towards the identification of sequences from the 3' ends of transcripts and thereby provides valuable information about the precise identity of these ends [105]. Some manipulations during library construction also complicate the analysis of RNA-seq results. For example, many shorts reads that are identical to each other can be obtained from cDNA libraries that have been amplified. These could be a genuine reflection of abundant RNA species, or they could be PCR artifacts. One way to discriminate between these possibilities is to determine whether the same sequences are observed in different biological replicates. Another key consideration concerning library construction is whether or not to prepare strand-specific libraries [33, 109]. These libraries have the advantage of yielding information about the orientation of transcripts, which is valuable for transcriptome annotation, especially for regions with overlapping transcription from opposite directions [39, 104, 113]; however, strand-specific libraries are currently laborious to produce because they require many steps [109] or direct RNA–RNA ligation [33], which is inefficient. Moreover, it is essential to ensure that the antisense transcripts are not artifacts of reverse transcription [114]. Because of these complications, most studies thus far have analyzed cDNAs without strand information.

Proteomics

In addition to genetic predispositions and markers, changes in expression and function of proteins in an individual are influenced by their complex interplay within cells and organs and by environmental factors throughout the total life span. Analyzing the proteomic changes in the context of diabetes and obesity thus promises to gain a direct access to perturbances in relevant protein networks on the level of single cells or subcellular compartments of tissues or on a systemic level.

The main challenge for proteomic studies, however, comes from the extreme dynamics of proteomic changes and of the very high complexity of proteomes. Consequently, depth and coverage of proteomic studies have been mainly driven by development of technologies during the past two decades. The key enabling technology for studying proteomes is high-resolution peptide mass spectrometry coupled to a variety of pre-fractionation methods in order to cope with the very high complexity of proteomes.

In early times, a popular pre-fractionation method, the two-dimensional gel electrophoresis (2DE), was used to separate intact proteins extracted from a given cell, tissue, or organ by means of isoelectric point and molecular mass, resulting in complex maps of protein expression snapshots. This was combined with methods for relative quantification, the most advanced being 2D fluorescence difference gel electrophoresis (2DE-DIGE), where proteins from different conditions are labeled with different fluorophores and combined before separation by 2DE. Inclusion of a standard labeled with a third fluorophore enabled to further control for technical variations across samples. As a result, differential expression of proteins or posttranslationally modified protein isoforms could be detected, and identification of the respective proteins was performed by excision of a protein spot from the gel, digestion with endoproteinase trypsin, which proteolyses amino acid chains with strict sequence specificity after glutamine and arginine residues, and thus produced a protein-specific pattern of peptide fragments. These masses are then detected by matrix-assisted laser desorption ionization mass spectrometry (MALDI-MS) and compared to "in silico digests" of known proteins deposited in public databases. While this method offered the advantage of monitoring potential isoforms of a given protein by detecting shifts in mass or charge on the 2DE maps, it is severely restricted with respect to sensitivity and throughput and thus has been outperformed by other mass spectrometry (MS)-based methods (see below) [115].

Large-scale MS approaches, specifically liquid chromatography-tandem mass spectrometry (LC-MSMS), are nowadays used for both discovery of novel biomedical knowledge ("shotgun proteomics") and for validation of potential biomarkers in high throughput. The typical discovery workflow using LC-MSMS comprises reproducible biological samples preparation potentially including pre-fractionation methods to reduce complexity of the proteome to be studied, protein digestion with trypsin, or other specific proteases, and then the resulting peptides are separated using liquid chromatography (so-called bottom-up approach). Separated peptides are typically directly injected into the mass spectrometer where the respective mass-over-charge ratios are detected. From these so-called survey scans, a subset of masses are selected for fragmentation and masses of fragments together with the "parent mass" are used to identify the respective peptide by searches against public databases. A key prerequisite to study proteomes, however, is the inclusion of relative or absolute quantification strategies, since only changes in proteomes in response to, e.g., environment or disease will enable advancement of systemic understanding. Several quantification methods for peptide-based proteomics are currently in place: stable isotope labeling by/with amino acids in cell culture (SILAC), which introduces metabolic labeling in appropriate biological samples, isotope-coded affinity tag (ICAT) and isotope-coded protein label (ICPL), which label intact proteins at specific sites, isobaric tags for relative and absolute quantitation (iTraq), which is used to label peptides and finally several label-free approaches [116]. A special and very successful variation of the shotgun proteomics approach is the combination of targeted purification of intact functional protein complexes with LC-MSMS with the aim to discover functions of novel proteins relevant for diseases ("interaction proteomics") [117]. Shotgun proteomics experiments have the capacity to simultaneously detect thousands of proteins and when combined with additional pre-fractionation strategies, e.g., strong cation exchange (SCX) chromatography or off-gel fractionation (OGE) of peptides based on isoelectric points, the complexity of cellular proteomes can be nearly fully covered [118, 119]. However, the time and cost efforts for such full coverage experiments are profound and thus throughput and applicability of shotgun proteomics is limited to discovery projects aiming to reveal proteomic changes in response to very specific systems perturbations. Another disadvantage of shotgun proteomics is the missing data points during data-dependent acquisition. While high sensitivity of mass spectrometry theoretically enables to fully cover complex proteomes, the speed of the MS instruments still limits the capacity of recorded sequence spectra resulting in a limited coverage of simultaneously analyzed peptide masses. Both limitations of shotgun proteomics are overcome by advancements in targeted MS approaches, which aim to increase speed and sensitivity of MS by preselection of monitored proteins/peptides relevant for a biological/clinical question and, in addition, enable to introduce methods for absolute quantification. Targeted MS is based on selected reaction monitoring (SRM) assays, a process which records predefined peptides and predefined fragment ions for each peptide simultaneously in triple quadrupole mass spectrometers [120]. The transitions between the peptide and its fragments are strictly co-eluting, and area under curves for the fragments can be used as measure for relative intensities. Those SRM assays are predefined, optimized, and multiplexed and thus can be tailored to monitor changes of few to hundreds of proteins of interest for a specific context. Since relevant peptides are predefined, stable isotope-labeled peptides at known concentrations can be spiked into the experimental samples and thus enable absolute quantification for all monitored peptides. Advantages of SRM-based targeted proteomics are very high sensitivity, specificity, and throughput, while development of tailored multiplexed SRM assays is still quite time-consuming. Any mass spectrometry-based method is currently still limited in sensitivity as compared to methods involving application of specific high-affinity binders [121].

In diabetes research, proteomics methods have mainly been applied for identification of disease relevant proteins/pathways in tissues from animal models, e.g., lep/lep [122, 123] and db/db mice [124] or high-fat-diet-induced obesity in BL6 mice [125–130] or type 2 diabetes patients [131–134]. These studies (and many additional studies not cited here) have resulted in a comprehensive list of proteins which have been rated as being central to the condition of diabetes and are currently collected and published in a publicly available database (http://www.hdpp.info/hdpp-1000/) through the Human Diabetes Proteome Project (HDPP). The HDPP initiative was founded to integrate international research expertise enabling to generate systems-level insights into cellular changes by gathering multivariate data sets over time from cells and organs of healthy subjects and patients with diabetes [135]. Since application of proteomics methods in diabetes research covers very different areas with inherent huge complexity of approaches reflecting the complexity of the proteome as such, the HDPP initiative has identified some focus areas where proteomics methods are especially well suited to advance target discovery and functional understanding of disease pathogenesis. These areas comprise the Islet Human Diabetes Proteome Project (i-HDPP) aiming at a comprehensive islet expression data set, the human blood glycated proteome database, collecting qualitative and quantitative data on glycated proteins in plasma, and functional analyses of mitochondria, beta cells, insulin-producing cell lines, as well as bioinformatics and network biology approaches for data integration and systemic analyses (http://www.hdpp.info).

Metabolomics

Modern metabolomics technologies that have been built on recent advances in nuclear magnetic resonance (NMR) spectroscopy, mass spectrometry, and high-performance liquid-phase chromatography (HPLC) can provide quantitative readouts for hundreds of small molecules. They can be used to detect these metabolites in large sets of biological samples and therefore are a prerequisite to conduct powerful studies in large epidemiological population-based cohorts. At present, more than 4,200 compounds have been annotated in human metabolite databases [136]. Such a wide-ranging metabolic characterization of biological samples generates a wealth of phenotypic data that has never been accessible before and has opened up unforeseen opportunities to the emerging field of metabolomics.

Before a metabolomics study can start, several important decisions have to be made which we describe in this chapter and can be found in more detail in Suhre and Gieger [137]. The first decision of a metabolomics study is the choice of measurement platform. Robust and high-throughput measurement capabilities are required to carry out analyses with metabolites. The technologies that are most often used in metabolomics experiments are based on either mass spectrometry or NMR spectroscopy. Mass-spectrometry-based methods characterize a metabolite by its molecular mass, its specific fractionation pattern (tandem mass spectrometry), and its retention time when liquid-phase or gas-phase chromatography separation is used. The most widely implemented NMR-based method in metabolomics is ^{1}H NMR. A small molecule is identified here by a specific pattern (called the chemical shift) in the resonance spectrum of its protons when excited by an oscillating magnetic field. The initial "raw" quantitative readout of a metabolic feature is a specific pattern of peaks in a mass spectrum or an NMR spectrum and related information, such as the elution time, when using a chromatography method. Ascertaining the biochemical identity of the metabolites that are represented by these raw data is sometimes an issue. Comparison with reference spectra that are obtained from pure substances or spiking experiments can provide such information. Nevertheless, many of the experimentally observed metabolites (or metabolic features) are currently not biochemically identified.

We thus distinguish between peak-based (or feature-based) metabolomics and metabolomics that uses annotated metabolite concentrations of known (and possibly also unknown) biochemical identity. The most notable advantage of mass-spectrometry-based methods compared with NMR methods is their higher sensitivity. However, this advantage comes at the cost of more complex demands in terms of sample preparation and in carrying out the actual measurement. NMR-based measurements, however, do not require the extraction of metabolites and leave the samples intact for further analysis. Also, absolute quantification with mass-spectrometry-based methods requires external reference standards for most of the measured metabolites, whereas NMR-based methods provide quantification with one or two references. Furthermore, the reproducibility of NMR experiments is excellent, whereas batch effects are often observed when mass spectrometry experiments are conducted at different times. Both methods thus have their strengths and weaknesses. If resources permit, a combination of both is worthwhile. The measurement setups of these platforms are complex and can rarely be fully replicated by any independent laboratory as reported in a pilot study on three different commercial metabolomics platforms [138]. Even if described in great detail, subtle differences in machine setup and sample processing may have a great impact on certain metabolic readouts. It is therefore essential to compare and to harmonize measurements taken from identical samples across platforms and to ensure that the final metabolomics readouts are within a well-defined range of experimental error. At this point, the choice of the metabolomics provider should be considered: relying on in-house methods has the advantage of providing full control over the measurements, but this comes with the requirement of having to build up and to maintain such a platform. Using a commercial provider is an alternative that can bring metabolomics experiments within the reach of groups that do not have access to local metabolomics core facilities. Potential drawbacks of this approach are the generally rather limited access to details of the implemented methods and also fewer options available for tweaking the experimental setup during the measurement process. Intermediate options are the use of commercial metabolomics kit technologies or out-licensing of proprietary know-how and software protocols on local platforms.

The second decision is that of which metabolites to study. Targeted methods study specific, in advance known, metabolites and thereby provide more precise measurements that are easy to replicate but are limited to analyzing only a subset of preselected compounds. Nontargeted metabolomics offers a wider and largely hypothesis-free approach. Additionally, targeted metabolomics methods are able to provide absolute quantification by comparison to isotope-labeled external standards, whereas nontargeted methods often only provide semiquantitative traits, such as ion counts per sampling time, which may vary extensively between experiments. This could limit the usability of the metabolomics data in some studies. In the choice of the metabolites to study, there is generally a trade-off to be made between a wide and largely nontargeted panel, which often comes at the cost of lower data quality, and a narrower targeted panel, which comes at the cost of missing potentially interesting metabolites. Bearing in mind that no single technique allows the measurement of all metabolites in one go, a nontargeted approach is currently more promising as it may allow the discovery of new associations with hitherto uncharacterized metabolites.

Studies have shown that complex disorders of the human organism, including type 2 diabetes and cardiovascular diseases, can be linked directly to metabolites and their corresponding biological pathways. On the other hand uncovering genetic, epigenetic, and transcriptomic influences on metabolic phenotypes is crucial to a systems-wide understanding of their interactions with environmental and lifestyle factors. Modern metabolomics techniques allow the genetics and genomics of large panels of metabolic traits to be explored by coupling genome-wide studies with metabolomics. Genetic and epigenetic association studies are beginning to unravel the genetic contribution to human metabolic individuality and thus to demonstrate its relevance for biomedical and pharmaceutical research. Wide-ranging metabolic phenotypes can be analyzed in association with genetic variants, disease-relevant phenotypes, and lifestyle and environmental parameters, allowing dissection of the relative influences of these factors. Now, wide GWAS can be carried out with broad panels of metabolite concentrations. The first GWAS with metabolic traits and with ratios between metabolite concentrations reported in Gieger et al. [139], investigated 276 metabolite covering 60 metabolic pathways. This paper reports 37 loci of human metabolic individuality and provides examples for a wide range of biomedical applications. Using this largely hypothesis-free approach, common genetic variants in genes encoding enzymes and transporter proteins have been identified that can have substantial influences on human metabolic traits. Knowledge of the genetic basis of human metabolic individuality is a key ingredient of emerging gene-based personalized therapies, including pharmacogenomics [140] and nutrigenomics [141, 142].

To gain the most from metabolic studies, it is necessary to use appropriate study designs and analytical tools. Below a definition of the metabolic phenotype and a description of the experimental methods that are available for high-throughput metabolic phenotyping and their application to larger human population studies are given. A few examples how recently discovered genetic variants with metabolic traits have provided new insights into the etiology of complex diseases will be highlighted. The focus lies on the design considerations that need to be kept in mind in future studies.

The metabolic phenotype (or metabotype) of an individual can be viewed as the ensemble state of the concentrations of all endogenous small molecules (metabolic traits) in all body organs and bodily fluids. In relation to a disease, a metabolic trait may be a functional intermediate trait or merely a correlated biomarker. In contrast to the genotype of an individual, which remains almost identical over their life span, the metabotype substantially varies with time and is influenced by a wide range of environmental and lifestyle factors, including fasting and feeding states, time of day, and menstrual cycle. Every metabolomic characterization of a biosample represents a snapshot of a part of that individual's present metabolic state at that particular time. It is important to note that every metabolite has specific properties: most of them are very sensitive to environmental influences, and their concentrations may vary over timescales of minutes, hours, or days. Nevertheless, their biochemical processing is controlled by enzymes and transporters, and thus they are influenced by the genetic variation that affects the expression or function of these proteins. GWAS have identified many genetic risk loci for complex disorders. The number of associations is increasing as more highly powered GWAS and meta-analyses are conducted. However, the effect sizes of genetic associations with complex disorders are generally small, and information on the underlying biological processes is often lacking. Therefore, the focus of GWAS is shifting increasingly away from studying associations with disease endpoints and towards studying associations with intermediate traits that are known risk factors of disease. Examples include GWAS for: blood triglyceride, cholesterol, and bilirubin levels, which are risk factors for cardiovascular disease; fasting blood glucose levels and fasting insulin levels, which are linked to diabetes; urate levels, which are linked to gout; and liver enzymes, which are indicators of liver disease. These studies have shown that genetic association with quantitative traits that are functional intermediates of complex disorders is often more highly powered, and furthermore they can provide information on the biological underpinning of the disease association. However, by studying only known risk factors of disease, it is unlikely that any new biological processes or pathways will be discovered that may be involved or disrupted in the etiology of the disease. Because metabolic phenotypes are important readouts of many biological processes, a largely hypothesis-free approach of GWAS with large panels of metabolic traits (metabolomics) may be used to respond to this challenge. The metabolic trait in a GWAS thus has the role of an intermediate phenotype that functionally links genetic variation to disease-predisposing factors and then to complex disease end points.

Most GWAS with metabolomics have so far been conducted in the general population, with participants mostly of European origin. It is therefore likely that many genetic effects that are specific to different ethnicities have not yet been discovered, calling for extended studies in other populations. Using samples from family-based studies and twin studies may allow for the familial component of variation in metabolite levels to be measured in addition to the heritability contribution [143]. If longitudinal data are available, the associations can be checked to verify that the genetic contribution to the metabolic phenotype of the individuals remains stable over a longer time period [144]. Most of the large-scale studies with metabolic traits conducted so far originated from epidemiological studies that had previously collected and stored sample aliquots. This strategy of collecting samples for future analysis in large national cohorts and biobanks, without the knowledge of the precise analysis techniques to be applied on them, made possible many of the present GWAS with metabolomics. Another source of valuable study material for GWAS with metabolomics is clinical case–control studies. Including individuals with disease in such studies allows the investigation of potentially extreme metabolic phenotypes and the discovery of genetic associations that are only revealed under disease conditions. However, ensuring standard operating procedures (SOPs) are followed in a clinical setting can be more challenging than in an epidemiological study. For example, whereas blood and urine samples taken under standardized conditions are generally available from epidemiological population studies, such conditions are more difficult to meet in a clinical setting. In particular, samples from cases and controls need to be treated identically as certain metabolites may be very susceptible to slight deviations from standard protocol. Strict SOPs need to be implemented, with a strong focus on homogeneous sample treatment, including sample storage at −80 °C and sample aliquoting at collection time to avoid any thawing of the samples between storage and measurement.

The beauty of the metabolic phenotype is that there is a rich knowledge base regarding many endogenous human metabolic pathways. In addition, more than 2,200 enzyme-coding genes are annotated in the human genome. This allows the corroboration of candidate associations with biological and functional arguments. Therefore, it is possible to analyze the association data from the point of view of a biochemist. Genes that are related to enzymatic and transport activities and that are located in regions in linkage disequilibrium with the lead SNP are prime candidates for harboring the causative variant. If such genes are present, researchers can then verify a biochemical link between these genes and the metabolic traits, using databases such as the Human Metabolome Database (HMDB) [145, 146]. Currently, this is mostly done manually; dedicated and automated network analysis methods with statistical evaluation tools need to be developed for this task.

Findings from GWAS with metabolomics have the potential to inform basic science. The field of functional genomics aims to identify the function of all genes in the human genome. To this end, an association of a poorly characterized enzyme or transporter gene with a metabolic trait may generate testable hypotheses on their substrate specificities. Following up on the predicted function of solute carrier family 16 member 9 (SLC16A9; also known as MCT9) as a carnitine transporter, on the basis of its association with serum carnitine concentrations, experiments using radiolabeled carnitine and SLC16A9-expressing *Xenopus laevis* oocytes showed that this transporter is indeed a carnitine efflux pump [144]. This concept can also be inversed. For around one-third of all measured metabolites, their biochemical identity is at present unknown. Association of a well-characterized enzyme or transporter gene with a metabolite of unknown identity may be used to infer its biochemical nature. We have recently applied this approach to predict and experimentally validate the identity of a number of unknown metabolites, such as dipeptides, on the basis of their association with the dipeptidase angiotensin-converting enzyme (ACE) [147].

There are current challenges that are briefly addressed here. Knowledge of the full set of genetic variation in human metabolism will have a wide range of biomedical and pharmaceutical applications. The genotype-metabolite-associations identified in GWAS can be used in clinical studies for association with response to drug treatment or with the development of particular complications during the course of a disease or treatment. Follow-up investigation of associations in their biochemical context is likely to provide a better understanding of the pathogenesis of common diseases. Furthermore, it can be expected that knowledge of the genetic basis of human metabolic individuality will allow the separation of genetic and environmental factors in complex gene-environment interactions and will provide a rational starting point for personalized and gene-based health-care and nutrition strategies.

Eventually, the epidemiological approach of a wide range of patient phenotyping and sample collection, using strict SOPs, needs to be translated to clinical studies, as studies that implement physiological challenges may provide access to perturbed systems [148]. The most useful approach for understanding the causal roles of the metabolites (on the pathways from genetic variants to intermediate traits to disease end points) would be to use prospective cohorts that allow for future disease risks to be evaluated on the basis of both genetic and metabolic information. Metabolic profiling of other biological samples, including saliva, cerebrospinal fluid, synovial fluid, semen, and tissue homogenates, should be investigated in the future but have so far not been used in high-throughput population-based studies [149]. Studies in stool samples may be particularly challenging. Here, the effect of the gut microbiome on human metabolism needs to be taken into account, and this requires the additional characterization of the bacterial communities in the samples.

To date, GWAS have mostly focused on common variants from chip-based genotyping arrays. However, with better coverage of low-frequency variants through sequencing or dense imputation reference panels, more associations with metabolites will most probably be uncovered. In cases in which a metabolite can be identified as being functionally relevant and an intermediate trait on a pathway to a complex disorder, its genetic association can be used to fine map the underlying disease risk locus to identify the disease-causing gene variant. For example, Tukiainen et al. [150] were able to fine map known lipid loci using a dense marker set and detailed metabolite profiles.

The future resides in the combination of data from multiple "omics" technologies. Inouye et al. [151] presented the first study of that kind by combining metabolomic, transcriptomic, and genomic variation in a large, population-based cohort. A major challenge is combining all of these data in what may be termed a genome-wide systems-biology approach.

Translating Results into Clinical Practice

Compared to the area of cancer research, where clinical applications are widely established from all omics fields, translation of omics-based results into clinical practice for type 2 diabetes and obesity is still developing slow mainly attributed to the complexity of these diseases. Figure 8.1 gives an overview of complex interplay between the omics areas and which technologies are applicable. In the past decade, applications of omics research have been pursued across the spectrum of disease management, ranging from diagnosis and prediction to treatment and personalized medicine.

Diagnostics

Up to now, only few candidates from thousands of proteins which had been identified by quantitative clinical proteomics have also been approved for clinical purposes as most of them have either not passed the verification stage or have not been validated in larger cohorts [153]. Recent results show that a panel of distinct biomarkers may be better suited for diagnosis and also for assessment of disease progression and response to therapy [153]. However, advances in RNA sequencing technology have already lead to a higher resolution view of the transcriptome, a progress which may facilitate the development of novel molecular diagnostics such as omics-based

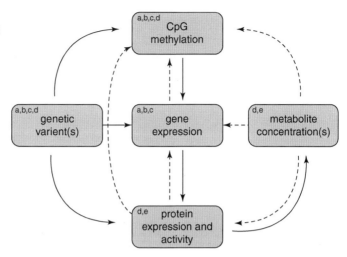

Fig. 8.1 Schematic view of the interactions between the targets addressed by the described omics technologies (Modified after Petersen et al. [152]). *Dashed lines* depict possible feedback mechanisms. *Lower case letters* indicate which technologies can be applied to measure omics targets: (**a**) PCR-based methods, (**b**) array technologies, (**c**) sequencing, (**d**) qualitative mass spectrometry, (**e**) quantitative mass spectrometry (Reprinted from Petersen et al. [152], by permission of Oxford University Press)

tests on the basis of small noncoding RNAs, RNA editing events or alternative splice variants that were not measured previously using hybridization-based technologies in the future. Similarly, DNA sequencing focusing on rare or previously unmeasured mutations may have important clinical implications. Next-generation sequencing technologies hold tremendous promise for the identification of complete DNA and RNA sequences, as well as a high-throughput identification of epigenetic and posttranscriptional modifications of DNA or RNA, respectively. For instance, new sequencing technologies are capable of monitoring a great variety of epigenetic changes at a genome-wide scale in addition to sequencing information. However, it is important to note that because next-generation RNA and DNA sequencing produce even more measurements per sample than traditional approaches, these new technologies add to the challenge of extremely high data dimensionality and the risks of overfitting computational models. Large meta-analyses of sequencing data sets collected at multiple sites may prove to be useful to overcome these risks and may help to develop clinically useful omics-based tests.

Prediction

Apart from more sensitive diagnoses, researchers in the field of type 2 diabetes and obesity facing the large amount of information and biomarkers generated by the newly developed omics technologies also hoped for an improved risk prediction which could be used in clinical practice. Particularly the introduction of GWAS technologies which lead to the discovery of several dozen genetic susceptibility loci for type 2 diabetes and obesity has nourished to hope of improving classical risk prediction models, and thus several studies have invested into this subject [154]. Most of the studies used genotype risk scores of either the unweighted or the weighted sum of total risk alleles in all subjects under investigation [155–158]. However, a comparison of the area under the curve of the receiver operating characteristics (C-statistics) indicated significantly higher C-statistics of type 2 diabetes prediction models composed of clinical risk factors such as family history, body mass index, blood pressure, and fasting plasma glucose than those of genotype risk score in isolation [155]. In addition, when genotype risk scores were included into clinical prediction models, the additional predictive value was only marginal [155]. There could be several explanations for these results. First, the minimal predictive value of genotype risk scores could result from the generally modest effect sizes of common genetic variants. Second, many of the clinical risk factors are thought to already reflect genetic effects of some genetic variants. Third, most studies involved middle-aged populations, and penetrance of genetic effects are more pronounced in subjects who develop type 2 diabetes at earlier age. At present, routine screening of genetic information to predict type 2 diabetes is not recommended [154]. Nevertheless, currently ongoing exome sequencing studies which increase the spectrum of measured genetic variants hold the promise of identifying low-frequency or rare functional variants with larger effect sizes and thus higher discriminative value. Furthermore, future research is warranted to assess the value of gene risk scores particularly in high-risk groups such as first degree relatives of type 2 diabetes patients in whom the precise genetic variants of their affected relative could be determined, as well as women with history of gestational diabetes. In addition, gene risk scores assessed in patients with early onset type 2 diabetes might further advance genetic risk prediction models. Studies evaluating the predictive value of results derived from other omics fields are currently on their way or need to be conducted in the near future. However, early studies in the field of metabolomics have already yielded some success. For example, Wang-Sattler et al. identified three metabolites (glycine, lysophosphatidylcholine (18:2), and acetylcarnitine) that in combination significantly improve prediction of type 2 diabetes and are connected to six known loci for type 2 diabetes [5]. Furthermore, branched-chain aminoacids (BCAAs) have been shown potential for screening marker for diabetes, insulin resistance, as well as cardiovascular disease [159]. The most promising approach to improve prediction is the combination of information of biomarkers derived from multiple omics studies. Beforehand, this, however, requires further developments in bioinformatics tools.

Novel Therapeutic Targets

At present, biomolecular functions of several identified genetic susceptibility variants for type 2 diabetes and obesity are mostly unknown. Therefore, many research groups are making efforts to clarify their role in the pathogenesis of type 2 diabetes which will hopefully reveal novel therapeutic targets of type 2 diabetes. One potential target for type 2 diabetes treatment could be melatonin receptor 1B (MTNR1B), because genetic variants impairing this receptors signaling were found to be associated with type 2 diabetes [160] and because melatonin itself is a strong antioxidant [161]. These findings have nourished the hope of melatonin being used as a treatment for diabetes [162]. Another potential target of type 2 diabetes that has been revealed through genetic research is cyclic adenosine monophosphate (AMP) response element-binding protein (CREBBP). In a recent GWA study, pathway analysis and protein–protein interaction analysis revealed that the transcriptional co-activator CREBBP was the main interacting protein variant associated with type 2 diabetes [10]. This suggests that CREBBP and its associated transcription factors are important in the pathogenesis of type 2 diabetes and should be investigated for potential modulation of pathogenic mechanisms. It is hoped that particularly further functional investigation of genes which may have been found to affect type 2 diabetes will help to uncover molecular mechanisms underlying these disease pathogenesis and serve as a starting point for development of novel drugs for type 2 diabetes. Furthermore, it is assumed that epigenetic therapies might provide more effective drugs with fewer adverse effects than currently available type 2 diabetes medication. Given the prevalence of epigenomic abnormalities in complex diseases, a better understanding of cause and consequence of these abnormalities may have a good prospect of translating into benefits in the clinic.

Pharmacogenomics

Today, the four most widely used classes of oral glucose-lowering medications include biguanides (represented by metformin), sulphonylureas, thiazolidinediones, and dipeptidyl peptidase (DPP)-4 inhibitors. There are individual variations in response to these medications, and genetic predisposition could be one of the factors influencing these variations. Regarding sulphonylureas, the rate-limiting enzyme of metabolism is *CYP2C9* [163]. It has been reported that loss-of-function variants of *CYP2C9* were associated with improved glycemic response presumably due to impaired sulphonylurea metabolism [164]. Several genetic variants like in *KCNJ11* and *ABCC8* have also been suggested to be associated with the glycemic response to sulphonylurea [165, 166]. Metformin is transported to hepatocytes via organic cation transporter 1 (OCT1) [167] and excreted to the bile through the multidrug and toxin extrusion 1 protein (MATE1) [168]. There are reports that variants in *OCT1* and *MATE1* genes influence the pharmacokinetics of metformin, affecting the glucose-lowering response [169, 170]. In case of metformin, the most noticeable finding regarding pharmacogenetics was derived from a GWA study. In 3,920 European subjects, the rs11212617 variant in the ataxia telangiectasia mutated gene (*ATM*) was significantly associated with better glycemic response to metformin [171]. As an explanation it was suggested that activation of AMP-activated protein kinase (AMPK), which is a target of metformin, through ATM is required for the glycemic response to metformin [171]. In a recent pharmacoproteomics approach, metformin treatment revealed only partial rescue of protein network perturbances in the retina providing an explanation for high prevalence of complications such as diabetic retinopathy despite treatment [172]. Pharmacogenetic information regarding thiazolidinediones and DPP-4 inhibitors is somewhat limited and further research is required. The incretin hormones glucagon-like peptide 1 (GLP-1) and glucose-dependent insulinotropic peptide 1 (GIP) both type 2 diabetes drugs can induce global changes in histone acetylation [173, 174]. The mechanism of GLP-1 and GIP action appears to be mediated through the ability of these compounds to increase histone H3 acetyltransferase activity and decrease histone deacetylase (HDAC) activity [173, 174]. Inappropriate chromatin remodelling and histone acetylation seem to contribute to the pathogenesis of diabetes and so HDAC inhibitors might have therapeutic potential for the treatment of diabetes [175].

Personalized Medicine

A major achievement of genetic research on type 2 diabetes would be to tailor a pharmacological therapy on an individual basis and optimize patient care. A recent study showed the possibility of incorporating the whole genome sequencing data of an individual into clinical decision making in terms of choosing an optimal medication with appropriate dosage [176]. This approach has been extended to multi-omics profiling combining genomics, transcriptomics, proteomics, and metabolomics in an individual in a time series of 14 months where the study subject experienced two viral infections and new onset of type 2 diabetes [177]. Results of this study suggest that multi-omics monitoring in an individual could help to interpret the physical condition of a patient. However, this study was only designed as proof of concept, and there are many hurdles before personalized genomic medicine is translated into clinical reality. First of all, the accuracy of omics derived data has to be improved for medical diagnostic purposes, and more solid information regarding genotype-phenotype relationship should be accumulated. In addition, the clinical utility and cost-effectiveness of novel omics tools in clinical practice should be evaluated. Based on growing literature on personalized medicine, the Clinical Pharmacogenetics Implementation Consortium (CPIC) has developed guidelines for application of pharmacogenetic information in the clinical setting [178]. As analytical approaches in the field of metabolomics move towards expanded metabolite identification and absolute quantitation, the technology can be envisioned as the opening of a vastly expanded clinical chemistry data set. One advantage of metabolomics-derived biomarkers is a potentially shorter path to clinically useful diagnostic assays than with markers derived from other omics fields. Metabolomics has clearly shown promise in both the preclinical and academic clinical settings, particularly in the areas of disease etiology and disease biomarkers [179]. For example, BCAAs were also postulated to predict response to bariatric surgery [159], and recent data suggest the promise of the technology for achieving patient stratification [180, 181]. However, clear evidence of the value of the technology in pharmaceutical development is still lacking. Replication and validation in additional population cohorts and through use of model systems and genomic approaches determining the mechanistic or causative role of these metabolites in disease are needed; these data are expected to be delivered in the near future. A more fundamental, and perhaps more difficult, challenge involves changing the perception of the technology as being complicated, unreliable, and remote from the clinical scientist to one of a tool that is readily available and readily understood in the evaluation of pharmaceutical agents within relevant patient populations. This transformation will take time and increasing familiarity with metabolomics data, but it needs to happen in order to make optimal use of this promising technology. As with other omics data types, a complex development path is necessary to establish a clinically relevant omics-based test from reports identifying metabolite concentration differences associated with a phenotype of interest [182]. New technologies emerge which are capable of assessing omics measurements on single cells [183, 184]. Such detailed molecular measurements provide deep insight into the underlying biology of tissues and potentially form a powerful basis for development of omics-based tests. However, in the same way as the resolution of these measurements increases so does the variability in the measurements due to the heterogeneity of cell states [185]. Thus, while emerging omics technologies hold great potential for the development of omics-based tests, they also may exacerbate dangers of overfitting the computational model (when the model describes random error or noise instead of the underlying relationship) to the data sets. Recent interest has focused on measuring multiple omics data types on a single set of samples, in order to integrate different types of molecular measurements into an omics-based test. Such multidimensional data sets have the potential to provide deep insight into biological mechanisms and networks, allowing for the development of more powerful clinical diagnostics.

Integrated Approach: Systems Approaches

Approaches that integrate multiple omics data types within the same clinical test are expected to grow in importance as the number of simultaneous measurements continues to increase. While it is relatively straightforward to raise the number of genomic and transcriptomic measurements (because DNA and RNA have complementary binding partners), increasing the number of protein measurements is more challenging because of the need for either high-affinity capture agents or other elaborate strategies to increase sensitivity of detection. Systems approaches that integrate multiple data types in functionally based models can be advantageous for the development of omics-based tests. For instance, the analysis of omics measurements in the context of biomolecular networks or pathways can help to reduce the number of variables in the data by constraining the possible relationships between variables, ultimately leading to more robust and clinically useful molecular tests. General approaches for using prior biological knowledge to enhance signals in omics data include removing measurements that are believed to be noise or for which there is no support in the published biological literature, using pathway databases or other sources to guide model construction, and aggregating individual measurements, often across data types, to integrate multiple sources of evidence to support conclusions [186]. Genomics, transcriptomics, proteomics, and metabolomics data can be combined with structural protein analysis in order to predict drug targets or even drug off-target effects [187]. An encouraging example of simultaneous measurement of multiple types of omics data is the DNA-encoded antibody libraries approach [188], which can measure DNA, RNA, and protein from the same sample.

During the past 10 years, much of the effort to identify genes linked to disease and other conditions of biological interest has focused on GWAS. However, more recent work has successfully identified disease-causal genes using whole genome or exome sequencing [189, 190]. Such studies may prove to be very beneficial for the development of omics-based tests, and indeed such strategies are being used clinically today for the identification of the causal gene mutation resulting in unidentified and uncommon inherited disease states.

Conclusions

Type 2 diabetes and obesity are closely related common complex diseases where genetic predisposition has a major role in their development. Recent advancement in GWAS, EWASs, and transcriptomics has significantly improved our knowledge regarding the genetic architecture and pathophysiology of type 2 diabetes and obesity. While in cancer research most omics fields have already shown their potential in clinical practice, translation of omics-based findings into clinical practice in case of type 2 diabetes and obesity though showing great potential is still just emerging. Likewise, early studies in the most recent omics fields, metabolomics and proteomics, have considerable potential for clinical application, although the latter is just starting to develop in this context. All omics technologies are still fast developing with a wide range of methods. In the fields of genomics, epigenomics, and transcriptomics, there are many locus-specific analysis methods and array technologies available while at the same time the importance of sequencing technologies constantly increases with dropping costs. In the future omics will generate complete profiles of each level. This information will be combined in systems approaches developing new methods in bioinformatics. Technologies continue to propel the fields forward, but translating discovery into clinical routine use is complex, requiring changes in the fundamental processes of regulation, reimbursement, and clinical practice. New omics-based tools have the potential to truly revolutionize patient care, but as with any great promise, they come with great responsibility. Progress is tempered by consideration of ethical issues and the need to fill the education gap that exists for health-care providers and consumers alike, which makes it difficult to keep pace with advances in the fields. Through all these efforts omics technologies will hopefully be used to optimize patient care and to improve outcomes and finally lead to new tests that are well integrated in routine medical care.

References

1. International Diabetes Federation (IDF) Diabetes atlas. Brussels: International Diabetes Federation; 2013. Available from: http://www.idf.org/diabetesatlas.
2. Lund E, Dumeaux V. Systems epidemiology in cancer. Cancer Epidemiol Biomarkers Prev. 2008;17(11):2954–7. Epub 2008/11/08.
3. Hu FB. Metabolic profiling of diabetes: from black-box epidemiology to systems epidemiology. Clin Chem. 2011;57(9):1224–6. Epub 2011/06/22.
4. McCarthy MI. Genomics, type 2 diabetes, and obesity. N Engl J Med. 2010;363(24):2339–50. Epub 2010/12/15.
5. Wang-Sattler R, Yu Z, Herder C, Messias AC, Floegel A, He Y, et al. Novel biomarkers for pre-diabetes identified by metabolomics. Mol Syst Biol. 2012;8:615. Epub 2012/09/27.
6. Wang TJ, Larson MG, Vasan RS, Cheng S, Rhee EP, McCabe E, et al. Metabolite profiles and the risk of developing diabetes. Nat Med. 2011;17(4):448–53. Epub 2011/03/23.
7. Mannino GC, Sesti G. Individualized therapy for type 2 diabetes: clinical implications of pharmacogenetic data. Mol Diagn Ther. 2012;16(5):285–302. Epub 2012/09/29.
8. Wheeler E, Barroso I. Genome-wide association studies and type 2 diabetes. Brief Funct Genomics. 2011;10(2):52–60.
9. Mahajan A, Go MJ, Zhang W, et al. Genome-wide trans-ancestry meta-analysis provides insight into the genetic architecture of type 2 diabetes susceptibility. Nat Genet. 2014;46(3):234–44. Epub 2014/02/11.
10. Morris AP, Voight BF, Teslovich TM, Ferreira T, Segre AV, Steinthorsdottir V, et al. Large-scale association analysis provides insights into the genetic architecture and pathophysiology of type 2 diabetes. Nat Genet. 2012;44(9):981–90. Epub 2012/08/14.
11. Locke AE, Kahali B, Berndt S, Justice AE, Pers TH, Day FR, et al. Large-scale genetic studies of body mass index provide insight into the biological basis of obesity. 2014 (in press).
12. Shungin D, Winkler TW, Croteau-Chonka DC, Ferreira T, Locke AE, Mägi R, et al. New genetic loci link adipocyte and insulin biology to body l fat distribution. 2014 (in press).
13. Evaluation of Genomic Applications in Practice and Prevention (EGAPP) Working Group. Recommendations from the EGAPP Working Group: does genomic profiling to assess type 2 diabetes risk improve health outcomes? Genet Med. 2013;15(8):612–7. Epub 2013/03/16.
14. Burke W, Psaty BM. Personalized medicine in the era of genomics. JAMA. 2007;298(14):1682–4. Epub 2007/10/11.
15. Maxam AM, Gilbert W. A new method for sequencing DNA. Proc Natl Acad Sci U S A. 1977;74(2):560–4. Epub 1977/02/01.

16. Sanger F, Nicklen S, Coulson AR. DNA sequencing with chain-terminating inhibitors. Proc Natl Acad Sci U S A. 1977;74(12):5463–7. Epub 1977/12/01.
17. Klein RJ, Zeiss C, Chew EY, Tsai JY, Sackler RS, Haynes C, et al. Complement factor H polymorphism in age-related macular degeneration. Science. 2005;308(5720):385–9. Epub 2005/03/12.
18. McCarthy JJ, McLeod HL, Ginsburg GS. Genomic medicine: a decade of successes, challenges, and opportunities. Sci Transl Med. 2013;5(189):189sr4. Epub 2013/06/14.
19. Lander ES. Initial impact of the sequencing of the human genome. Nature. 2011;470(7333):187–97. Epub 2011/02/11.
20. Boyd SD. Diagnostic applications of high-throughput DNA sequencing. Annu Rev Pathol. 2013;8:381–410. Epub 2012/11/06.
21. Abecasis GR, Auton A, Brooks LD, DePristo MA, Durbin RM, Handsaker RE, et al. An integrated map of genetic variation from 1,092 human genomes. Nature. 2012;491(7422):56–65. Epub 2012/11/07.
22. Dudley JT, Sirota M, Shenoy M, Pai RK, Roedder S, Chiang AP, et al. Computational repositioning of the anticonvulsant topiramate for inflammatory bowel disease. Sci Transl Med. 2011;3(96):96ra76. Epub 2011/08/19.
23. Sanseau P, Agarwal P, Barnes MR, Pastinen T, Richards JB, Cardon LR, et al. Use of genome-wide association studies for drug repositioning. Nat Biotechnol. 2012;30(4):317–20. Epub 2012/04/12.
24. Sirota M, Dudley JT, Kim J, Chiang AP, Morgan AA, Sweet-Cordero A, et al. Discovery and preclinical validation of drug indications using compendia of public gene expression data. Sci Transl Med. 2011;3(96):96ra77. Epub 2011/08/19.
25. Portela A, Esteller M. Epigenetic modifications and human disease. Nat Biotechnol. 2010;28(10):1057–68. Epub 2010/10/15.
26. Feil R, Fraga MF. Epigenetics and the environment: emerging patterns and implications. Nat Rev Genet. 2011;13(2):97–109. Epub 2012/01/05.
27. Herceg Z, Vaissiere T. Epigenetic mechanisms and cancer: an interface between the environment and the genome. Epigenetics: Off J DNA Methylation Soc. 2011;6(7):804–19. Epub 2011/07/16.
28. Sandoval J, Heyn H, Moran S, Serra-Musach J, Pujana MA, Bibikova M, et al. Validation of a DNA methylation microarray for 450,000 CpG sites in the human genome. Epigenetics: Off J DNA Methylation Soc. 2011;6(6):692–702. Epub 2011/05/20.
29. Bibikova M, Barnes B, Tsan C, Ho V, Klotzle B, Le JM, et al. High density DNA methylation array with single CpG site resolution. Genomics. 2011;98(4):288–95. Epub 2011/08/16.
30. Harris RA, Wang T, Coarfa C, Nagarajan RP, Hong C, Downey SL, et al. Comparison of sequencing-based methods to profile DNA methylation and identification of monoallelic epigenetic modifications. Nat Biotechnol. 2010;28(10):1097–105. Epub 2010/09/21.
31. Baylin SB, Jones PA. A decade of exploring the cancer epigenome – biological and translational implications. Nat Rev Cancer. 2011;11(10):726–34. Epub 2011/09/24.
32. Cokus SJ, Feng S, Zhang X, Chen Z, Merriman B, Haudenschild CD, et al. Shotgun bisulphite sequencing of the Arabidopsis genome reveals DNA methylation patterning. Nature. 2008;452(7184):215–9. Epub 2008/02/19.
33. Lister R, O'Malley RC, Tonti-Filippini J, Gregory BD, Berry CC, Millar AH, et al. Highly integrated single-base resolution maps of the epigenome in Arabidopsis. Cell. 2008;133(3):523–36. Epub 2008/04/22.
34. Lister R, Pelizzola M, Dowen RH, Hawkins RD, Hon G, Tonti-Filippini J, et al. Human DNA methylomes at base resolution show widespread epigenomic differences. Nature. 2009;462(7271):315–22. Epub 2009/10/16.
35. Schweighoffer F, Ait-Ikhlef A, Resink AL, Brinkman B, Melle-Milovanovic D, Laurent-Puig P, et al. Qualitative gene profiling: a novel tool in genomics and in pharmacogenomics that deciphers messenger RNA isoforms diversity. Pharmacogenomics. 2000;1(2):187–97. Epub 2001/03/21.
36. Yamada K, Lim J, Dale JM, Chen H, Shinn P, Palm CJ, et al. Empirical analysis of transcriptional activity in the Arabidopsis genome. Science. 2003;302(5646):842–6. Epub 2003/11/01.
37. Cheng J, Kapranov P, Drenkow J, Dike S, Brubaker S, Patel S, et al. Transcriptional maps of 10 human chromosomes at 5-nucleotide resolution. Science. 2005;308(5725):1149–54. Epub 2005/03/26.
38. Bertone P, Stolc V, Royce TE, Rozowsky JS, Urban AE, Zhu X, et al. Global identification of human transcribed sequences with genome tiling arrays. Science. 2004;306(5705):2242–6. Epub 2004/11/13.
39. David L, Huber W, Granovskaia M, Toedling J, Palm CJ, Bofkin L, et al. A high-resolution map of transcription in the yeast genome. Proc Natl Acad Sci U S A. 2006;103(14):5320–5. Epub 2006/03/30.
40. Okoniewski MJ, Miller CJ. Hybridization interactions between probesets in short oligo microarrays lead to spurious correlations. BMC Bioinformatics. 2006;7:276. Epub 2006/06/06.
41. Royce TE, Rozowsky JS, Gerstein MB. Toward a universal microarray: prediction of gene expression through nearest-neighbor probe sequence identification. Nucleic Acids Res. 2007;35(15):e99. Epub 2007/08/10.
42. Wolf-Yadlin A, Sevecka M, MacBeath G. Dissecting protein function and signaling using protein microarrays. Curr Opin Chem Biol. 2009;13(4):398–405. Epub 2009/08/08.
43. Ahrens CH, Brunner E, Qeli E, Basler K, Aebersold R. Generating and navigating proteome maps using mass spectrometry. Nat Rev Mol Cell Biol. 2010;11(11):789–801. Epub 2010/10/15.
44. Picotti P, Rinner O, Stallmach R, Dautel F, Farrah T, Domon B, et al. High-throughput generation of

selected reaction-monitoring assays for proteins and proteomes. Nat Methods. 2010;7(1):43–6. Epub 2009/12/08.
45. Omenn GS, Baker MS, Aebersold R. Recent Workshops of the HUPO Human Plasma Proteome Project (HPPP): a bridge with the HUPO CardioVascular Initiative and the emergence of SRM targeted proteomics. Proteomics. 2011;11(17):3439–43. Epub 2011/08/19.
46. Farrah T, Deutsch EW, Omenn GS, Campbell DS, Sun Z, Bletz JA, et al. A high-confidence human plasma proteome reference set with estimated concentrations in PeptideAtlas. Mol Cell Proteomics. 2011;10(9), M110 006353. Epub 2011/06/03.
47. Fagerberg L, Stromberg S, El-Obeid A, Gry M, Nilsson K, Uhlen M, et al. Large-scale protein profiling in human cell lines using antibody-based proteomics. J Proteome Res. 2011;10(9):4066–75. Epub 2011/07/06.
48. Ayoglu B, Haggmark A, Neiman M, Igel U, Uhlen M, Schwenk JM, et al. Systematic antibody and antigen-based proteomic profiling with microarrays. Expert Rev Mol Diagn. 2011;11(2):219–34. Epub 2011/03/17.
49. Legrain P, Aebersold R, Archakov A, Bairoch A, Bala K, Beretta L, et al. The human proteome project: current state and future direction. Mol Cell Proteomics. 2011;10(7):M111 009993. Epub 2011/07/12.
50. Gold L, Ayers D, Bertino J, Bock C, Bock A, Brody EN, et al. Aptamer-based multiplexed proteomic technology for biomarker discovery. PLoS One. 2010;5(12):e15004. Epub 2010/12/18.
51. Service RF. Chemistry. Click chemistry clicks along. Science. 2008;320(5878):868–9. Epub 2008/05/20.
52. Weckwerth W. Metabolomics in systems biology. Annu Rev Plant Biol. 2003;54:669–89. Epub 2003/09/25.
53. Zhang GF, Sadhukhan S, Tochtrop GP, Brunengraber H. Metabolomics, pathway regulation, and pathway discovery. J Biol Chem. 2011;286(27):23631–5. Epub 2011/05/14.
54. Seppanen-Laakso T, Oresic M. How to study lipidomes. J Mol Endocrinol. 2009;42(3):185–90. Epub 2008/12/09.
55. Masoodi M, Eiden M, Koulman A, Spaner D, Volmer DA. Comprehensive lipidomics analysis of bioactive lipids in complex regulatory networks. Anal Chem. 2010;82(19):8176–85. Epub 2010/09/11.
56. Drexler DM, Reily MD, Shipkova PA. Advances in mass spectrometry applied to pharmaceutical metabolomics. Anal Bioanal Chem. 2011;399(8):2645–53. Epub 2010/11/26.
57. Lewis GD, Gerszten RE. Toward metabolomic signatures of cardiovascular disease. Circ Cardiovasc Genet. 2010;3(2):119–21. Epub 2010/04/22.
58. Arrell DK, Zlatkovic Lindor J, Yamada S, Terzic A. K(ATP) channel-dependent metaboproteome decoded: systems approaches to heart failure prediction, diagnosis, and therapy. Cardiovasc Res. 2011;90(2):258–66. Epub 2011/02/16.
59. Millis MP. Medium-throughput SNP, genotyping using mass spectrometry: multiplex SNP genotyping using the iPLEX(R) Gold assay. Methods Mol Biol. 2011;700:61–76. Epub 2011/01/05.
60. Johnson JA, Burkley BM, Langaee TY, Clare-Salzler MJ, Klein TE, Altman RB. Implementing personalized medicine: development of a cost-effective customized pharmacogenetics genotyping array. Clin Pharmacol Ther. 2012;92(4):437–9. Epub 2012/08/23.
61. Kim KK, Won HH, Cho SS, Park JH, Kim MJ, Kim S, et al. Comparison of identical single nucleotide polymorphisms genotyped by the GeneChip Targeted Genotyping 25K, Affymetrix 500K and Illumina 550K platforms. Genomics. 2009;94(2):89–93. Epub 2009/04/28.
62. Zagursky RJ, McCormick RM. DNA sequencing separations in capillary gels on a modified commercial DNA sequencing instrument. Biotechniques. 1990;9(1):74–9. Epub 1990/07/01.
63. Kircher M, Kelso J. High-throughput DNA sequencing – concepts and limitations. BioEssays. 2010;32(6):524–36. Epub 2010/05/21.
64. Kircher M, Stenzel U, Kelso J. Improved base calling for the Illumina Genome Analyzer using machine learning strategies. Genome Biol. 2009;10(8):R83. Epub 2009/08/18.
65. Emond MJ, Louie T, Emerson J, Zhao W, Mathias RA, Knowles MR, et al. Exome sequencing of extreme phenotypes identifies DCTN4 as a modifier of chronic Pseudomonas aeruginosa infection in cystic fibrosis. Nat Genet. 2012;44(8):886–9. Epub 2012/07/10.
66. Schnabel RB, Baccarelli A, Lin H, Ellinor PT, Benjamin EJ. Next steps in cardiovascular disease genomic research – sequencing, epigenetics, and transcriptomics. Clin Chem. 2012;58(1):113–26. Epub 2011/11/22.
67. Umer M, Herceg Z. Deciphering the epigenetic code: an overview of DNA methylation analysis methods. Antioxid Redox Signal. 2013;18(15):1972–86. Epub 2012/11/06.
68. Herman JG, Graff JR, Myohanen S, Nelkin BD, Baylin SB. Methylation-specific PCR: a novel PCR assay for methylation status of CpG islands. Proc Natl Acad Sci U S A. 1996;93(18):9821–6. Epub 1996/09/03.
69. Eads CA, Danenberg KD, Kawakami K, Saltz LB, Blake C, Shibata D, et al. MethyLight: a high-throughput assay to measure DNA methylation. Nucleic Acids Res. 2000;28(8):E32. Epub 2000/03/29.
70. Warnecke PM, Stirzaker C, Melki JR, Millar DS, Paul CL, Clark SJ. Detection and measurement of PCR bias in quantitative methylation analysis of bisulphite-treated DNA. Nucleic Acids Res. 1997;25(21):4422–6. Epub 1997/10/23.
71. Uhlmann K, Brinckmann A, Toliat MR, Ritter H, Nurnberg P. Evaluation of a potential epigenetic biomarker by quantitative methyl-single nucleotide polymorphism analysis. Electrophoresis. 2002;23(24):4072–9. Epub 2002/12/14.

72. Dejeux E, El Abdalaoui H, Gut IG, Tost J. Identification and quantification of differentially methylated loci by the pyrosequencing technology. Methods Mol Biol. 2009;507:189–205. Epub 2008/11/07.
73. Tost J, El Abdalaoui H, Gut IG. Serial pyrosequencing for quantitative DNA methylation analysis. Biotechniques. 2006;40(6):721–2. 4, 6. Epub 2006/06/16.
74. Ehrich M, Nelson MR, Stanssens P, Zabeau M, Liloglou T, Xinarianos G, et al. Quantitative high-throughput analysis of DNA methylation patterns by base-specific cleavage and mass spectrometry. Proc Natl Acad Sci U S A. 2005;102(44):15785–90. Epub 2005/10/26.
75. Weber M, Davies JJ, Wittig D, Oakeley EJ, Haase M, Lam WL, et al. Chromosome-wide and promoter-specific analyses identify sites of differential DNA methylation in normal and transformed human cells. Nat Genet. 2005;37(8):853–62. Epub 2005/07/12.
76. Rauch TA, Wu X, Zhong X, Riggs AD, Pfeifer GP. A human B cell methylome at 100-base pair resolution. Proc Natl Acad Sci U S A. 2009;106(3):671–8. Epub 2009/01/14.
77. Laird PW. Principles and challenges of genome-wide DNA methylation analysis. Nat Rev Genet. 2010;11(3):191–203. Epub 2010/02/04.
78. Bibikova M, Fan JB. GoldenGate assay for DNA methylation profiling. Methods Mol Biol. 2009;507:149–63. Epub 2008/11/07.
79. Bibikova M, Le J, Barnes B, Saedinia-Melnyk S, Zhou L, Shen R, et al. Genome-wide DNA methylation profiling using Infinium(R) assay. Epigenomics. 2009;1(1):177–200. Epub 2009/10/01.
80. Frommer M, McDonald LE, Millar DS, Collis CM, Watt F, Grigg GW, et al. A genomic sequencing protocol that yields a positive display of 5-methylcytosine residues in individual DNA strands. Proc Natl Acad Sci U S A. 1992;89(5):1827–31. Epub 1992/03/01.
81. Lister R, Ecker JR. Finding the fifth base: genome-wide sequencing of cytosine methylation. Genome Res. 2009;19(6):959–66. Epub 2009/03/11.
82. Oda M, Glass JL, Thompson RF, Mo Y, Olivier EN, Figueroa ME, et al. High-resolution genome-wide cytosine methylation profiling with simultaneous copy number analysis and optimization for limited cell numbers. Nucleic Acids Res. 2009;37(12):3829–39. Epub 2009/04/24.
83. Brunner AL, Johnson DS, Kim SW, Valouev A, Reddy TE, Neff NF, et al. Distinct DNA methylation patterns characterize differentiated human embryonic stem cells and developing human fetal liver. Genome Res. 2009;19(6):1044–56. Epub 2009/03/11.
84. Meissner A, Mikkelsen TS, Gu H, Wernig M, Hanna J, Sivachenko A, et al. Genome-scale DNA methylation maps of pluripotent and differentiated cells. Nature. 2008;454(7205):766–70. Epub 2008/07/05.
85. Park JH, Park J, Choi JK, Lyu J, Bae MG, Lee YG, et al. Identification of DNA methylation changes associated with human gastric cancer. BMC Med Genomics. 2011;4:82. Epub 2011/12/03.
86. Down TA, Rakyan VK, Turner DJ, Flicek P, Li H, Kulesha E, et al. A Bayesian deconvolution strategy for immunoprecipitation-based DNA methylome analysis. Nat Biotechnol. 2008;26(7):779–85. Epub 2008/07/10.
87. Brinkman AB, Simmer F, Ma K, Kaan A, Zhu J, Stunnenberg HG. Whole-genome DNA methylation profiling using MethylCap-seq. Methods. 2010;52(3):232–6. Epub 2010/06/15.
88. Serre D, Lee BH, Ting AH. MBD-isolated genome sequencing provides a high-throughput and comprehensive survey of DNA methylation in the human genome. Nucleic Acids Res. 2010;38(2):391–9. Epub 2009/11/13.
89. Heyn H, Esteller M. DNA methylation profiling in the clinic: applications and challenges. Nat Rev Genet. 2012;13(10):679–92. Epub 2012/09/05.
90. Bernstein BE, Stamatoyannopoulos JA, Costello JF, Ren B, Milosavljevic A, Meissner A, et al. The NIH Roadmap Epigenomics Mapping Consortium. Nat Biotechnol. 2010;28(10):1045–8. Epub 2010/10/15.
91. Adams D, Altucci L, Antonarakis SE, Ballesteros J, Beck S, Bird A, et al. BLUEPRINT to decode the epigenetic signature written in blood. Nat Biotechnol. 2012;30(3):224–6. Epub 2012/03/09.
92. Holloway AJ, van Laar RK, Tothill RW, Bowtell DD. Options available – from start to finish–for obtaining data from DNA microarrays II. Nat Genet. 2002;32(Suppl):481–9. Epub 2002/11/28.
93. Schulze A, Downward J. Navigating gene expression using microarrays–a technology review. Nat Cell Biol. 2001;3(8):E190–5. Epub 2001/08/03.
94. Kane MD, Jatkoe TA, Stumpf CR, Lu J, Thomas JD, Madore SJ. Assessment of the sensitivity and specificity of oligonucleotide (50mer) microarrays. Nucleic Acids Res. 2000;28(22):4552–7. Epub 2000/11/10.
95. Gerhard DS, Wagner L, Feingold EA, Shenmen CM, Grouse LH, Schuler G, et al. The status, quality, and expansion of the NIH full-length cDNA project: the Mammalian Gene Collection (MGC). Genome Res. 2004;14(10B):2121–7. Epub 2004/10/19.
96. Boguski MS, Tolstoshev CM, Bassett Jr DE. Gene discovery in dbEST. Science. 1994;265(5181):1993–4. Epub 1994/09/30.
97. Velculescu VE, Zhang L, Vogelstein B, Kinzler KW. Serial analysis of gene expression. Science. 1995;270(5235):484–7. Epub 1995/10/20.
98. Harbers M, Carninci P. Tag-based approaches for transcriptome research and genome annotation. Nat Methods. 2005;2(7):495–502. Epub 2005/06/24.
99. Shiraki T, Kondo S, Katayama S, Waki K, Kasukawa T, Kawaji H, et al. Cap analysis gene expression for high-throughput analysis of transcriptional starting point and identification of promoter usage. Proc Natl Acad Sci U S A. 2003;100(26):15776–81. Epub 2003/12/10.
100. Kodzius R, Kojima M, Nishiyori H, Nakamura M, Fukuda S, Tagami M, et al. CAGE: cap analysis of gene expression. Nat Methods. 2006;3(3):211–22. Epub 2006/02/21.

101. Reinartz J, Bruyns E, Lin JZ, Burcham T, Brenner S, Bowen B, et al. Massively parallel signature sequencing (MPSS) as a tool for in-depth quantitative gene expression profiling in all organisms. Brief Funct Genomic Proteomic. 2002;1(1):95–104. Epub 2004/07/15.
102. Peiffer JA, Kaushik S, Sakai H, Arteaga-Vazquez M, Sanchez-Leon N, Ghazal H, et al. A spatial dissection of the Arabidopsis floral transcriptome by MPSS. BMC Plant Biol. 2008;8:43. Epub 2008/04/23.
103. Brenner S, Johnson M, Bridgham J, Golda G, Lloyd DH, Johnson D, et al. Gene expression analysis by massively parallel signature sequencing (MPSS) on microbead arrays. Nat Biotechnol. 2000;18(6):630–4. Epub 2000/06/03.
104. Wilhelm BT, Marguerat S, Watt S, Schubert F, Wood V, Goodhead I, et al. Dynamic repertoire of a eukaryotic transcriptome surveyed at single-nucleotide resolution. Nature. 2008;453(7199):1239–43. Epub 2008/05/20.
105. Nagalakshmi U, Wang Z, Waern K, Shou C, Raha D, Gerstein M, et al. The transcriptional landscape of the yeast genome defined by RNA sequencing. Science. 2008;320(5881):1344–9. Epub 2008/05/03.
106. Mortazavi A, Williams BA, McCue K, Schaeffer L, Wold B. Mapping and quantifying mammalian transcriptomes by RNA-Seq. Nat Methods. 2008;5(7):621–8. Epub 2008/06/03.
107. Morin R, Bainbridge M, Fejes A, Hirst M, Krzywinski M, Pugh T, et al. Profiling the HeLa S3 transcriptome using randomly primed cDNA and massively parallel short-read sequencing. Biotechniques. 2008;45(1):81–94. Epub 2008/07/10.
108. Marioni JC, Mason CE, Mane SM, Stephens M, Gilad Y. RNA-seq: an assessment of technical reproducibility and comparison with gene expression arrays. Genome Res. 2008;18(9):1509–17. Epub 2008/06/14.
109. Cloonan N, Forrest AR, Kolle G, Gardiner BB, Faulkner GJ, Brown MK, et al. Stem cell transcriptome profiling via massive-scale mRNA sequencing. Nat Methods. 2008;5(7):613–9. Epub 2008/06/03.
110. Holt RA, Jones SJ. The new paradigm of flow cell sequencing. Genome Res. 2008;18(6):839–46. Epub 2008/06/04.
111. Vera JC, Wheat CW, Fescemyer HW, Frilander MJ, Crawford DL, Hanski I, et al. Rapid transcriptome characterization for a nonmodel organism using 454 pyrosequencing. Mol Ecol. 2008;17(7):1636–47. Epub 2008/02/13.
112. Emrich SJ, Barbazuk WB, Li L, Schnable PS. Gene discovery and annotation using LCM-454 transcriptome sequencing. Genome Res. 2007;17(1):69–73. Epub 2006/11/11.
113. Dutrow N, Nix DA, Holt D, Milash B, Dalley B, Westbroek E, et al. Dynamic transcriptome of Schizosaccharomyces pombe shown by RNA-DNA hybrid mapping. Nat Genet. 2008;40(8):977–86. Epub 2008/07/22.
114. Wu JQ, Du J, Rozowsky J, Zhang Z, Urban AE, Euskirchen G, et al. Systematic analysis of transcribed loci in ENCODE regions using RACE sequencing reveals extensive transcription in the human genome. Genome Biol. 2008;9(1):R3. Epub 2008/01/05.
115. Scott EM, Carter AM, Findlay JB. The application of proteomics to diabetes. Diab Vasc Dis Res. 2005;2(2):54–60. Epub 2005/11/25.
116. Bantscheff M, Schirle M, Sweetman G, Rick J, Kuster B. Quantitative mass spectrometry in proteomics: a critical review. Anal Bioanal Chem. 2007;389(4):1017–31. Epub 2007/08/02.
117. Paul FE, Hosp F, Selbach M. Analyzing protein-protein interactions by quantitative mass spectrometry. Methods. 2011;54(4):387–95. Epub 2011/03/09.
118. Picotti P, Bodenmiller B, Mueller LN, Domon B, Aebersold R. Full dynamic range proteome analysis of S. cerevisiae by targeted proteomics. Cell. 2009;138(4):795–806. Epub 2009/08/12.
119. Schafer A, von Toerne C, Becker S, Sarioglu H, Neschen S, Kahle M, et al. Two-dimensional peptide separation improving sensitivity of selected reaction monitoring-based quantitative proteomics in mouse liver tissue: comparing off-gel electrophoresis and strong cation exchange chromatography. Anal Chem. 2012;84(20):8853–62. Epub 2012/09/22.
120. Mallick P, Schirle M, Chen SS, Flory MR, Lee H, Martin D, et al. Computational prediction of proteotypic peptides for quantitative proteomics. Nat Biotechnol. 2007;25(1):125–31. Epub 2007/01/02.
121. Huttenhain R, Malmstrom J, Picotti P, Aebersold R. Perspectives of targeted mass spectrometry for protein biomarker verification. Curr Opin Chem Biol. 2009;13(5–6):518–25. Epub 2009/10/13.
122. Edvardsson U, von Lowenhielm HB, Panfilov O, Nystrom AC, Nilsson F, Dahllof B. Hepatic protein expression of lean mice and obese diabetic mice treated with peroxisome proliferator-activated receptor activators. Proteomics. 2003;3(4):468–78. Epub 2003/04/11.
123. Sanchez JC, Converset V, Nolan A, Schmid G, Wang S, Heller M, et al. Effect of rosiglitazone on the differential expression of obesity and insulin resistance associated proteins in lep/lep mice. Proteomics. 2003;3(8):1500–20. Epub 2003/08/19.
124. Kim GH, Park EC, Yun SH, Hong Y, Lee DG, Shin EY, et al. Proteomic and bioinformatic analysis of membrane proteome in type 2 diabetic mouse liver. Proteomics. 2013;13(7):1164–79. Epub 2013/01/26.
125. von Toerne C, Kahle M, Schafer A, Ispiryan R, Blindert M, Hrabe De Angelis M, et al. Apoe, Mbl2, and Psp plasma protein levels correlate with diabetic phenotype in NZO mice–an optimized rapid workflow for SRM-based quantification. J Proteome Res. 2013;12(3):1331–43.
126. Schmid GM, Converset V, Walter N, Sennitt MV, Leung KY, Byers H, et al. Effect of high-fat diet on the expression of proteins in muscle, adipose tissues, and liver of C57BL/6 mice. Proteomics. 2004;4(8):2270–82. Epub 2004/07/27.

127. Sabido E, Wu Y, Bautista L, Porstmann T, Chang CY, Vitek O, et al. Targeted proteomics reveals strain-specific changes in the mouse insulin and central metabolic pathways after a sustained high-fat diet. Mol Syst Biol. 2013;9:681. Epub 2013/07/19.
128. Qiu L, List EO, Kopchick JJ. Differentially expressed proteins in the pancreas of diet-induced diabetic mice. Mol Cell Proteomics. 2005;4(9):1311–8. Epub 2005/06/18.
129. Kirpich IA, Gobejishvili LN, Bon Homme M, Waigel S, Cave M, Arteel G, et al. Integrated hepatic transcriptome and proteome analysis of mice with high-fat diet-induced nonalcoholic fatty liver disease. J Nutr Biochem. 2011;22(1):38–45. Epub 2010/03/23.
130. Guo Y, Darshi M, Ma Y, Perkins GA, Shen Z, Haushalter KJ, et al. Quantitative proteomic and functional analysis of liver mitochondria from high fat diet (HFD) diabetic mice. Mol Cell Proteomics. 2013;12(12):3744–58. Epub 2013/09/14.
131. Hwang H, Bowen BP, Lefort N, Flynn CR, De Filippis EA, Roberts C, et al. Proteomics analysis of human skeletal muscle reveals novel abnormalities in obesity and type 2 diabetes. Diabetes. 2010;59(1):33–42. Epub 2009/10/17.
132. Thingholm TE, Bak S, Beck-Nielsen H, Jensen ON, Gaster M. Characterization of human myotubes from type 2 diabetic and nondiabetic subjects using complementary quantitative mass spectrometric methods. Mol Cell Proteomics. 2011;10(9):M110 006650. Epub 2011/06/24.
133. Hojlund K, Wrzesinski K, Larsen PM, Fey SJ, Roepstorff P, Handberg A, et al. Proteome analysis reveals phosphorylation of ATP synthase beta-subunit in human skeletal muscle and proteins with potential roles in type 2 diabetes. J Biol Chem. 2003;278(12):10436–42. Epub 2003/01/18.
134. Giebelstein J, Poschmann G, Hojlund K, Schechinger W, Dietrich JW, Levin K, et al. The proteomic signature of insulin-resistant human skeletal muscle reveals increased glycolytic and decreased mitochondrial enzymes. Diabetologia. 2012;55(4):1114–27. Epub 2012/01/28.
135. Topf F, Schvartz D, Gaudet P, Priego-Capote F, Zufferey A, Turck N, et al. The Human Diabetes Proteome Project (HDPP): from network biology to targets for therapies and prevention. Trans Proteomics. 2013;1(1):3–11.
136. Psychogios N, Hau DD, Peng J, Guo AC, Mandal R, Bouatra S, et al. The human serum metabolome. PLoS One. 2011;6(2):e16957. Epub 2011/03/02.
137. Suhre K, Gieger C. Genetic variation in metabolic phenotypes: study designs and applications. Nat Rev Genet. 2012;13(11):759–69. Epub 2012/10/04.
138. Suhre K, Meisinger C, Doring A, Altmaier E, Belcredi P, Gieger C, et al. Metabolic footprint of diabetes: a multiplatform metabolomics study in an epidemiological setting. PLoS One. 2010;5(11):e13953. Epub 2010/11/19.
139. Gieger C, Geistlinger L, Altmaier E, Hrabe de Angelis M, Kronenberg F, Meitinger T, et al. Genetics meets metabolomics: a genome-wide association study of metabolite profiles in human serum. PLoS Genet. 2008;4(11):e1000282.
140. Link E, Parish S, Armitage J, Bowman L, Heath S, Matsuda F, et al. SLCO1B1 variants and statin-induced myopathy – a genomewide study. N Engl J Med. 2008;359(8):789–99. Epub 2008/07/25.
141. Lu Y, Feskens EJ, Dolle ME, Imholz S, Verschuren WM, Muller M, et al. Dietary n-3 and n-6 polyunsaturated fatty acid intake interacts with FADS1 genetic variation to affect total and HDL-cholesterol concentrations in the Doetinchem Cohort Study. Am J Clin Nutr. 2010;92(1):258–65. Epub 2010/05/21.
142. Dumont J, Huybrechts I, Spinneker A, Gottrand F, Grammatikaki E, Bevilacqua N, et al. FADS1 genetic variability interacts with dietary alpha-linolenic acid intake to affect serum non-HDL-cholesterol concentrations in European adolescents. J Nutr. 2011;141(7):1247–53. Epub 2011/05/20.
143. Nicholson G, Rantalainen M, Li JV, Maher AD, Malmodin D, Ahmadi KR, et al. A genome-wide metabolic QTL analysis in Europeans implicates two loci shaped by recent positive selection. PLoS Genet. 2011;7(9):e1002270. Epub 2011/09/21.
144. Suhre K, Wallaschofski H, Raffler J, Friedrich N, Haring R, Michael K, et al. A genome-wide association study of metabolic traits in human urine. Nat Genet. 2011;43(6):565–9. Epub 2011/05/17.
145. Wishart DS, Knox C, Guo AC, Eisner R, Young N, Gautam B, et al. HMDB: a knowledgebase for the human metabolome. Nucleic Acids Res. 2009;37(Database issue):D603–10. Epub 2008/10/28.
146. Kanehisa M, Goto S, Sato Y, Furumichi M, Tanabe M. KEGG for integration and interpretation of large-scale molecular data sets. Nucleic Acids Res. 2012;40(Database issue):D109–14. Epub 2011/11/15.
147. Krumsiek J, Suhre K, Evans AM, Mitchell MW, Mohney RP, Milburn MV, et al. Mining the unknown: a systems approach to metabolite identification combining genetic and metabolic information. PLoS Genet. 2012;8(10):e1003005. Epub 2012/10/25.
148. Krug S, Kastenmuller G, Stuckler F, Rist MJ, Skurk T, Sailer M, et al. The dynamic range of the human metabolome revealed by challenges. FASEB J. 2012;26(6):2607–19. Epub 2012/03/20.
149. Zhang A, Sun H, Wang P, Han Y, Wang X. Recent and potential developments of biofluid analyses in metabolomics. J Proteomics. 2012;75(4):1079–88. Epub 2011/11/15.
150. Tukiainen T, Kettunen J, Kangas AJ, Lyytikainen LP, Soininen P, Sarin AP, et al. Detailed metabolic and genetic characterization reveals new associations for 30 known lipid loci. Hum Mol Genet. 2012;21(6):1444–55. Epub 2011/12/14.
151. Inouye M, Kettunen J, Soininen P, Silander K, Ripatti S, Kumpula LS, et al. Metabonomic, transcriptomic, and genomic variation of a population cohort. Mol Syst Biol. 2010;6:441. Epub 2010/12/24.

152. Petersen AK, Zeilinger S, Kastenmuller G, Romisch-Margl W, Brugger M, Peters A, et al. Epigenetics meets metabolomics: an epigenome-wide association study with blood serum metabolic traits. Hum Mol Genet. 2014;23(2):534–45. Epub 2013/09/10.
153. Matafora V, Bachi A, Capasso G. Genomics and proteomics: how long do we need to reach clinical results? Blood Purif. 2013;36(1):7–11. Epub 2013/06/06.
154. Vassy JL, Meigs JB. Is genetic testing useful to predict type 2 diabetes? Best Pract Res Clin Endocrinol Metab. 2012;26(2):189–201. Epub 2012/04/14.
155. Meigs JB, Shrader P, Sullivan LM, McAteer JB, Fox CS, Dupuis J, et al. Genotype score in addition to common risk factors for prediction of type 2 diabetes. N Engl J Med. 2008;359(21):2208–19. Epub 2008/11/21.
156. Lyssenko V, Jonsson A, Almgren P, Pulizzi N, Isomaa B, Tuomi T, et al. Clinical risk factors, DNA variants, and the development of type 2 diabetes. N Engl J Med. 2008;359(21):2220–32. Epub 2008/11/21.
157. de Miguel-Yanes JM, Shrader P, Pencina MJ, Fox CS, Manning AK, Grant RW, et al. Genetic risk reclassification for type 2 diabetes by age below or above 50 \ using 40 type 2 diabetes risk single nucleotide polymorphisms. Diabetes Care. 2011;34(1):121–5. Epub 2010/10/05.
158. Muhlenbruch K, Jeppesen C, Joost HG, Boeing H, Schulze MB. The value of genetic information for diabetes risk prediction - differences according to sex, age, family history and obesity. PLoS One. 2013;8(5):e64307. Epub 2013/05/24.
159. Roberts LD, Koulman A, Griffin JL. Towards metabolic biomarkers of insulin resistance and type 2 diabetes: progress from the metabolome. Lancet Diabetes Endocrinol. 2014;2(1):65–75.
160. Bonnefond A, Clement N, Fawcett K, Yengo L, Vaillant E, Guillaume JL, et al. Rare MTNR1B variants impairing melatonin receptor 1B function contribute to type 2 diabetes. Nat Genet. 2012;44(3):297–301. Epub 2012/01/31.
161. Hardeland R. Antioxidative protection by melatonin: multiplicity of mechanisms from radical detoxification to radical avoidance. Endocrine. 2005;27(2):119–30. Epub 2005/10/12.
162. Korkmaz A, Ma S, Topal T, Rosales-Corral S, Tan DX, Reiter RJ. Glucose: a vital toxin and potential utility of melatonin in protecting against the diabetic state. Mol Cell Endocrinol. 2012;349(2):128–37. Epub 2011/11/15.
163. Kirchheiner J, Brockmoller J, Meineke I, Bauer S, Rohde W, Meisel C, et al. Impact of CYP2C9 amino acid polymorphisms on glyburide kinetics and on the insulin and glucose response in healthy volunteers. Clin Pharmacol Ther. 2002;71(4):286–96. Epub 2002/04/17.
164. Zhou K, Donnelly L, Burch L, Tavendale R, Doney AS, Leese G, et al. Loss-of-function CYP2C9 variants improve therapeutic response to sulfonylureas in type 2 diabetes: a Go-DARTS study. Clin Pharmacol Ther. 2010;87(1):52–6. Epub 2009/10/02.
165. Sesti G, Laratta E, Cardellini M, Andreozzi F, Del Guerra S, Irace C, et al. The E23K variant of KCNJ11 encoding the pancreatic beta-cell adenosine 5′-triphosphate-sensitive potassium channel subunit Kir6.2 is associated with an increased risk of secondary failure to sulfonylurea in patients with type 2 diabetes. J Clin Endocrinol Metab. 2006;91(6):2334–9.
166. Feng Y, Mao G, Ren X, Xing H, Tang G, Li Q, et al. Ser1369Ala variant in sulfonylurea receptor gene ABCC8 is associated with antidiabetic efficacy of gliclazide in Chinese type 2 diabetic patients. Diabetes Care. 2008;31(10):1939–44. Epub 2008/07/05.
167. Wang DS, Jonker JW, Kato Y, Kusuhara H, Schinkel AH, Sugiyama Y. Involvement of organic cation transporter 1 in hepatic and intestinal distribution of metformin. J Pharmacol Exp Ther. 2002;302(2):510–5. Epub 2002/07/20.
168. Tanihara Y, Masuda S, Sato T, Katsura T, Ogawa O, Inui K. Substrate specificity of MATE1 and MATE2-K, human multidrug and toxin extrusions/H(+)-organic cation antiporters. Biochem Pharmacol. 2007;74(2):359–71. Epub 2007/05/19.
169. Shu Y, Sheardown SA, Brown C, Owen RP, Zhang S, Castro RA, et al. Effect of genetic variation in the organic cation transporter 1 (OCT1) on metformin action. J Clin Invest. 2007;117(5):1422–31. Epub 2007/05/04.
170. Becker ML, Visser LE, van Schaik RH, Hofman A, Uitterlinden AG, Stricker BH. Genetic variation in the multidrug and toxin extrusion 1 transporter protein influences the glucose-lowering effect of metformin in patients with diabetes: a preliminary study. Diabetes. 2009;58(3):745–9. Epub 2009/02/21.
171. Zhou K, Bellenguez C, Sutherland C, Hardie G, Palmer C, Donnelly P, et al. The role of ATM in response to metformin treatment and activation of AMPK. Nat Genet. 2012;44(4):361–2. Epub 2012/03/30.
172. Ly A, Scheerer MF, Zukunft S, Muschet C, Merl J, Adamski J, et al. Retinal proteome alterations in a mouse model of type 2 diabetes. Diabetologia. 2014;57(1):192–203. Epub 2013/10/01.
173. Kim SJ, Nian C, McIntosh CH. Glucose-dependent insulinotropic polypeptide and glucagon-like peptide-1 modulate beta-cell chromatin structure. J Biol Chem. 2009;284(19):12896–904. Epub 2009/03/13.
174. Pinney SE, Simmons RA. Epigenetic mechanisms in the development of type 2 diabetes. Trends Endocrinol Metab. 2010;21(4):223–9. Epub 2009/10/30.
175. Christensen DP, Dahllof M, Lundh M, Rasmussen DN, Nielsen MD, Billestrup N, et al. Histone deacetylase (HDAC) inhibition as a novel treatment for diabetes mellitus. Mol Med. 2011;17(5–6):378–90. Epub 2011/01/29.
176. Ashley EA, Butte AJ, Wheeler MT, Chen R, Klein TE, Dewey FE, et al. Clinical assessment incorporating a personal genome. Lancet. 2010;375(9725):1525–35. Epub 2010/05/04.
177. Chen R, Mias GI, Li-Pook-Than J, Jiang L, Lam HY, Miriami E, et al. Personal omics profiling reveals

dynamic molecular and medical phenotypes. Cell. 2012;148(6):1293–307. Epub 2012/03/20.
178. Whirl-Carrillo M, McDonagh EM, Hebert JM, Gong L, Sangkuhl K, Thorn CF, et al. Pharmacogenomics knowledge for personalized medicine. Clin Pharmacol Ther. 2012;92(4):414–7. Epub 2012/09/21.
179. Collino S, Martin FP, Rezzi S. Clinical metabolomics paves the way towards future healthcare strategies. Br J Clin Pharmacol. 2013;75(3):619–29. Epub 2012/02/22.
180. Trupp M, Zhu H, Wikoff WR, Baillie RA, Zeng ZB, Karp PD, et al. Metabolomics reveals amino acids contribute to variation in response to simvastatin treatment. PLoS One. 2012;7(7):e38386. Epub 2012/07/19.
181. Ji Y, Hebbring S, Zhu H, Jenkins GD, Biernacka J, Snyder K, et al. Glycine and a glycine dehydrogenase (GLDC) SNP as citalopram/escitalopram response biomarkers in depression: pharmacometabolomics-informed pharmacogenomics. Clin Pharmacol Ther. 2011;89(1):97–104. Epub 2010/11/26.
182. Koulman A, Lane GA, Harrison SJ, Volmer DA. From differentiating metabolites to biomarkers. Anal Bioanal Chem. 2009;394(3):663–70. Epub 2009/03/12.
183. Teague B, Waterman MS, Goldstein S, Potamousis K, Zhou S, Reslewic S, et al. High-resolution human genome structure by single-molecule analysis. Proc Natl Acad Sci U S A. 2010;107(24):10848–53. Epub 2010/06/11.
184. Tang F, Lao K, Surani MA. Development and applications of single-cell transcriptome analysis. Nat Methods. 2011;8(4 Suppl):S6–11. Epub 2011/04/01.
185. Ma C, Fan R, Ahmad H, Shi Q, Comin-Anduix B, Chodon T, et al. A clinical microchip for evaluation of single immune cells reveals high functional heterogeneity in phenotypically similar T cells. Nat Med. 2011;17(6):738–43. Epub 2011/05/24.
186. Ideker T, Dutkowski J, Hood L. Boosting signal-to-noise in complex biology: prior knowledge is power. Cell. 2011;144(6):860–3. Epub 2011/03/19.
187. Chang RL, Xie L, Bourne PE, Palsson BO. Drug off-target effects predicted using structural analysis in the context of a metabolic network model. PLoS Comput Biol. 2010;6(9):e1000938. Epub 2010/10/20.
188. Bailey RC, Kwong GA, Radu CG, Witte ON, Heath JR. DNA-encoded antibody libraries: a unified platform for multiplexed cell sorting and detection of genes and proteins. J Am Chem Soc. 2007;129(7):1959–67. Epub 2007/01/31.
189. Roach JC, Glusman G, Smit AF, Huff CD, Hubley R, Shannon PT, et al. Analysis of genetic inheritance in a family quartet by whole-genome sequencing. Science. 2010;328(5978):636–9. Epub 2010/03/12.
190. Ng SB, Bigham AW, Buckingham KJ, Hannibal MC, McMillin MJ, Gildersleeve HI, et al. Exome sequencing identifies MLL2 mutations as a cause of Kabuki syndrome. Nat Genet. 2010;42(9):790–3. Epub 2010/08/17.

Part II

Emerging and Complementary Research Methods; Ethical and Regulatory Considerations

Early Phase Metabolic Research with Reference to Special Populations

9

Linda A. Morrow and Andrew J. Krentz

Abstract

Well-designed and expertly executed early phase clinical trials can provide valuable information that may accelerate 'go, no go' decisions, thereby potentially shortening the time of access to new, more efficacious treatments. While first-in-human studies have conventionally been performed in healthy volunteers, there is a move towards increasing use of patients with the disease of interest. In the context of developing new drugs for the treatment of diabetes and obesity, this paradigm shift requires consideration of the risks, benefits, and practical challenges of studying patients with obesity, glucose intolerance, type 1 diabetes, and type 2 diabetes. Within these disorders, issues of renal impairment, fatty liver disease, the metabolic syndrome, and cognitive impairment demand additional consideration. In addition, safe and ethical inclusion of patients with special characteristics, e.g. the paediatric and adolescent age groups, older subjects, and women of childbearing potential, in early phase studies mandates specific risk management strategies.

Keywords

Early phase clinical trials • Obesity • Cardiovascular disease • Fatty liver disease • Diabetic nephropathy • Type 1 diabetes • Type 2 diabetes • Impaired glucose tolerance • Older people • Women of childbearing potential • Diabetes in childhood

Introduction

The progress of drug development is dependent upon the extension of preclinical trials in animal species into human studies. In the era when clinical trials were unregulated, there were multiple

L.A. Morrow, MD (✉) • A.J. Krentz, MD, FRCP
Profil Institute for Clinical Research,
Chula Vista, CA, USA
e-mail: linda.morrow@profilinstitute.com

well-documented violations of ethical principles leading to egregious abuses of human subjects [1–3]. Over the past seven decades, the principles for the participation of human subjects in clinical trials have been codified into several key documents:
- Declaration of Helsinki [4]
- Belmont Report [5]
- International Conference on Harmonization of Technical Requirements for Registration of Pharmaceuticals for Human Use guidelines [6]

The cornerstones of these documents, which are now widely accepted by both the scientific community and the regulatory authorities, are the protection of human subjects' rights and validity of the data. Also included are concerns around the protection of vulnerable populations and sharing of the burden of participation in clinical trials across the entire population. As such, the participation of patients (as opposed to healthy volunteers) in early clinical development of new metabolic compounds has been the basis for ongoing discussion. The ethical debate on the use of patients in first-in-human and other phase 1 clinical trials is centred on the issue of justice – should patients with metabolic disease bear all of the burden of study participation in early clinical trials that will be of no benefit to them personally [7, 8]?

However, the other central tenets of ethics in clinical trials are those of respect for subjects and beneficence. The use of healthy volunteers, particularly for evaluation of glucose-lowering compounds, places them at risk for hypoglycaemia that would be perhaps greater than that for a diabetic population. The contra-argument to this is, of course, that unexpected or unanticipated adverse events might be better tolerated in a healthy population as opposed to a diseased one that might have undiagnosed underlying comorbidities, particularly cardiac disease [9]. The current accepted approach, particularly for first-in-human studies, has varied between different regulatory environments. In the USA the participation of patients with the target disease in first-in-human studies has been accepted by the Food and Drug Administration (FDA); however, other regulatory bodies have been more reticent and continue to allow only healthy volunteers to participate in these trials.

First-in-Human Studies

While healthy volunteers have traditionally been the population used in early phase (first-in-human, phase 1) clinical trials of new therapies for diabetes, there is precedence for the use of patients with the disease of interest as volunteers in trials outside the metabolic arena. Certainly, treatments for malignancies are rarely, if ever, tested in healthy volunteers, as safety and risk issues make this argument essentially moot in this clinical scenario [10]. In this context, it has been proposed that phase 1 clinical studies should be governed by three guiding principles: safety, ethical conduct, and efficiency [10]; in oncology the ethics of including vulnerable severely ill patients in phase 1 trials has been the subject of debate [7, 8]. The use of populations with the target metabolic disease in early clinical trials commenced during the past few years. There are several sound arguments for the continuation of this practice. These include:
- First, safety: the risk for hypoglycaemia during the development of compounds to treat diabetes may be significantly lower, particularly in subjects with type 2 diabetes who tend to be insulin resistant [11].
- Second, the lack of a signal for drug efficacy may be apparent, potentially reducing the unnecessary exposure of other subjects to investigational products. A non-efficacy signal may be less readily confirmed in nondiabetic subjects.
- Third, patients may benefit from receiving diabetes education around standard of care treatment while participating in a clinical trial that they might not otherwise receive, depending on the local provision of diabetes healthcare.

Well-designed and expertly executed first-in-human, first-in-patient clinical trials can provide substantial information that can shorten the clinical development of therapeutic compounds in metabolic diseases and accelerate 'go, no go' decisions, thereby potentially reducing the time of access to new, more efficacious treatments [12].

When evaluating the use of special populations in early clinical trials, it is useful to subdivide them into two groups: the patient group, i.e. subjects with the disease under consideration for treatment, and those with additional special characteristics, i.e. features that require careful risk management when these individuals are included in clinical trials. For the purposes of this discussion, the disease groups that will be addressed in the context of metabolic clinical trials are those patients with obesity, glucose intolerance, type 1 diabetes, and type 2 diabetes. Within these groups, individuals with renal impairment, fatty liver disease, the metabolic syndrome, and cognitive impairment merit additional consideration. The special characteristics groups include the paediatric and adolescent age groups, older subjects, and women of childbearing potential.

Disease Populations

Obesity

In the USA, obesity has recently been recognized as a disease by the American Medical Association [13]. The characterization of obesity has been classified most uniformly by body mass index (BMI = wt (kg)/ht (m^2)), with obesity being defined as a BMI $\geq$30 and overweight being defined as BMI $\geq$25. BMI cutoffs have been defined based on risk, with the prevalence of diabetes-related diseases rising with increasing BMI. While widely accepted, this can be problematic in individuals where a high BMI is related to large muscle mass (body-builders, athletes) or ethnic groups where the classification of individuals as 'overweight' or 'obese' may be more appropriately defined at lower BMI levels (i.e. Asian populations). However, the World Health Organization (WHO) reviewed this issue for Asian and Pacific populations and recommended that the ranges defined above be retained globally, because of regional differences among these populations [14, 15].

The participation of obese subjects in early phase clinical trials, particularly in first-in-human trials, has both advantages and challenges that must be considered in the design of these studies. Specific characteristics of the compound in development, particularly related to absorption, distribution, and metabolism as well as the early formulation of the compound, must be considered. For example, one might anticipate different pharmacokinetics in an obese population versus a nonobese population for a compound that was highly lipophilic [16] or hepatically metabolized or for a compound where a subcutaneous dose must be administered based on mg/kg dosing. In the obese population, a larger volume would be required to be delivered into the subcutaneous space, potentially impacting drug absorption. The dose volume could be so large that it would need to be administered as two or more injections, raising considerations around the injection site, i.e. one site versus more than one. The area under the curve and duration of action of long- and rapid-acting insulin analogues generally increases with dose elevation [17]. Furthermore, the pharmacokinetics (PK) and pharmacodynamics (PD) of subcutaneous insulin therapy are altered in obese patients with diabetes [17, 18].

Because of the prevalence of obesity worldwide, the pool of obese subjects available to participate in early phase trials is large and recruitment of obese subjects for early clinical trials usually proceeds smoothly. Nonetheless, several considerations may impact subject selection. Desirable subjects for early clinical trials are considered to be those with no comorbidities and no concomitant medications – the so-called 'healthy obese' population. While this concept is controversial [19], perhaps 10–25 % of the obese population are considered to be metabolically healthy, defined as having a BMI $\geq$30 kg/m^2 and less than three criteria of the metabolic syndrome [20, 21]. The converse suggests that the majority of obese individuals will have one or more metabolic derangements and careful screening is required to assure that the subject population is indeed metabolically healthy, if this is part of the trial design. Minimum screening assessments would include height, weight, calculation of BMI, blood pressure, waist measurement, fasting plasma glucose, and measurement of high-density lipoprotein (HDL) cholesterol and triglycerides; other authors have suggested the addition of an assessment of insulin sensitivity using homeostasis model assessment (HOMA-IR) [22] (see Chap. 1) or assessment of inflammation using high-sensitivity C-reactive protein [23]. Alternatively, including obese individuals with other comorbidities may be much more representative of the target population. Metabolic comorbidities in the obese population should be anticipated in at least 70 % of individuals screening for a trial; hypertension, dyslipidemias, and/or disorders of carbohydrate metabolism (insulin resistance, glucose intolerance, or even frank diabetes) may have been undiagnosed until the point of screening. Careful consideration must be given to allowing individuals with these other chronic disorders to enter a trial – the presence of features of the metabolic syndrome implies the need to allow certain concomitant medications during the trial (e.g. glucose-lowering agents, antihypertensive drugs, lipid-modifying agents, and aspirin) for which there may be little or no information regarding drug-drug interactions with the compound under investigation. Candidates for trial participation should also be queried regarding their use of over-the-counter (OTC) preparations, including vitamins or herbal preparations, particularly those marketed as weight-loss products. The inclusion of individuals on concomitant medications may be safe, depending upon the safety profile of the compound, the outcome measures under investigation in the trial, and the degree of metabolic derangement within the specific subject. One possible alternative for managing concomitant medications is to make provisions within the protocol for wash-off of medications, both prescribed and OTC, particularly if these medications are being utilized for prophylaxis and the duration of the wash-off period is not excessive. The wash-off period should take into account the half-life of the medication(s) in question, and most protocols will require 7–14-day wash-off periods. Additionally, safety parameters need to be included in the protocol, defining criteria for when a study participant would be discontinued from the study and returned to his/her pre-trial medication.

Some subjects with obesity may have physical characteristics that make them poorer candidates for early clinical trials, such as difficult venous access. Body size may be too large to fit into magnetic resonance imaging (MRI) machines or onto dual-energy X-ray absorptiometry (DXA) tables (see Chap. 6), unless arrangements are made during trial planning for access to equipment that can accommodate larger subjects. Special beds may be required for overnight stays and additional consideration should be given to be sure that larger study participants can be made comfortable with the available bathroom facilities. Impaired mobility related to obesity and its complications (e.g. degenerative joint disease) may impact the ability of subjects to complete assessments that can be routine parts of early clinical trials (e.g. exercise tolerance tests, study exercise requirements).

Certainly in most early phase trials, safety and tolerability are the primary objectives and the most important evaluation in the early clinical development of a new compound. However, the use of obese individuals as a target population may allow for an early read on efficacy, an important signal to move a new drug forward in development. Trial designs that include early efficacy assessments have become increasingly common as have trials of increasing complexity e.g. combined single ascending dose (SAD) and multiple ascending dose (MAD) trials into single protocol, adaptive design protocols [24]. The management of diet during early phase clinical trials is a major challenge for obesity trials, particularly when weight loss is one of the primary or secondary objectives of the study. Life within a phase 1 clinical trial unit is considerably different for most subjects compared to their routine, out-of-clinic existence – everything from changes in sleep-wake cycle, to alterations in activity level, to meal schedules and composition are likely to be somewhat altered. While most Americans eat more than three times per day [25], the timing and composition of the diet (caloric distribution, salt content) may be significantly different when domiciled in a research unit. Additionally, the act of observing food intake may have an impact on what and how much a subject in a trial consumes [26]. Numerous approaches have been suggested to estimate caloric requirements for weight maintenance, including multiples of the Harris-Benedict equation (men: basal metabolic rate = 88.36 + (13.397 × weight in kg) + (4.799 × height in cm) – (5.677 x age in years); women: basal metabolic rate = 447.593 + (9.247 × weight in kg) + 3.098 × height in cm) – 4.330 × age in years)), multiples of measures from indirect calorimetry (resting energy expenditure, REE), or even straightforward BMI – or body weight-based caloric ranges (see Chap. 7). The last approach is the most fraught, particularly if women are included; some women have difficulty completing meals that may contain more than 3,000 kcal/day. One approach that has been used in a specialized early phase metabolic research unit (Profil Institute for Clinical Research, Chula Vista, CA, USA) is a multiple of the Harris-Benedict equation, specifically 1.55× (Harris-Benedict equation). This approach has been shown to maintain weight with <3 % weight loss over an 8-week in-house trial (unpublished data). However, this issue mandates the use of control subjects in trials of this design; duration and period effects make crossover designs generally untenable for testing the efficacy of weight-loss drugs.

Diabetes Mellitus

As mentioned earlier, the participation of individuals with diabetes in early phase clinical trials has become increasingly common. Even first-in-human trials in the USA are currently being designed as first-in-human, first-in-patient trials and are becoming more widely accepted. Certainly, clinical trials with products such as novel insulins are most appropriately conducted in patients with diabetes (see above), and similar arguments can be made for other glucose-lowering compounds. However, trials must be carefully designed to protect the safety of study participants, and a number of factors must be considered in the patient selection process. A primary purpose of the inclusion and exclusion criteria in a clinical trial protocol is to ensure that study participants are not unnecessarily exposed to risk. Table 9.1 outlines some factors that

Table 9.1 Considerations for inclusion/exclusion criteria for study participants with type 1 and type 2 diabetes in early phase clinical trials

1. Disease status
   (a) How was the diagnosis made?
   (b) Consideration of variant forms of diabetes (e.g. pancreatic insufficiency secondary to pancreatic disease, MODY, etc.)
   (c) Duration of disease
      i. Pancreatic functional reserve
      ii. Serum C-peptide level
   (d) Complications
      i. Retinopathy
      ii. Nephropathy
      iii. Neuropathy
      iv. Macrovascular disease
   (e) Current control – HbA_{1c}
   (f) History of hypoglycaemia
2. Comorbidities
   (a) Metabolic syndrome
      i. Hypertension
      ii. Dyslipidaemia
   (b) Fatty liver disease
   (c) Depression
   (d) Degenerative joint disease
   (e) Hypothyroidism
   (f) Sleep apnoea
3. Current diabetes therapy
   (a) Diet and exercise controlled
   (b) Monotherapy
   (c) Insulin therapy
4. Concomitant medications
   (a) Antihypertensive agents
      i. Diuretics
      ii. β-adrenergic blockers
      iii. ACE inhibitors
      iv. ARBs
   (b) Treatments for dyslipidemia
      i. Statins
      ii. Fibrates
      iii. Fish oil
   (c) Aspirin
   (d) Pain medication (NSAIDs, opiates)
   (e) Antidepressants
      i. SSRIs
   (f) Hormonal therapy
      i. Thyroid hormone replacement
      ii. Oestrogen/progesterone replacement
      iii. Oral/implantable contraceptives
      iv. Testosterone replacement
   (g) Nutraceuticals/vitamins/herbal treatments

See text for definitions of abbreviations

should be considered for both patients with type 1 and type 2 diabetes.

Assessment of disease status is the first criterion. For most patients, differentiating between type 1 and type 2 diabetes is straightforward. A well-performed medical history, conducted by qualified medical personnel ad accompanied by supporting medical evidence (use of glucose-lowering medication, laboratory findings consistent with the diagnosis of diabetes mellitus, or medical records), is usually sufficient. While medical records can be very helpful, obtaining such records in a timely fashion can be challenging in early phase clinical trials. Additionally, medical records not infrequently contain information that is discrepant to that obtained from the patient; the judgement of the investigator is necessary to determine whether or not a patient is eligible for participation in a particular study. Occasionally, the diagnosis of diabetes is in question – particularly for individuals who have achieved excellent metabolic control through non-pharmacological methods, i.e. diet and exercise, and no longer appear to meet diagnostic criteria for diabetes. The success of gastric bypass surgery on remission of diabetes is relevant, although patients with a history of bariatric surgery would be excluded from most early phase diabetes drug studies because of the potential impact of the surgery on absorption of the investigational product and the known impact of these procedures of the gastrointestinal hormonal milieu and glucose metabolism [27]. Additionally, the category of diabetes is sometimes in question, e.g. in individuals with type 1 diabetes mellitus who may be initially misdiagnosed as having type 2 diabetes, particularly if they are older at the time of diagnosis [28]. Alternatively, individuals with maturity-onset diabetes of the young (MODY) may be misdiagnosed as having type 1 diabetes [29]. Measurements of islet autoantibodies, both glutamate decarboxylase (GAD) and islet antigen-2 (IA-2) autoantibodies, highly prevalent in type 1 diabetes and not usually present in MODY, can be helpful in differentiating these forms of diabetes [30, 31].

Additionally, the presence of GAD antibodies in individuals with previously diagnosed type 2 diabetes mellitus (perhaps as high as 10–25 %) who did not require insulin therapy in the first 6 months after diagnosis suggests that the correct diagnosis is latent autoimmune diabetes in adults (LADA) [32]. Including these assessments can be useful if the differentiation of the subtypes of diabetes is critical. Additionally, the measurement of serum C-peptide can be of value in helping to support the diagnosis of type 1 diabetes mellitus or the lack of residual β-cell function [33]. Low fasting serum C-peptide levels (<0.3 nmol/L) are indicative of absolute insulin deficiency and type 1 diabetes mellitus. The use of serum C-peptide measurement in studies involving patients with type 2 diabetes is more useful in determining residual β-cell function than using duration of diagnosis, as the date of diagnosis poorly reflects duration of disease [34].

Included in the assessment of disease status is an assessment of the presence or absence of long-term vascular and neurological complications of diabetes [35]. The presence of advanced complications, particularly proliferative retinopathy; diabetic nephropathy with significant proteinuria or renal insufficiency; diabetic neuropathy, particularly with impaired gastric emptying; or clinically significant macrovascular disease are likely to be exclusionary conditions for individuals with diabetes wishing to participate in early phase clinical trials. The lack of experience with patient exposures to the new investigational product may place these more vulnerable patients at increased levels of risk. Impairment of drug absorption, metabolism, or excretion because of underlying complications of diabetes could have substantial impact on initial assessments of drug pharmacokinetics, from which many early decisions in drug development are made. Additionally, the occurrence of a serious or severe adverse event, which may or may not be related to the compound under investigation, in a subject participating in an early phase trial can significantly delay or even curtail drug development.

Glycaemic Control

Essentially every volunteer participating in an early phase clinical trial involved with carbohydrate metabolism has an assessment of his/her glycated haemoglobin (HbA_{1c}) level. Figure 9.1 demonstrates the ranges of HbA_{1c} for our volunteer database; only about one quarter of volunteers with type 1 diabetes have an HbA_{1c} of <7.0 % (<53 mmol/mol) and only about one third of volunteers with type 2 diabetes are similarly well controlled. Most clinical trials have defined upper and lower boundaries for inclusion in studies. These cutoffs serve several purposes: safety, uniformity of effects on outcome measures, and efficacy assessments. Most safety considerations are concerned with putting trial participants at risk for hypoglycaemia if they enter studies with a normal or only modestly elevated HbA_{1c}. Lower cutoffs are usually at 6.5 or 7 % (48–53 mmol/mol) whereas upper boundaries are generally in the 10–11 % (86–97 mmol/mol) range. Individuals who are above these levels are excluded for ethical reasons – these patients should receive an urgent referral for appropriate healthcare. Such patients face risks for worsening hyperglycaemia should the compound under study be ineffective or the subject is randomized to a placebo treatment arm. This risk can be accentuated for proof-of-concept studies where the participation period of any given subject could extend to 3 months or more. Additionally, concerns of detrimental effects on islet β cells from hyperglycaemia (so-called glucotoxicity) [36] and variable treatment effects because of variability in the level of metabolic control contribute to these limits. While the primary purpose of early phase studies, particularly first-in-human, single ascending dose, and multiple ascending dose studies, is assessment of safety and tolerability, increasingly, sponsors look to these studies to provide early efficacy signals. In general, HbA_{1c} is a poor indicator of efficacy in these early trials because of the treatment time needed to see improvements in HbA_{1c}. For trials that extend over several weeks, an alternative measure of glycaemic control (1,5 anhydroglucitol, fructosamine) may be of value [37, 38].

Risk of Hypoglycaemia

A related factor to diabetes control that must be assessed in the medical evaluation is the patient's history regarding hypoglycaemia. It is well documented that the risk for hypoglycaemia often rises in concert with attempts to lower HbA_{1c}. Individuals with tighter diabetes control and longer duration of disease tend to have more

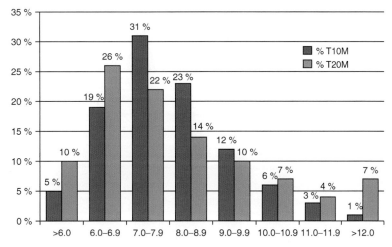

Fig. 9.1 HbA_{1c} distribution derived from a subset of US database of early phase trial volunteers. Data represents a subset of patients with type 1 diabetes ($n=874$, 53 % of total population) and a subset of patients with type 2 diabetes ($n=2{,}889$, 33 % of total population) for whom clinic-measured HbA_{1c} results were available

episodes of hypoglycaemia [39], and recurrent bouts of hypoglycaemia put patients at risk for so-called hypoglycaemia unawareness [40]. Most protocols appropriately exclude individuals with recent episodes of severe hypoglycaemia (defined as hypoglycaemia rendering the patient unable to treat himself/herself), and individuals with hypoglycaemic unawareness must be excluded from early clinical trials where the glucose-lowering capabilities of new compounds are not yet defined. Because investigators and study staff (as well as the participating subjects) are usually blinded to treatment randomization and potentially unblinding pharmacodynamic results, subjects must be able to alert staff promptly to symptoms of hypoglycaemia.

Cardiovascular Disease

Enrolling patients into clinical trials implies the willingness to consider the presence of comorbidities related to the disease state under investigation and the concomitant medications that might be required to treat either the primary disease or the comorbidities. Frequent comorbidities in individuals with diabetes are the known associated complications of diabetes as discussed above, many of which could exclude a patient from participating in an early phase trial by virtue of the unacceptable safety risk. Other comorbidities, particularly in patients with type 2 diabetes, include those related to the metabolic syndrome – obesity, hypertension, and dyslipidaemia (see below). Of particular importance in patients with any disorder of carbohydrate metabolism is atherosclerotic coronary heart disease. It is known that any abnormality in glucose tolerance increases the risk of coronary heart disease along a continuum [41], even without the presence of diabetes mellitus. As a minimum, individuals must be screened with a careful medical history and a 12-lead electrocardiograph (ECG). Any suggestion of previously undiagnosed disease (chest pain, both typical and atypical, shortness of breath, exercise intolerance, signs of congestive heart failure, or resting ECG abnormalities suggestive of ischaemia or prior myocardial infarction) requires further evaluation. For patients with a known history of coronary heart disease, relevant medical records must be obtained. While a history of a cardiac event does not invariably lead to exclusion from participation in all early phase trials, such individuals should be excluded from first-in-human studies until there is a greater understanding of the risk associated with the compound under development. Alterations in routine laboratory measurements (e.g. platelet counts, lipid profiles, clotting function), evidence of ECG conduction defects, and individual risk for hypoglycaemia need to be carefully considered on an individual basis. One of the potential benefits for individuals screening for trials is that previously undiagnosed comorbidities can be revealed and then the patient referred for additional evaluation and treatment.

Prolongation of the electrocardiographic QT/QTc interval is a standard exclusion criterion for early phase studies of new diabetes drugs. The need to ensure cardiovascular safety of novel glucose-lowering drugs, as is the case for all new non-antiarrhythmic drugs, starts with the 'thorough QT/QTc' study [42]. The 'International Conference on Harmonization of Technical Requirements for Registration of Pharmaceuticals for Human Use' (ICH) issued the E14 clinical guidance in 2005 which was quickly implemented in the USA and Europe [43]. The thorough QT/QTc study has become a standard component of the clinical development for new molecular entities. The link between QT prolongation and drug therapies was established following reports of deaths in patients treated with cisapride, a gastrointestinal prokinetic drug that was widely used in the treatment of diabetic gastroparesis [44, 45]. With some exceptions, such as cytotoxic cancer drugs, thorough QT/QTc studies are usually performed in healthy volunteers. The QT interval, which is measured from the beginning of the QRS complex to the end of the T wave, represents the duration of ventricular depolarization and subsequent repolarization. A delay in cardiac repolarization creates an electrophysiological environment that favours the development of cardiac arrhythmias, most clearly torsade de pointes [44]. QTc refers to the correction of QT interval for heart rate [42]. Cardiovascular toxicity is a major concern for many classes of drugs during preclinical and clinical development and may lead to post-approval withdrawal of medicines [46]. Since 2008, in the wake of the controversy concerning a reported increase in myocardial infarction with rosiglitazone [47, 48], the FDA has mandated rigorous demonstration of cardiovascular safety of new diabetes drugs [49, 50]. Before rosiglitazone, the cardiovascular safety of diabetes drugs had not been closely scrutinized [51]. While the FDA subsequently rescinded its restrictions on the use of rosiglitazone [51, 52], a major change in policy towards the assessment of cardiovascular risk of new diabetes drugs was already firmly in place. The European Medicines Agency (EMA) has also issued guidance on cardiovascular safety requirements of diabetes drugs [53]. New therapies directed towards glycaemic control may have cardiovascular benefits; however, a reduction in clinical events remains to be proven [54]. According to the 2008 FDA guidance, phase 2 clinical studies may be included in a meta-analysis of premarketing cardiovascular safety studies [55]. The cautious new regulatory environment has increased awareness of the need to de-risk new drugs for cardiometabolic disorders. This needs to happen before expensive late phase clinical studies are initiated [12]. Early phase clinical studies offer an opportunity to identify early signals of cardiovascular effects of new drugs for diabetes and obesity that may inform clinical development decisions. Differences in risk of diabetes-associated cardiovascular disease outcomes between men and women are recognized and remain incompletely understood [56, 57]. Recent data suggest heterogeneity in the effects of certain glucose-lowering drugs on cardiac metabolism and function between men and women [58]; this observation merits further study.

Fatty Liver Disease

While the presence of fatty liver within the obese and type 2 diabetes populations is well known, patients with type 1 diabetes may also have an increased prevalence of fatty liver [59, 60]. Elevations in transaminases are commonly seen in individuals with diabetes [61] and are seen frequently in those screening for participation in early phase clinical trials. Other causes of elevated liver function tests need to be excluded (e.g. alcohol, hepatitis, human immunodeficiency infection). Careful consideration is needed concerning the inclusion of subjects with modest elevations of transaminases in first-in-human trials. Since Hy's law [62, 63] is commonly utilized to assess the risk of liver injury from a new compound in development, subjects should not be included in early phase studies with transaminases >3× upper limit of normal (ULN) as defined by the particular laboratory service provider; consideration should be given to setting the limit for inclusion to <1.5 or 2× ULN. Enrolling subjects with higher transaminases risks exceeding the limits included in Hy's law related to variability that is commonly seen with transaminases and might not be attributable to the compound under investigation. One additional abnormality this is commonly seen is an elevation in indirect bilirubin levels in Gilbert's syndrome, a variant of glucuronyl transferase that affects ~5–10 % of the total population. Most commonly, this is initially noted as an elevation in total bilirubin concentration since fractionation of bilirubin is frequently omitted in screening panels. Fasting or even modest dehydration can raise the level of indirect bilirubin in individuals with Gilbert's syndrome. Fractionation of bilirubin can be helpful in excluding more serious disorders. Most early phase studies allow subjects with Gilbert's syndrome with modest elevations in indirect bilirubin unless there are specific compound-related effects under consideration.

Diabetic Nephropathy

Diabetic nephropathy is the most common cause of chronic kidney disease in the USA [64]. Patients with either long-duration type 1 diabetes or type 2 diabetes may be affected. Depending on factors including age, duration of diabetes, and long-term glycaemic control, approximately 20–40 % of patients with type 2 diabetes may incur a moderate or severe deterioration of renal function. The clinical stages range from degrees of albuminuria to end-stage chronic kidney disease. Albuminuria not only is regarded as a marker and predictor of progressive renal disease but also denotes an increased risk of cardiovascular events [65]. A decline in glomerular filtration is not invariably paralleled by the emergence and increase of urinary albumin excretion; dissociations between albuminuria and decreased glomerular filtration rates (GFR) may be observed [66], Unless testing a new therapy that is focused on preventing, retarding, or reversing nephropathy, good renal function, i.e. estimated GFR (eGFR) calculated by the Modification of Diet in Renal Disease (MDRD) [67], is usually specified as an inclusion criterion for participation in early phase studies of new treatments for diabetes. Renal impairment necessitates dose reduction or avoidance of most classes of glucose-lowering agents to maintain a favourable risk-benefit equation, primarily with respect to the risk of hypoglycaemia [68]. Studies of PK in subgroups of patients with varying degrees of renal impairment will usually form part of the clinical development programme of a novel glucose-lowering drug [69].

Other Comorbidities

Additional clinically evident or subclinical comorbidities commonly encountered in diabetes populations screening for clinical trials are degenerative joint disease, hypothyroidism, sleep apnoea, and depression. Each of these, apart from the associated concomitant medications, has potentially important practical implications for participants in early phase trials. Patients with degenerative joint disease may have mobility issues that make completing study assessments more challenging; affected patients may need special accommodations when resident to manage their disabilities. Subjects with hypothyroidism need to be tested to be sure that their thyroid function tests are within an acceptable range and that their medication regimen is stable. Patients with sleep apnoea who require continuous positive airway pressure (CPAP) or other support will need to have this treatment provided while accommodated in a clinical trial unit, assuming that the therapy is compatible with the protocol. Depression is common among individuals with diabetes, with a meta-analysis revealing an overall prevalence of depression of ~25 %, twice that of the nondiabetic population [70]. This has at least two significant implications for early clinical trials: firstly, many of these patients will be using antidepressant medication, most commonly selective serotonin reuptake inhibitors (SSRIs), and secondly, changes in mood are of particular interest for compounds that could act centrally to control appetite, obesity, and even glucose counter-regulation [71]. The demise of the first selective endocannabinoid receptor antagonist, rimonabant, as a treatment for obesity resulted from adverse effects on mood and increased risk of suicidal ideation [72]. Patients with a past or current history of depression should be excluded from early trials where these issues might be anticipated; early trials should also be designed to include assessments for central effects of novel therapies.

Concomitant Medications

While it is not possible to cover all of the concomitant medications that patients with type 1 or type 2 diabetes might be taking at the time of screening, the majority of individuals volunteering for clinical trials will be taking some concomitant therapy, particularly those with type 2 diabetes. In our database of >20,000 active research subjects with maintained medical records, only 7 % of patients with type 2 diabetes take no medications whereas 64 % of patients with type 1 diabetes take no medication in addition to their insulin. As noted above, comorbidities are commonplace in these populations and medications are often recommended for prophylaxis of such comorbidities for all patients with diabetes, principally statins and other lipid-modifying agents, angiotensin converting enzyme (ACE) inhibitors, angiotensin receptor blockers (ARBs), and aspirin. Table 9.1 contains the classes of medications that are commonly encountered. These should be considered for every protocol written for early phase metabolic trials including patient populations as well as healthy volunteers. Exclusion of these medications significantly affects the ability of clinical sites to enrol subjects in trials; additionally, these medications will be used by the target population, and issues with drug-drug interactions should be identified as early as possible.

However, drugs known to be strong inducers or inhibitors or substrates for metabolic pathways utilized by the compound in development are usually excluded from early phase trials. The FDA has provided guidance for these issues, along with tables of substrates, inhibitors, and inducers [73, 74]. A few medications deserve special mention: oral or injectable corticosteroids are usually excluded if patients have had recent exposure (usually within 3 months of study drug dosing) because of the well-recognized adverse effects on insulin sensitivity and carbohydrate metabolism [75]. Inhaled or topical corticosteroids can usually be allowed because the very low circulating levels that are achieved by these routes are not considered to have any significant impact on glucose tolerance. β-adrenergic blockers are also frequently excluded because of concerns, focused on non-selective agents, that include impairment of glucose and lipid metabolism and masking symptoms of iatrogenic hypoglycaemia [76, 77]. Acetaminophen is generally allowed as needed up to certain doses (usually 1,000–1,500 mg/day) to manage headache or other common discomforts that can be present during participation in a clinical trial, as are routine vitamin therapies at therapeutic doses (e.g. once-a-day multiple vitamin preparations). Most other vitamin and herbal preparations can and probably should be discontinued after screening until study end.

Type 1 Diabetes

Patients with type 1 diabetes mellitus commonly participate in very early development of new insulins and new devices that are developed for assessment and treatment of diabetes (insulin pumps, continuous glucose monitors, and blood glucose meters). The lack of, or very low levels of, endogenous insulin makes the interpretation of studies much simpler, as PK assessments reflect only exogenously administered insulin, and there is no risk of stimulation of endogenous insulin secretion during glucose clamp studies, for example. While the type 1 diabetes study population tends to skew towards the younger age range, the risk for hypoglycaemia and hyperglycaemia is much greater in this patient population; clinical trials must be carefully designed to take due account of these risks. When a new insulin is being evaluated, care must be taken to avoid any interference from routine insulin therapy. Long-acting basal insulin preparations must be discontinued 48 or more hours (depending on the half-life of the basal insulin currently being used by the patient) prior to study dosing. This can be accomplished by initially switching the patient from a basal/bolus regimen to one using isophane (NPH, neutral protamine Hagedorn) insulin and a rapid-acting insulin analogue and then admitting the patient to the clinical unit at least 24 h prior to planned study drug dosing. The last dose of NPH should be administered subcutaneously no later than 24 h prior to study drug dosing, and the last dose of rapid-acting insulin should be administered no later than 6 h prior to dosing. Patients with type 1 diabetes using continuous subcutaneous insulin infusion pumps should discontinue their pumps at this time. Whenever insulin therapy is altered, careful supervision, close monitoring, and ready access to expert advice must be in place to avoid metabolic decompensation. Competence in managing insulin therapy is a prerequisite for investigators supervising clinical trials of diabetic patients.

Two other critical factors in designing studies with patients with type 1 diabetes are ensuring comparability of baseline measurements of glucose and a stable metabolic milieu. Both of these can be accomplished by admission of patients to the study unit at least 24 h prior to important study procedures, which allows for tight control of meals and blood glucose. By giving the last dose of NPH insulin 24 h prior to study drug dosing, administering rapid-acting insulin prandially and as needed until ~12 h prior to study drug dosing, and then instituting an overnight intravenous insulin infusion along with the fasting state, good control can usually be accomplished with modest amounts of insulin. The intravenous insulin infusion can be discontinued at or prior to study drug dosing or with the apparent onset of study drug action or even maintained at a stable infusion rate, depending upon the study design and compound under investigation. Care should be taken to avoid discontinuation of intravenous insulin prior to the onset of study drug action since it may result in hyperglycaemia with unstable baseline conditions.

Maintenance of diabetes control in an early phase clinical trial unit can be a complex undertaking, depending on the compound under study and the particulars of the trial protocol. Use of standardized diets, with known nutrient content, can simplify prandial insulin dosing, particularly for those patients who utilize insulin-to-carbohydrate ratios to determine their mealtime doses. Input from the patients themselves regarding appropriate dosing for meal coverage will usually be helpful for the investigators; this information should be sought unless the protocol dictates the dosing. Upon release from the clinical unit, study volunteers are usually returned to their usual insulin regimen. Frequent monitoring should be performed and adjustments to insulin dosing should be made as needed to accommodate any lingering drug and/or diet effects. Follow-up of the patients should continue until their metabolic control is back to their individual baseline and can usually be accomplished by telephone contact; avoidance of hypoglycaemia is the prime consideration.

Type 2 Diabetes

Patients with type 2 diabetes are frequent participants in clinical trials, beginning with first-in-human trials. However, recruitment of these subjects can be challenging as inclusion/exclusion criteria can eliminate most study volunteers. Common reasons for excluding these volunteers include HbA_{1c} out of range for the trial, exclusionary comorbidities, and exclusionary concomitant medications, including glucose-lowering therapies. Patients whose diabetes is managed with diet and exercise alone are frequently desired participants for first-in-human or SAD and MAD studies. However, it is often difficult to recruit these patients in the numbers needed. In the USA, while diet and exercise have conventionally been recommended as initial interventions, many patients are either commenced on metformin either at or shortly after diagnosis [78]. Potential trial participants who have subscribed to volunteer databases are frequently found to no longer be 'naïve' to pharmacotherapy when contacted about possible participation in a study.

For the majority of trials with patients with type 2 diabetes, the question of temporarily withdrawing routine glucose-lowering agents will be posed. Many new drug therapies to treat type 2 diabetes are being developed as add-on therapy to metformin; in such cases, the maintenance of metformin monotherapy is designed into the protocol. In circumstances when addition of an investigative drug to other ongoing oral glucose-lowering drugs is not required, patient enrolment may be accelerated by allowing washout of therapies, i.e. metformin monotherapy or washing out second-line therapies such as sulphonylureas or dipeptidyl-peptidase (DPP)-4 inhibitors. Oral glucose-lowering drugs can often be withdrawn temporarily for patients on metformin monotherapy or metformin-sulphonylurea dual therapy, with the achievement of stable blood glucose within 2 weeks [79]. These data are supported by modelling work, projecting that fasting plasma glucose concentration is stable within 30 days of washout of metformin monotherapy, sulphonylurea monotherapy, or combination of metformin and sulphonylurea-metformin dual therapy [80]. While safety parameters and glucose monitoring instructions must be built into protocols where glucose-lowering drug washout is included, if subjects are selected with HbA_{1c} values that are less than 10 % (86 mmol/mol), the number of subjects whose fasting plasma glucose will exceed 270 mg/dL (15 mmol/L) (FDA-specified limits for trials less than 6 weeks in duration) [69] will be small, and thus, the numbers of subjects lost during washout will also be small. In addition to considering the pharmacological half-life of the drug(s) to be washed out, one should also consider the biological half-life. Most trials will exclude prior therapy with thiazolidinediones for at least 6 months because of concerns around persistence of metabolic effects long after the drug is discontinued. This reflects the genomic effects of thiazolidinediones [81].

Because other features of the metabolic syndrome are common among subjects with type 2 diabetes, issues surrounding these comorbidities should be considered. Hypertension is present in

50 % or more of individuals with type 2 diabetes [82, 83] and may or may not be well controlled at the time of screening for entry into a clinical trial. Blood pressure, if elevated, should be assessed on multiple occasions, usually after a resting period in the sitting or supine position, as individuals may be anxious when screening for study participation. An appropriate-sized cuff should be used in obese patients [84]. Patients should be questioned as to their most recent dose of medications – patients will frequently hold their medications prior to a screening visit, in spite of instructions to the contrary. Similar caveats apply when subjects check in to an inpatient unit. Generally, persistent blood pressure >160 mmHg systolic and >95 mmHg diastolic is exclusionary in most trials and should necessitate referral of the patient to a physician for further assessment and treatment.

Dyslipidaemia is another common feature of patients with type 2 diabetes [85]. This is frequently evident as increases in plasma triglycerides and decreases in HDL cholesterol compared to the nondiabetic population, although total cholesterol and low-density lipoprotein (LDL) levels are generally similar [85]. While no significant clinical effects are known for acute changes in high-density lipoprotein (HDL) cholesterol, marked elevations in triglycerides exceeding 11 mmol/L (1,000 mg/dL) are considered a risk for the development of acute pancreatitis [86] and most trials exclude patients with triglyceride levels >4.5 or 5.1 mmol/L (>400 or 450 mg/dL) if there is concern for rising triglyceride levels during the trial. Gemfibrozil, because of its potential for drug-drug interactions secondary to CYP2C8 inhibition [87], is a frequently excluded concomitant medication during metabolic trials. While LDL cholesterol concentrations are not usually elevated in patients with diabetes, the current US American College of Cardiology (ACC) and American Heart Association (AHA) guidelines recommend moderate-intensive statin therapy for all patients with diabetes between the ages of 40–75 to reduce the risk of cardiovascular events [88]. While not all trial volunteers with diabetes will be on statin therapy, many will, and careful consideration should be given to continuing these medications throughout the trial as background therapy or washing them out for subjects where statins are being used as prophylaxis. For patients with a history of known coronary heart disease, statins should not be discontinued.

Impaired Glucose Tolerance and Impaired Fasting Glucose

Situated between normal glucose tolerance and diabetes are the diagnostic categories of impaired glucose tolerance (IGT) and impaired fasting glucose (IFG) [89, 90]. These intermediate states of glucose intolerance, which may be stable, progress to type 2 diabetes, or revert to normal glucose tolerance, usually result from a combination of insulin resistance and insulin secretion [89]. Interest in enrolling individuals with IGT or IFG in clinical trials results from an interest in developing therapies that could be preventative and/or therapeutic for diabetes mellitus. Definitions of both IGT and IFG have been established by both the WHO [91] and American Diabetes Association (ADA) [92].

Impaired Glucose Tolerance

WHO and ADA define IGT as a fasting plasma glucose <7.0 mmol/L (126 mg/dL), 2-h plasma glucose ≥7.8 mmol/L (≥140 mg/dL), and <11.1 mmol/L (<200 mg/dL).

Impaired Fasting Glucose

The ADA defines IFG as fasting plasma glucose ≥5.6 mmol/L (≥100 mg/L) and <7.0 mmol/L (<126 mg/dL), whereas the WHO criteria define IFG as fasting plasma glucose ≥6.1 mmol/L (≥110 mg/dL) and ≤6.9 mmol/L (≤125 mg/dL).

More recently, the use of HbA_{1c} has been sanctioned enabling subjects to be classified as normal <5.7 (<39 mmol/mol), prediabetes 5.7–6.4 % (39–46 mmol/mol), and diabetes ≥6.5 % (>48 mmol/mol) [92]. HbA_{1c} methods must be certified by the National Glycohemoglobin Standardization Program (NGSP) and standardized or traceable to the Diabetes Control and Complications Trial reference assay. A test result diagnostic of diabetes should be repeated to rule out laboratory error, unless the diagnosis is clear on clinical grounds, e.g. in a patient with classic symptoms of diabetes. When two different tests are available in an individual and the results are discordant, the test whose result is above the diagnostic cut point should be repeated, and the diagnosis is made on the basis of the confirmed test [92].

The diagnosis of insulin resistance is less precise and is dependent upon the methodology used. The accepted gold standard for the assessment of whole body insulin sensitivity is the hyperinsulinaemic euglycaemic glucose clamp technique (see Chap. 1) [93]. However, other approaches such as modified insulin suppression test have been utilized [94]. Both of these techniques are technically challenging and labour intensive. Other less rigorous methods based on measures of fasting plasma glucose and insulin, e.g. homeostasis model assessment (HOMA-IR) [95] and quantitative insulin sensitivity check index (QUICKI) [96], have been used for studies requiring larger numbers of subjects, where a simpler technique is required.

While data vary on the numbers of individuals falling within these categorical definitions (ranging from approximately 10 % to 30 % depending on age range and ethnic group), the relative numbers of individuals in each of these diagnostic categories are insulin resistance > impaired glucose tolerance > impaired fasting glucose for a generally healthy, previously unscreened population. In addition, this population can be challenging to recruit from the perspective of meeting inclusion and exclusion criteria for clinical trials. There are two major issues: the first is that the majority of individuals who meet these criteria are unaware that they have impaired carbohydrate metabolism and the second is that these are not stable states. The reproducibility for the impaired glucose tolerance test is less than 50 %, even if the repeat test is performed within 6 weeks of the first. A significant proportion (up to half) will be 'normal' on repeat, whereas another 6–10 % will be classified as having diabetes mellitus [97]. This discrepancy poses substantial challenges for quickly enrolling individuals in early phase research studies, where timelines are critical. Studies designed to assess these populations should expect large screen failure rates, even if potentially eligible subjects have been identified from previously known abnormal tests.

Groups with Special Characteristics

Older People

The inclusion of older adults in studies with metabolic compounds is particularly important as the prevalence of disorders of carbohydrate metabolism rises with increasing age [98]. The paucity of information on the PK/PD of glucose-lowering drugs in older patients with diabetes has long been recognized [99–101]. The standard inclusion/exclusion criteria in the past have arbitrarily excluded volunteers above a certain age (usually 65 years but occasionally even 55 or 45), in spite of rigorous inclusion and exclusion criteria regarding comorbidities and concomitant medications. One important comorbidity in this group is mild cognitive impairment, a precursor of dementia in older adults [102]. This is particularly relevant in studies of older adults with diabetes, as diabetes has been shown in multiple studies to increase the risk of mild cognitive impairment [103] as well as the risk for both Alzheimer's disease and vascular dementia [104, 105]. However, an argument can be made for removing any age-related criteria and allowing an individual to participate in early phase clinical studies, regardless of age, if he or she is able to meet the other inclusion and exclusion criteria with careful screening. Granted, this would skew the population under evaluation towards the 'fit' elderly, but this would at least start to provide some representation of older adults in these trials. Recommendations have been proposed to address some of the shortcomings related to the participation of older subjects in clinical trials [106].

Children and Adolescents

The increasing incidence of both type 1 and type 2 diabetes in children and adolescents has fuelled interest in the development of new treatments for these populations [107–109]. The FDA has addressed this issue briefly in its guidance materials [69] but the inclusion of these populations in early studies will need to be addressed on a case-by-case basis. The ethical guidelines around enrolment of vulnerable populations must be followed, and issues around informed consent (and assent) are paramount. Research with these populations should be performed at centres with special expertise and the resources to sensitively manage children and their parents or guardians through these studies.

Women of Childbearing Potential

Women of childbearing potential are routinely excluded from early phase drug trials because of concerns about risks to the fetus should there be accidental fetal exposure if pregnancy occurs during study treatment. This occurs despite the 1993 FDA guidance that changed the previous guidance from 1977 that generally excluded women of childbearing potential from early clinical drug development. The aim was to encourage participation of women with appropriate precautions to avoid pregnancy and fetal exposure. Most early clinical development programmes continue to exclude these women, although participation is occasionally allowed with extreme precaution to avoid pregnancy (use of hormonal contraception and double-barrier method, contraception plus tubal ligation, continued use of protocol-mandated contraception for 90 days post study, etc.). More recently, concerns have been raised regarding pregnancy or exposure of the fetus through seminal fluid while the father has been a study participant. Protocols increasingly mandate contraception for male participants in early phase trials as well.

References

1. Hornblum AM, Newman JL, Dober GJ. Against their will: the secret history of medical experimentation on children in cold war America. New York: Palgrave Macmillan; 1997.
2. Pellegrino ED. The Nazi doctors and Nuremberg: some moral lessons revisited. Ann Intern Med. 1997;127(4):307–8.
3. Resnick DB. Research ethics timeline (1932–present). Available from: http://www.niehs.nih.gov/research/resources/bioethics/timeline/.
4. WMA Declaration of Helsinki – ethical principles for medical research involving human subjects. 2014. Available from: http://www.wma.net/en/30publications/10policies/b3/. Accessed 10 June 2014.
5. Belmont report: ethical principles and guidelines for the protection of human subjects of research, report of the National Commission for the Protection of Human Subjects of Biomedical and Behavioral Research. Available from: http://www.hhs.gov/ohrp/humansubjects/guidance/belmont.html.
6. International conference on harmonisation of technical requirements for registration of pharmaceuticals for human use. Available from: http://www.ich.org/fileadmin/Public_Web_Site/ICH_Products/Guidelines/Efficacy/E2F/Step4/E2F_Step_4.pdf.
7. Markman M. The ethical dilemma of phase I clinical trials. CA Cancer J Clin. 1986;36(6):367–9.
8. Dresser R. First-in-human trial participants: not a vulnerable population, but vulnerable nonetheless. J Law Med Ethics. 2009;37(1):38–50.
9. Grundy SM, Benjamin IJ, Burke GL, Chait A, Eckel RH, Howard BV, et al. Diabetes and cardiovascular disease: a statement for healthcare professionals from the American Heart Association. Circulation. 1999;100(10):1134–46.
10. Ivy SP, Siu LL, Garrett-Mayer E, Rubinstein L. Approaches to phase 1 clinical trial design focused on safety, efficiency, and selected patient populations: a report from the clinical trial design task force of the national cancer institute investigational drug steering committee. Clin Cancer Res. 2010;16(6):1726–36.
11. Kahn SE, Cooper ME, Del Prato S. Pathophysiology and treatment of type 2 diabetes: perspectives on the past, present, and future. Lancet. 2014;383(9922):1068–83.
12. Krentz AJ, Morrow L, Hompesch M. Developing new drugs for diabetes and cardiometabolic disorders: a changing paradigm. Drugs. 2012;72(13):1709–11.
13. American Medical Association. Available from: http://www.ama-assn.org/ama/pub/news/news/2013/2013-06-18-new-ama-policies-annual-meeting.page.
14. WHO/IASO/IOTF. The Asia-Pacific perspective: redefining obesity and its treatment. Melbourne: Health Communications Australia; 2000.
15. James WP, Chunming C, Inoue S. Appropriate Asian body mass indices? Obes Rev. 2002;3(3):139.
16. Blouin RA, Warren GW. Pharmacokinetic considerations in obesity. J Pharm Sci. 1999;88(1):1–7.
17. Morello CM. Pharmacokinetics and pharmacodynamics of insulin analogs in special populations with type 2 diabetes mellitus. Int J Gen Med. 2011;4:827–35.
18. Barnett AH. How well do rapid-acting insulins work in obese individuals? Diabetes Obes Metab. 2006;8(4):388–95.
19. Chang Y, Kim BK, Yun KE, Cho J, Zhang Y, Rampal S, et al. Metabolically healthy obesity and coronary artery calcification. J Am Coll Cardiol. 2014;63:2679–86.

20. Bluher M. The distinction of metabolically 'healthy' from 'unhealthy' obese individuals. Curr Opin Lipidol. 2010;21(1):38–43.
21. Karelis AD. To be obese – does it matter if you are metabolically healthy? Nat Rev Endocrinol. 2011;7(12):699–700.
22. Karelis AD, Brochu M, Rabasa-Lhoret R. Can we identify metabolically healthy but obese individuals (MHO)? Diabetes Metab. 2004;30(6):569–72.
23. Hamer M, Stamatakis E. Metabolically healthy obesity and risk of all-cause and cardiovascular disease mortality. J Clin Endocrinol Metab. 2012;97(7):2482–8.
24. Chow SC, Chang M. Adaptive design methods in clinical trials – a review. Orphanet J Rare Dis. 2008;3:11.
25. Ma Y, Bertone ER, Stanek 3rd EJ, Reed GW, Hebert JR, Cohen NL, et al. Association between eating patterns and obesity in a free-living US adult population. Am J Epidemiol. 2003;158(1):85–92.
26. Herman CP, Roth DA, Polivy J. Effects of the presence of others on food intake: a normative interpretation. Psychol Bull. 2003;129(6):873–86.
27. Laferrere B, Teixeira J, McGinty J, Tran H, Egger JR, Colarusso A, et al. Effect of weight loss by gastric bypass surgery versus hypocaloric diet on glucose and incretin levels in patients with type 2 diabetes. J Clin Endocrinol Metab. 2008;93(7):2479–85.
28. Stone MA, Camosso-Stefinovic J, Wilkinson J, de Lusignan S, Hattersley AT, Khunti K. Incorrect and incomplete coding and classification of diabetes: a systematic review. Diabet Med. 2010;27(5):491–7.
29. Thanabalasingham G, Pal A, Selwood MP, Dudley C, Fisher K, Bingley PJ, et al. Systematic assessment of etiology in adults with a clinical diagnosis of young-onset type 2 diabetes is a successful strategy for identifying maturity-onset diabetes of the young. Diabetes Care. 2012;35(6):1206–12.
30. McDonald TJ, Colclough K, Brown R, et al. Islet autoantibodies can discriminate maturity-onset diabetes of the young (MODY) from type 1 diabetes. Diabet Med. 2011;28(9):1028–33.
31. Zinman B, Kahn SE, Haffner SM, O'Neill MC, Heise MA, Freed MI, ADOPT Study Group. Phenotypic characteristics of GAD antibody-positive recently diagnosed patients with type 2 diabetes in North America and Europe. Diabetes. 2004;53(12):3193–200.
32. Stenstrom G, Gottsater A, Bakhtadze E, Berger B, Sundkvist G. Latent autoimmune diabetes in adults: definition, prevalence, beta-cell function, and treatment. Diabetes. 2005;54 Suppl 2:S68–72.
33. Jones AG, Hattersley AT. The clinical utility of C-peptide measurement in the care of patients with diabetes. Diabet Med. 2013;30(7):803–17.
34. Harris MI, Klein R, Welborn TA, Knuiman MW. Onset of NIDDM occurs at least 4–7 yr before clinical diagnosis. Diabetes Care. 1992;15(7):815–9.
35. Nathan DM. Long-term complications of diabetes mellitus. N Engl J Med. 1993;328(23):1676–85.
36. Robertson RP, Harmon J, Tran PO, Tanaka Y, Takahashi H. Glucose toxicity in beta-cells: type 2 diabetes, good radicals gone bad, and the glutathione connection. Diabetes. 2003;52(3):581–7.
37. Narbonne H, Renacco E, Pradel V, Portugal H, Vialettes B. Can fructosamine be a surrogate for HbA(1c) in evaluating the achievement of therapeutic goals in diabetes? Diabetes Metab. 2001;27(5 Pt 1):598–603.
38. Koga M. Glycated albumin; clinical usefulness. Clin Chim Acta. 2014;433:96–104.
39. Cryer PE, Davis SN, Shamoon H. Hypoglycemia in diabetes. Diabetes Care. 2003;26(6):1902–12.
40. Cryer PE. Mechanisms of hypoglycemia-associated autonomic failure in diabetes. N Engl J Med. 2013;369(4):362–72.
41. Donahue RP, Abbott RD, Reed DM, Yano K. Postchallenge glucose concentration and coronary heart disease in men of Japanese ancestry. Honolulu Heart Program. Diabetes. 1987;36(6):689–92.
42. Guidance for industry. E14 clinical evaluation of QT/QTc interval prolongation and proarrhythmic potential for non-antiarrhythmic drugs. Available from: http://www.fda.gov/downloads/Drugs/GuidanceComplianceRegulatoryInformation/Guidances/ucm073153.pdf.
43. Darpo B. The thorough QT/QTc study 4 years after the implementation of the ICH E14 guidance. Br J Pharmacol. 2010;159(1):49–57.
44. Watters K, Munro N, Feher M. QTc prolongation and diabetes therapies. Diabet Med. 2012;29(3):290–2.
45. Evans AJ, Krentz AJ. Should cisapride be avoided in patients with diabetic gastroparesis? J Diabetes Complications. 1999;13(5–6):314–5.
46. Ferri N, Siegl P, Corsini A, Herrmann J, Lerman A, Benghozi R. Drug attrition during pre-clinical and clinical development: understanding and managing drug-induced cardiotoxicity. Pharmacol Ther. 2013;138(3):470–84.
47. Nissen SE, Wolski K. Effect of rosiglitazone on the risk of myocardial infarction and death from cardiovascular causes. N Engl J Med. 2007;356(24):2457–71.
48. Krentz AJ. Rosiglitazone: trials, tribulations and termination. Drugs. 2011;71(2):123–30.
49. Guidance for industry. Diabetes mellitus—evaluating cardiovascular risk in new antidiabetic therapies to treat type 2 diabetes. Available from: http://www.fda.gov/downloads/Drugs/GuidanceComplianceRegulatoryInformation/Guidances/UCM071627.pdfeutm_term=guidance.
50. Adler AI. Drugs and diabetes: understanding the new breed of cardiovascular safety trials. Lancet Diabetes Endocrinol. 2013;1(3):175–7.
51. Hiatt WR, Kaul S, Smith RJ. The cardiovascular safety of diabetes drugs – insights from the rosiglitazone experience. N Engl J Med. 2013;369(14):1285–7.
52. Nissen SE. Rosiglitazone: a case of regulatory hubris. BMJ. 2013;347:f7428.
53. Guideline on clinical investigation of medicinal products in the treatment or prevention of diabetes mellitus. Available from: http://www.ema.europa.eu/docs/en_GB/document_library/Scientific_guideline/2012/06/WC500129256.pdf.

54. Joshi PH, Kalyani RR, Blumenthal RS, Donner TW. Cardiovascular effects of noninsulin, glucose-lowering agents: need for more outcomes data. Am J Cardiol. 2012;110(9 Suppl):32B–42.
55. Krentz AJ, Hompesch M. Cardiovascular safety of new drugs for diabetes: getting the balance right? Pharm Med. 2014;28:109–17.
56. Kanaya AM, Grady D, Barrett-Connor E. Explaining the sex difference in coronary heart disease mortality among patients with type 2 diabetes mellitus: a meta-analysis. Arch Intern Med. 2002;162(15):1737–45.
57. Miller TM, Gilligan S, Herlache LL, Regensteiner JG. Sex differences in cardiovascular disease risk and exercise in type 2 diabetes. J Investig Med. 2012;60(4):664–70.
58. Lyons MR, Peterson LR, McGill JB, Herrero P, Coggan AR, Saeed IM, et al. Impact of sex on the heart's metabolic and functional responses to diabetic therapies. Am J Physiol Heart Circ Physiol. 2013;305(11):H1584–91.
59. Targher G, Bertolini L, Padovani R, Rodella S, Zoppini G, Pichiri I, et al. Prevalence of non-alcoholic fatty liver disease and its association with cardiovascular disease in patients with type 1 diabetes. J Hepatol. 2010;53(4):713–8.
60. Smith BW, Adams LA. Nonalcoholic fatty liver disease and diabetes mellitus: pathogenesis and treatment. Nat Rev Endocrinol. 2011;7(8):456–65.
61. Salmela PI, Sotaniemi EA, Niemi M, Maentausta O. Liver function tests in diabetic patients. Diabetes Care. 1984;7(3):248–54.
62. Food and Drug Administration. Guidance for industry drug-induced liver injury: premarketing clinical evaluation. 2009. Available from: http://www.fda.gov/downloads/Drugs/.../Guidances/UCM174090.pdf.
63. Lewis JH. 'Hy's law', the 'Rezulin Rule', and other predictors of severe drug-induced hepatotoxicity: putting risk-benefit into perspective. Pharmacoepidemiol Drug Saf. 2006;15(4):221–9.
64. Gosmanov AR, Wall BM, Gosmanova EO. Diagnosis and treatment of diabetic kidney disease. Am J Med Sci. 2014;347(5):406–13.
65. Karalliedde J, Viberti G. Proteinuria in diabetes: bystander or pathway to cardiorenal disease? J Am Soc Nephrol. 2010;21(12):2020–7.
66. Halimi JM. The emerging concept of chronic kidney disease without clinical proteinuria in diabetic patients. Diabetes Metab. 2012;38(4):291–7.
67. Levey AS, Coresh J, Greene T, Stevens LA, Zhang YL, Hendriksen S, et al. Using standardized serum creatinine values in the modification of diet in renal disease study equation for estimating glomerular filtration rate. Ann Intern Med. 2006;145(4):247–54.
68. Bailey C, Day C. Diabetes therapies in renal impairment. Br J Diabetes Vasc Dis. 2012;12:167–71.
69. Food and Drug Administration. Guidance for industry. Diabetes mellitus: developing drugs and therapeutic biologics for treatment and prevention. 2008. http://www.fda.gov/downloads/Drugs/Guidances/ucm071624.pdf. Accessed 1 June 2014.
70. Anderson RJ, Freedland KE, Clouse RE, Lustman PJ. The prevalence of comorbid depression in adults with diabetes: a meta-analysis. Diabetes Care. 2001;24(6):1069–78.
71. Norjavaara E, Ericsson H, Sjoberg F, Leonsson-Zachrisson M, Sjöstrand M, Morrow LA, et al. Glucokinase activators AZD6370 and AZD1656 do not affect the central counterregulatory response to hypoglycemia in healthy males. J Clin Endocrinol Metab. 2012;97(9):3319–25.
72. Butler H, Korbonits M. Cannabinoids for clinicians: the rise and fall of the cannabinoid antagonists. Eur J Endocrinol. 2009;161(5):655–62.
73. Food and Drug Administration. Drug development and drug interactions. Updated 2011. Available from: http://www.fda.gov/Drugs/DevelopmentApprovalProcess/DevelopmentResources/DrugInteractionsLabeling/ucm080499.htm. Accessed 8 June 2014.
74. Food and Drug Administration. Drug development and drug interactions: table of substrates, inhibitors and inducers. Available from: http://www.fda.gov/Drugs/DevelopmentApprovalProcess/DevelopmentResources/DrugInteractionsLabeling/ucm093664.htm. Accessed 30 May 2014.
75. Kauh EA, Mixson LA, Shankar S, McCarthy J, Maridakis V, Morrow L, et al. Short-term metabolic effects of prednisone administration in healthy subjects. Diabetes Obes Metab. 2011;13(11):1001–7.
76. White JR, Campbell RK. Dangerous and common drug interactions in patients with diabetes mellitus. Endocrinol Metab Clin North Am. 2000;29(4):789–802.
77. Fonseca VA. Effects of beta-blockers on glucose and lipid metabolism. Curr Med Res Opin. 2010;26(3):615–29.
78. Inzucchi SE, Bergenstal RM, Buse JB, Diamant M, Ferrannini E, Nauck M, et al. Management of hyperglycemia in type 2 diabetes: a patient-centered approach: position statement of the American Diabetes Association (ADA) and the European Association for the Study of Diabetes (EASD). Diabetes Care. 2012;35(6):1364–79.
79. Schott R, Angeles J, Larrabee H, Humphreys C, Shott K, Morrow L, Hompesch M. Effect of discontinuing oral anti-diabetic drugs (OADs) prior to enrollment in a phase 1 trial. Clin Pharmacol Ther. 2012;91 Suppl 1:S52.
80. Wald J, Bush M, Young M, O'Connor-Semmes R, Hastie P, Schibler T. Model-based approach to study fasting plasma glucose during washout of prior antidiabetic therapy. Clin Pharmacol Ther. 2008;83 Suppl 1:S79.
81. Yki-Jarvinen H. Thiazolidinediones. N Engl J Med. 2004;351(11):1106–18.
82. Hypertension in Diabetes Study (HDS): I. Prevalence of hypertension in newly presenting type 2 diabetic patients and the association with risk factors for cardiovascular and diabetic complications. J Hypertens. 1993;11(3): 309–17.
83. Colosia AD, Palencia R, Khan S. Prevalence of hypertension and obesity in patients with type 2 diabetes mellitus in observational studies: a systematic literature review. Diabetes Metab Syndr Obes. 2013;6:327–38.

84. Mancia G, Fagard R, Narkiewicz K, Redón J, Zanchetti A, Böhm M, et al. 2013 ESH/ESC Guidelines for the management of arterial hypertension: the Task Force for the management of arterial hypertension of the European Society of Hypertension (ESH) and of the European Society of Cardiology (ESC). J Hypertens. 2013;31(7):1281–357.
85. Mooradian AD. Dyslipidemia in type 2 diabetes mellitus. Nat Clin Pract Endocrinol Metab. 2009;5(3):150–9.
86. Berglund L, Brunzell JD, Goldberg AC, Goldberg IJ, Sacks F, Murad MH, et al. Evaluation and treatment of hypertriglyceridemia: an Endocrine Society clinical practice guideline. J Clin Endocrinol Metab. 2012;97(9):2969–89.
87. Ogilvie BW, Zhang D, Li W, Rodrigues AD, Gipson AE, Holsapple J, et al. Glucuronidation converts gemfibrozil to a potent, metabolism-dependent inhibitor of CYP2C8: implications for drug-drug interactions. Drug Metab Dispos. 2006;34(1):191–7.
88. Stone NJ, Robinson J, Lichtenstein AH, Bairey Merz CN, Blum CB, Eckel RH, et al. 2013 ACC/AHA guideline on the treatment of blood cholesterol to reduce atherosclerotic cardiovascular risk in adults: a report of the American College of Cardiology/American Heart Association Task Force on Practice Guidelines. Circulation. 2014;63(25 Pt B):2889–934.
89. Nathan DM, Davidson MB, DeFronzo RA, Heine RJ, Henry RR, Pratley R, et al. Impaired fasting glucose and impaired glucose tolerance: implications for care. Diabetes Care. 2007;30(3):753–9.
90. Alberti KG. Impaired glucose tolerance: what are the clinical implications? Diabetes Res Clin Pract. 1998;40(Suppl):S3–8.
91. Alberti KG, Zimmet PZ. Definition, diagnosis and classification of diabetes mellitus and its complications. Part 1: diagnosis and classification of diabetes mellitus provisional report of a WHO consultation. Diabet Med. 1998;15(7):539–53.
92. American Diabetes Association. Diagnosis and classification of diabetes mellitus. Diabetes Care. 2013;36 Suppl 1:S67–74.
93. DeFronzo RA, Tobin JD, Andres R. Glucose clamp technique: a method for quantifying insulin secretion and resistance. Am J Physiol. 1979;237(3):E214–23.
94. Pei D, Jones CN, Bhargava R, Chen YD, Reaven GM. Evaluation of octreotide to assess insulin-mediated glucose disposal by the insulin suppression test. Diabetologia. 1994;37(8):843–5.
95. Matthews DR, Hosker JP, Rudenski AS, Naylor BA, Treacher DF, Turner RC. Homeostasis model assessment: insulin resistance and beta-cell function from fasting plasma glucose and insulin concentrations in man. Diabetologia. 1985;28(7):412–9.
96. Katz A, Nambi SS, Mather K, Baron AD, Follmann DA, Sullivan G, et al. Quantitative insulin sensitivity check index: a simple, accurate method for assessing insulin sensitivity in humans. J Clin Endocrinol Metab. 2000;85(7):2402–10.
97. Santaguida PL, Balion C, Hunt D, Morrison K, Gerstein H, Raina P, Booker L, Yazdi H. Diagnosis, prognosis, and treatment of impaired glucose tolerance and impaired fasting glucose. Evidence report/Technology Assessment No. 128. 2005. Agency for Healthcare Research and Quality. Rockville, USA.
98. International Diabetes Federation. IDF global guideline for managing older people with type 2 diabetes. Brussels: International Diabetes Federation; 2013.
99. Turnheim K. When drug therapy gets old: pharmacokinetics and pharmacodynamics in the elderly. Exp Gerontol. 2003;38(8):843–53.
100. Doucet J. Use of antidiabetic drugs in elderly patients. Diabetes Metab. 2005;31(Spec No 2):5S98–104.
101. Pratley RE, Gilbert M. Clinical management of elderly patients with type 2 diabetes mellitus. Postgrad Med. 2012;124(1):133–43.
102. Visser PJ, Kester A, Jolles J, Verhey F. Ten-year risk of dementia in subjects with mild cognitive impairment. Neurology. 2006;67(7):1201–7.
103. Cheng G, Huang C, Deng H, Wang H. Diabetes as a risk factor for dementia and mild cognitive impairment: a meta-analysis of longitudinal studies. Intern Med J. 2012;42(5):484–91.
104. Strachan MW, Reynolds RM, Marioni RE, Price JF. Cognitive function, dementia and type 2 diabetes mellitus in the elderly. Nat Rev Endocrinol. 2011;7(2):108–14.
105. Ninomiya T. Diabetes mellitus and dementia. Curr Diab Rep. 2014;14(5):487.
106. Herrera AP, Snipes SA, King DW, Torres-Vigil I, Goldberg DS, Weinberg AD. Disparate inclusion of older adults in clinical trials: priorities and opportunities for policy and practice change. Am J Public Health. 2010;100 Suppl 1:S105–12.
107. Aguayo-Mazzucato C, Bonner-Weir S. Stem cell therapy for type 1 diabetes mellitus. Nat Rev Endocrinol. 2010;6(3):139–48.
108. Copeland KC, Silverstein J, Moore KR, Prazar GE, Raymer T, Shiffman RN, et al. Management of newly diagnosed type 2 Diabetes Mellitus (T2DM) in children and adolescents. Pediatrics. 2013;131(2):364–82.
109. Pulgaron ER, Delamater AM. Obesity and type 2 diabetes in children: epidemiology and treatment. Curr Diab Rep. 2014;14(8):508.

Quantitative Approaches in Translational Research: An Overview

10

Puneet Gaitonde, Shannon A. Miller, Mirjam N. Trame, and Stephan Schmidt

Abstract

Cardiometabolic diseases are a group of complex and highly intertwined disorders that contribute significantly to healthcare expenditures. Despite the substantial efforts made for making safe and effective treatment options available to patients, cardiometabolic diseases are still a leading cause of death worldwide. This is in part due to the apparent disconnect between drug development and clinical application of medications. In order to bridge this gap, translational research approaches are needed which allow for integration of available knowledge and transition of drugs from bench to bedside. These translational research approaches further allow to feedback the lessons learned during the development of one drug into the development of next-in-pipeline drugs, which improves their chances to successfully make it to the market. Ultimately, these quantitative approaches can also serve as a knowledge platform for bedside-ready decision support tools that can guide the clinician's choice of the most appropriate drug and/or dosing regimen.

Keywords

Diabetes • Obesity • Cardiometabolic • Translational • Modelling and simulation • Quantitative pharmacology • Bench to bedside • Drug development • Top down • Bottom up • Genomics • Personalized medicine

P. Gaitonde, PhD • M.N. Trame, PharmD, PhD
S. Schmidt, PhD (✉)
Department of Pharmaceutics, College of Pharmacy, University of Florida, Orlando, FL, USA
e-mail: sschmidt@cop.ufl.edu

S.A. Miller, PharmD, BCACP
Department of Pharmacotherapy and Translational Research, College of Pharmacy, University of Florida, Orlando, FL, USA

Background and Clinical Relevance

Cardiometabolic diseases are a group of complex interrelated diseases affecting millions of people worldwide. Together, they constitute the leading cause of morbidity and mortality. The group is largely comprised of diseases associated with the cardiovascular system (e.g., myocardial infarction, atherosclerosis, thromboembolism,

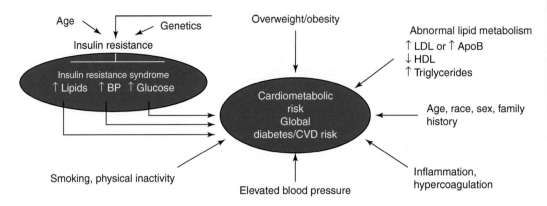

Fig. 10.1 Modifiable and non-modifiable cardiometabolic risk factors (Reprinted by permission from Macmillan Publishers Ltd.: Vlasakakis et al. [3], copyright 2013)

hypertension, dyslipidemia, diabetes mellitus, and obesity). These diseases are highly interlinked, share common pathogenetic features, and often occur in combination in affected individuals [1]. According to the Centers for Disease Control (CDC) [2], approximately one-third of American adults have hypertension, and more than a third of American adults are obese. In addition, 71 million American adults have high levels of low-density lipoproteins (LDL), and roughly 26 million Americans are diagnosed with diabetes mellitus. In 2012, the cost of treatment and care for hypertension was close to US$50 billion, whereas the cost of diabetes mellitus was US$245 billion. Treatment and cost of care are becoming prohibitively expensive precipitating insurmountable financial burden.

Risk factors associated with the development of cardiometabolic diseases can be categorized as either non-modifiable (e.g., age, gender, ethnicity, family history) or modifiable (e.g., smoking, high-fat and cholesterol diet, sedentary lifestyle, state of mental health) [3] (Fig. 10.1). In order to tackle this goliath plaguing today's society, innovative approaches involving interdisciplinary teams are needed to understand the disease as to cause and effect and to translate the acquired knowledge into actionable preventative and therapeutic measures. In addition, it is important to raise public awareness of effective health and wellness strategies in order to slow down the onset or halt or even prevent these diseases.

In pharmacotherapy, there is often an apparent disconnect between physicochemical, biological (e.g., protein targets, transporters, enzymes, and pathways), system/patient-specific properties, treatment effects, and long-term clinical outcome. In order to overcome this limitation and to enable optimal treatment for each individual patient, it is important to integrate these different pieces of information into a harmonized approach [4]. Patient safety should here be of utmost priority provided that numerous observational studies have reported that adverse drug events (ADEs) account for a significant percentage of patient hospitalizations and inpatient morbidity and mortality, and they add a significant financial burden to healthcare costs [4]. Adverse drug reactions are often not discovered until late in the drug development process, particularly during phase 3 pivotal clinical trials. Attrition due to drug safety at this stage of development is a multimillion dollar loss to the company but also significantly contributes to the cost of new medicines or therapies to the patient. Even in the case of regulatory approval, ADEs may limit the clinical use of an otherwise efficacious medicine in either parts or the entire patient population. Pharmaceutical companies and regulatory agencies are consequently increasingly challenged to improve their risk-assessment strategies for novel and existing medicines. Mathematical and experimental models support this effort by establishing a strictly quantitative link between drug administration and effect at various levels of biological/organizational complexity (Fig. 10.2), using either a "reductionist" (top-down) or an "integrative" (bottom-up) approach. Top-down approaches usually

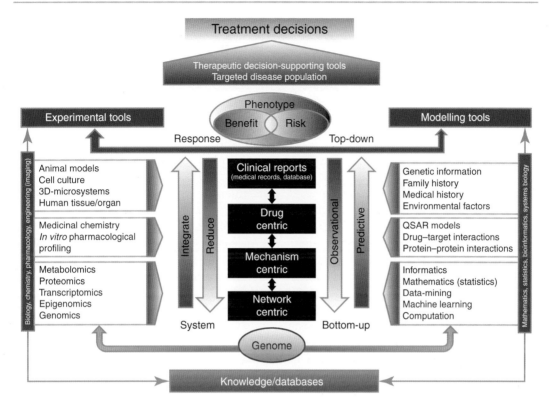

Fig. 10.2 Framework of the vertical integration of top-down and bottom-up approaches and the various levels at which different types of quantitative approaches could be applied (Reprinted by permission from Macmillan Publishers Ltd: Lesko et al. [4], copyright 2013)

start at a high level of organization (e.g., the patient level) and become increasingly more complex in order to better understand and characterize the underlying biological system. In contrast, bottom-up approaches start with the "bottom" elements of the organism (e.g., genes or proteins and their known interactions) and work their way up to the patient-phenotype level. Both of these approaches have advantages and limitations. Top-down approaches have usually a drug- and/or patient-centric focus and evaluate exposure-response relationships, i.e., dose/response or pharmacokinetics (PK)/pharmacodynamics (PD), which are then used to define exposure limits, both in terms of efficacy and safety, for acceptable benefit/risk profiles in different patient cohorts. The main limitation of the top-down approach is that the clinical studies used to inform it typically focus only on one or few covariate(s) at a time and thus represent a methodological reductionist approach. Completely mechanistic bottom-up approaches, on the other hand, are network or pathway centric and may face problems with the translation of the vast amounts of data generated into clinically actionable strategies. The advantages and limitations of both approaches have given rise to mechanism-based hybrid approaches, which represent a compromise between the "reductionist view" of the top-down approach and the "elementary view" of the bottom-up approach. They also serve as a link ("link models") between the next lower and next higher levels of structural complexity and, thus, enable a bidirectional, quantitative flow of information between the different stages of drug development.

Overview of Translational Research

The National Institutes of Health (NIH) defines translational research as the process of applying discoveries generated during research in the laboratory and preclinical studies to the development of trials and studies in humans.

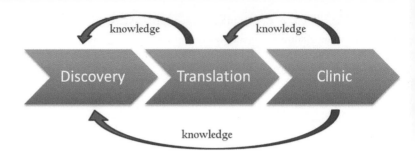

Fig. 10.3 Translational research triad

This research is directed toward enhancing the adoption of best practices in the community and, thus, toward enhancing the cost-effectiveness of prevention and therapeutic strategies [5]. In simple terms research findings are moved from "bench to bedside" to ultimately support the translation of preclinical and clinical study results into everyday clinical practice and decision making [6]. The importance of translational research is evident from the NIH design centres of translational research, as well as the NIH's initiation of the Clinical and Translational Science Institute (CTSI) Award program [6]. Translational research enables exchange of ideas and scientific knowledge between disciplines, such as biochemistry, cell biology, genetics, and immunology, as well as between scientists of different backgrounds to further the development of novel and effective therapies. Thus, translational research in essence, can be described as a triad feedback loop between research, investigation, and discovery, clinical trials and finally with medical treatment (Fig. 10.3).

The American Diabetes Association (ADA) recently published a report on the Standard of Care in Diabetes [7], which focuses on a patient-centred approach balancing choice of pharmacological agents with respect to efficacy, cost, and potential impact on cardiovascular disease. In a separate document, Jain and colleagues [8] reviewed labeling summaries of a vast number of therapeutic products to determine if obesity is a factor that affects drug PK, PD, efficacy, or safety (Table 10.1). Improving the treatment and management of diabetes, its comorbidities and associated complications, is an important focus of pharmaceutical research and development (R&D). Additionally, the assessment of benefit and risk must be the goal when developing a plan for therapeutic interventions [9].

This chapter presents an overview on the use of quantitative analysis tools for assessing drug efficacy and safety during drug development and regulatory decision-making. Examples of specific model applications at different stages of the development process are also provided.

Role of Quantifiable and Accurate Biomarkers

The predictive performance of the earlier mentioned hybrid models relies to a large extent on the use of biomarkers. The Biomarkers Definitions Working Group (BDWG) defined a biomarker as a characteristic that is objectively measured and evaluated as an indicator of normal biological processes, pathogenic processes, or pharmacological responses to a therapeutic intervention [9]. Thus, a biomarker is a laboratory measurement or clinical phenotype that reflects the activity of a disease process. These markers quantitatively correlate (either directly or inversely) with disease progression. Surrogate endpoints are a subset of biomarkers that are used to establish therapeutic efficacy in registration trials. It is defined as a biomarker that is intended to substitute for a clinical endpoint and is expected to predict clinical benefit or harm or lack of benefit or harm – based on epidemiological, therapeutic, pathophysiological, or other scientific evidence [9].

Further, intermediate biomarkers are routinely used at different stages of the drug development process [10] (Fig. 10.4). For practical implementation of this biomarker classification system, some of the biomarker types may be combined in the

Table 10.1 Review of pharmaceutical product labels listing link with obesity

Description	Drugs
Obesity listed as a risk factor for cardiovascular adverse events such as CAD, hypertension, MI, and thromboembolic events	Dalteparin, estradiol, estrone, follitropin, fondaparinux, frovatriptan, iloperidone, naratriptan, progesterone, rizatriptan, sumatriptan, synthetic conjugated estrogens, zolmitriptan, FDC (drospirenone, levonorgestrel/ethinyl estradiol, norelgestromin/estradiol, sumatriptan/naproxen), others (etonogestrel implant, conjugated estrogen vaginal cream, ring delivers)
Obesity listed as risk factor for lactic acidosis	Abacavir, adefovir, emtricitabine, entecavir, lamivudine, metformin, tenofovir, zidovudine, FDC (abacavir/lamivudine, abacavir/lamivudine/zidovudine, lamivudine/zidovudine, pioglitazone/metformin, rosiglitazone/metformin, sitagliptin/metformin, tenofovir/emtricitabine)
Obesity listed as an adverse event	Atazanavir, dexlansoprazole, efavirenz, fosamprenavir, paroxetine, ritonavir, FDC (crixivan/indinavir, lopinavir/ritonavir)
Obesity listed as a risk factor for diabetes	Acitretin, asenapine, paliperidone, quetiapine, risperidone, somatropin, ziprasidone
Impact of obesity or BMI on PK or PK/PD	Cisatracurium, insulin aspart, insulin glulisine, FDC (quinupristin/dalfopristin, insulin lispro [MIX50/50])
Obesity listed as a caution without any specifics	Oxymorphone, tapentadol
Obesity does not change efficacy	Atorvastatin, FDC (amlodipine/atorvastatin)
Obesity does not change efficacy and safety	Insulin glargine
Dosage and administration for obesity	Rocuronium
Obesity listed as a miscellaneous risk factor (i.e., respiratory depression, apnea)	Aripiprazole, buprenorphine (transdermal), somatropin
Obesity listed as miscellaneous information	Rosuvastatin, valsartan, levothyroxine, sibutramine, thyroid, liothyronine, octreotide

Reprinted by permission from Macmillan Publishers Ltd: Jain et al. [8], copyright 2011
BMI body mass index, *CAD* coronary artery disease, *FDC* fixed-dose combination, *MI* myocardial infarction, *PD* pharmacodynamics, *PDR* Physician's Desk Reference

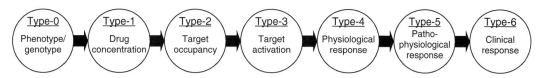

Fig. 10.4 Schematic of in vivo drug effects on the basis of intermediary biomarker responses (With kind permission from Springer Science+Business Media: Danhof et al. [10])

context of risk assessment in order to appropriately reflect their position in the causal chain between drug administration and effect. For example, types 2 and 3 are largely reflective of target occupancy and upstream transduction, whereas types 4–6 are reflective of downstream events.

Specifically, biomarkers for diabetes can be categorized according to their turnover half-lives as fast (minutes–hours), intermediate (hours–days), or slow biomarkers (days–weeks). Plasma glucose, C-peptide, and insulin are examples for fast biomarkers, whereas glycated haemoglobin [HbA_{1c}] is considered a slow biomarker. The latter also serves as the clinical surrogate endpoint for glucose-lowering drugs due to its proximity to clinical outcome relative to plasma glucose. Other biomarkers, such as glucagon, dipeptidyl peptidase (DPP)-4 enzyme inhibition, glucagon-like peptide-1 (GLP-1), glucose-dependent insulinotropic peptide (GIP), and other hormones may also be used to make inferences about drug-target engagement. It should be noted at this point that drug-centric models frequently rely on measures of one or few biomarkers, whereas systems pharmacology/network-based models attempt to link biomarkers at different temporal and spatial levels (e.g. plasma cholesterol, fatty acids, blood pressure, heart rate) on a mechanistic/physiological basis.

Role of Quantitative Approaches in Various Stages of Drug Development

Quantitative approaches are a set of particularly valuable tools within the translational medicine arena as they combine computational with experimental methods to elucidate, validate, and apply new pharmacological concepts to the development and use of small molecule and biologic drugs [11]. They also enable the integration of information on a systems level to determine the mechanisms of action of new and existing drugs in preclinical and animal models and to subsequently apply this knowledge to patients.

The drug development process can generally be divided into preclinical and clinical stages. These stages are tightly interlinked as the information gathered during one phase is carried forward into the next to gain confidence in the drug's ability to treat a certain disease, in other words to de-risk the drug for the patient by reducing uncertainty. Despite the fact that a drug typically passes through one development phase at a time, the process of "learning and confirming" is by no means linear. Lessons learned during one phase may feed back into the development stream to inform the next steps to be taken for the drug(s) in the development pipeline. Mathematical and statistical models are ideally suited to serve as the knowledge platform for this "learn, confirm, and apply" cycle as they allow the integration of the available information into a single, unifying approach [12] (Fig. 10.5). To avoid late-stage development failures in large and expensive clinical trials, it is imperative to learn as much as possible about a particular drug candidate as early as possible in the discovery and development process. The identification of the correct target for a given disease is consequently critical, followed by the optimization of lead compounds as well as preclinical proof of concept, PK/PD, and safety-toxicity studies. As a drug candidate traverses from preclinical to clinical stages (see Fig. 10.5), there is a high degree of uncertainty surrounding the probability of success at the preclinical stage. Very little is known about the drug and its potential effect in the disease area at this point. To build the knowledge base and enhance predictability at each step of the drug development process, quantitative tools are employed to analyze and interpret experimental data. System, (semi-)

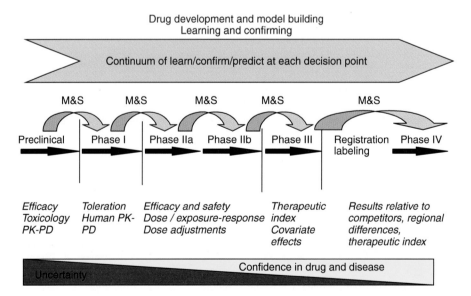

Fig. 10.5 Predictive model-guided preclinical and clinical drug development (M&S: Modelling and Simulation) (Reprinted by permission from Macmillan Publishers Ltd: LaLonde et al. [12])

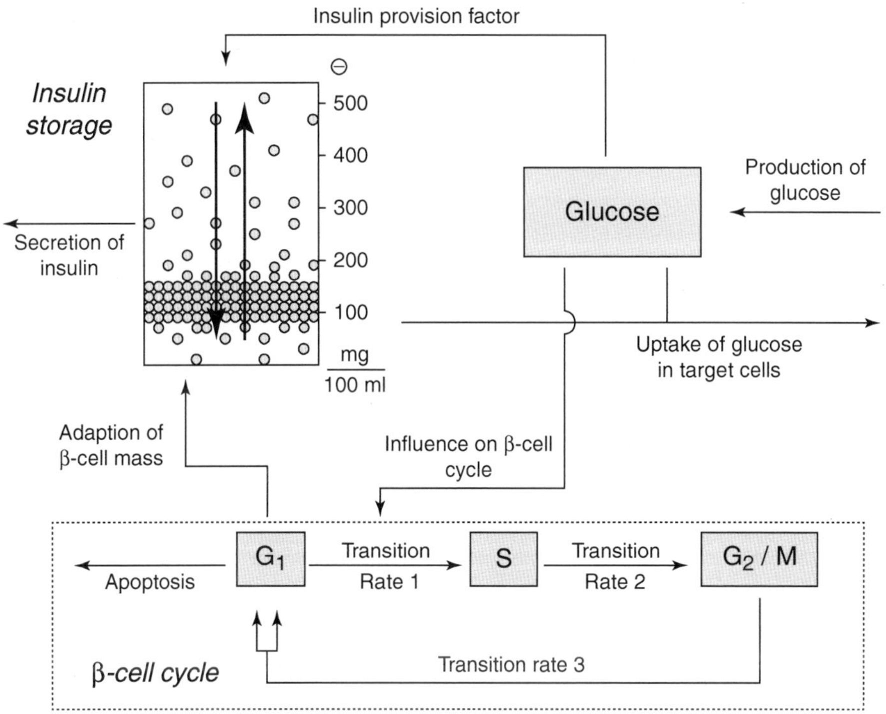

Fig. 10.6 Schematic concept of Gallenberger et al. [17] model. Glucose enters the system at a constant production rate mainly by the liver. Elevated blood glucose levels lead to immediate release of stored insulin and an enhanced provision of insulin. Also, glucose influences the transition rate between phases G_1 and S of the cell cycle. Insulin regulates the uptake of glucose in target cells. The molecules are stored in packets with different release thresholds. These packets can be redistributed within the storage (Reprinted with permission from Gallenberger et al. [17]. This is an open access article distributed under the terms of the Creative Commons Attribution License (http://creativecommon.org/licenses/by/2.0), which permits unrestricted use, distribution, and reproduction in any medium, provided original work is properly cited)

mechanistic, empirical, and trial-outcome models are developed to describe various aspects of the physiology, sites, and mechanisms of drug action and probability of success of a clinical trial, as well as treatment outcomes and patient-benefit analysis.

Within the purview of translational research, physiologically and mechanism-based models have gained momentum in the pharmaceutical drug development arena. During the translational phase of development, the choice of animal models for a particular disease is important. This is often dependent on the mechanism of action of the pharmacological agent and known interspecies differences in target expression and biomarker response [13, 14]. Disease progression models, for example, enable the understanding of the pathophysiology of the disease and the impact of treatment interventions. Alternatively, disease processes can also be characterized based on a complete mechanistic description of the biological system, starting at the molecular/tissue level [15, 16].

System-Centric Modelling

In diabetes drug development, quantitative approaches have been applied to identify the relationship between glucose, insulin, glucagon, β-cell cycle dynamics, incretin-responsive insulin secretion, homeostatic feedback conversion of glycogen and glucose in the liver, with the interplay between different organs at the whole-body level. To this end, a system-centric model was developed to describe the pancreatic β-cell cycle and impact of glucose challenge on insulin production as shown in Fig. 10.6 [17]. In

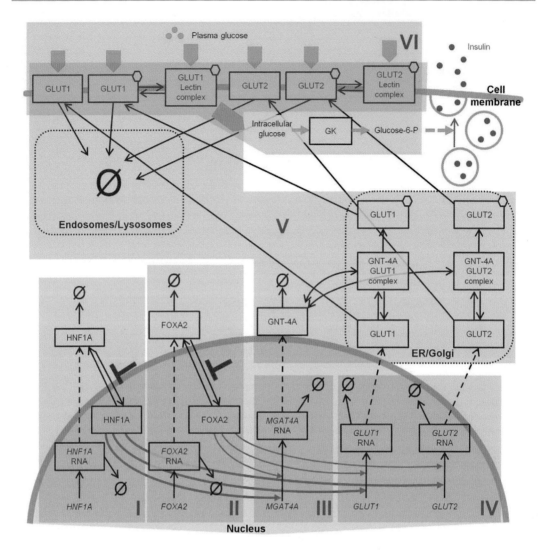

Fig. 10.7 Conceptual model by Luni et al. [18] depicting the various signaling steps involved in the secretion of insulin at the cellular level (Reprinted with permission from Luni et al. [18]. Copyright: 2012 Luni et al. This is an open access article distributed under the terms of the Creative Commons Attribution License, which permits unrestricted use, distribution, and reproduction in any medium, provided the original author and source are credited)

this model, the β-cell cycle is characterized by a three-compartment model,

$$G_1(t) = 2p3G_2/M(t) - \left[p1[1+p5G(t)] + p4\right] \times G_1(t) \quad (10.1)$$

$$S(t) = p1[1+p5G(t)]G_1(t) - p2S(t) \quad (10.2)$$

$$G_2/M(t) = p2S(t) - p3G_2/M(t) \quad (10.3)$$

where the factor 2 in Eq. 10.1 accounts for cell division in the transition from G_2/M to G_1-phase. Under physiological conditions, the β-cell cycle is very slow in adults but can adjust to metabolic demands. Changes in glucose levels (Eq. 10.2) drive the transition rate $p1$ from G_1- to S-phase and, thus, regulate the β-cell cycle. The way glucose stimuli are handled here has wide-ranging implications on the overall system. For example, if the system is triggered by increased glucose concentrations, and neither immediate release of stored insulin nor enhanced insulin provision

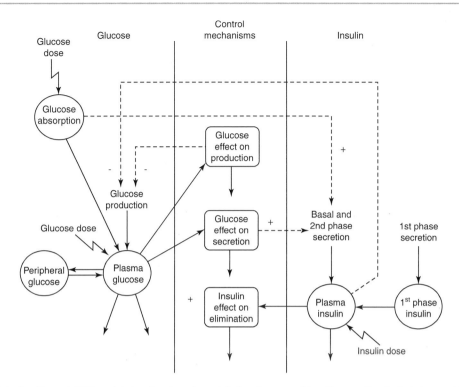

Fig. 10.8 Jauslin et al. [19] model showing the sub-models for glucose and insulin as well as included control mechanism (Reprinted with permission from Jauslin et al. [19]. Copyright © 2007 American College of Pharmacology)

is able to normalize blood glucose levels, it will respond by accelerating the cell cycle.

Similarly, glucose transport in pancreatic islet β-cells is thought to set metabolic thresholds and serves as a therapeutic target in diabetes as shown in Fig. 10.7 [18]. Under normal conditions, there is limited glucose transport across the plasma membrane of β-cells. The model identified a metabolic threshold that limits intracellular glucose-6-phosphate production by glucokinase. Thresholds are of general importance in disease systems analysis because they allow a system to maintain balance and function properly within certain physiological limits. The maintenance of these thresholds is typically accomplished via homeostatic feedback control. Once a system becomes unresponsive to a stimulus, such as elevated glucose concentrations even with the release of insulin, it progressively spins out of control resulting in β-cell dysfunction and loss of glucose-stimulated insulin secretion.

Figures 10.8 [19] and 10.9 [20] present further examples of system-centric models that are intended to describe a network of processes responsible for maintaining glucose homeostasis. The model presented in Fig. 10.8 developed by Jauslin et al. [19] represents an integrated glucose-insulin model that integrates the sequence of insulin secretion, glucose-insulin feedback, and natural control mechanisms (see Fig. 10.8), whereas Fig. 10.9 focuses on the various physiological processes contributing to glucose homeostasis on a cell and organ level. In this spatial representation of glucose homeostasis, green arrows depict pathways that have already been incorporated into currently available models, whereas red arrows pinpoint to pathways where these models could be expanded. While Figs. 10.8 and 10.9 focus either on the temporal or spatial characterization of the system, Fig. 10.10 represents a combination of the two [21]. This model places the mechanisms responsible for glucose homeostasis in a whole-body context, which then allows to accounting for the route of intake as well as elimination of glucose. Ultimately, these models are intended to reflect the clinical situation as close as possible and may serve as a virtual patient for hypothesis testing and generation in the future.

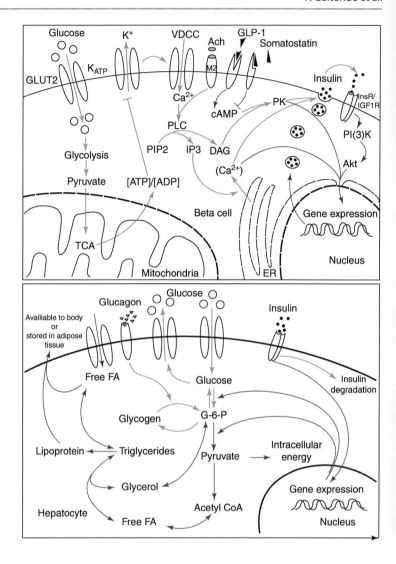

Fig. 10.9 Schematic representing the current stage of quantitative modelling to describe the various signalling mechanisms (Reprinted with permission from Ajmera et al. [20]. Copyright © 2013 American Society for Clinical Pharmacology and Therapeutics)

Mechanism-Centric Modelling

Once the mechanism and site of drug action is determined, the focus of preclinical modeling and simulation shifts toward gaining confidence in the drug effect(s), both in terms of efficacy and safety, and the establishment of a dose-response relationship. Once established and qualified, such mechanism-centric models allow for comparing and contrasting multiple drug candidates within the same drug class or with similar mechanisms of action. This enables the identification of lead compound with desirable therapeutic properties alongside with an opportunity to identify key rate-limiting steps, which aids decision making at the next juncture in the development process, e.g., when switching from preclinical to clinical development. In addition, these models are frequently used to evaluate the impact of disease progression on the underlying biological system and its ability to respond to therapeutic interventions. Cao et al. [22] developed a mathematical model to describe the PK and PD of a GLP-1 agonist following parenteral route of administration. GLP-1 agonists are incretin mimetics that enhance glucose-dependent insulin secretion (Fig. 10.11). Models like these can be beneficial not only to characterize the drug effect but also to evaluate the impact of factors such as routes of administration, formulation, organ impairment, etc. on the PK/PD of the drug.

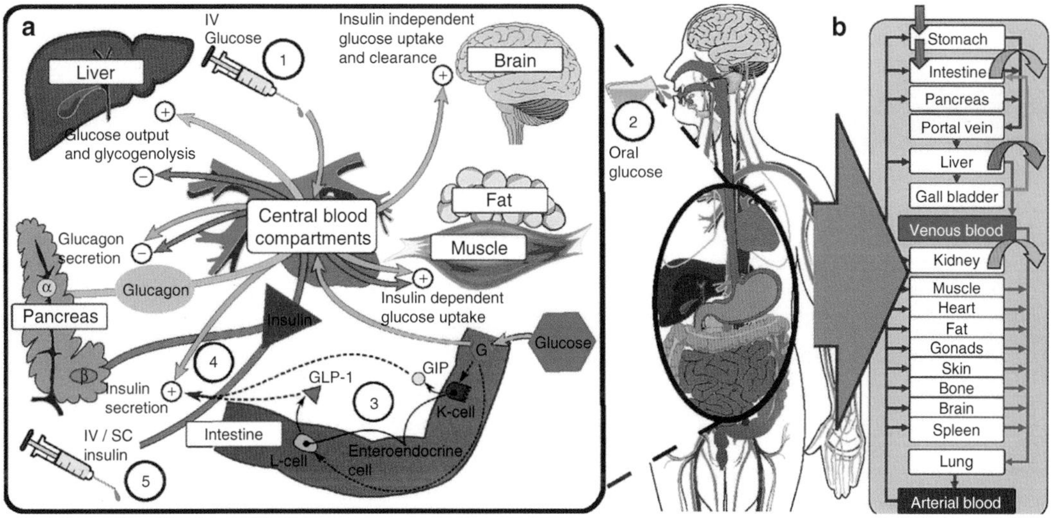

Fig. 10.10 (**a**) Multi-organ pharmacodynamic interaction of glucose and insulin (**b**) Whole-body physiological modelling with organ-level integration. *IV* intravenous, *SC* subcutaneous, *GLP* glucagon-like peptide, *GIP* glucagon inhibitory peptide (Reprinted with permission from Schaller et al. [21]. Copyright © 2013 American Society for Clinical Pharmacology and Therapeutics)

$$\frac{dA_p}{dt} = k_0 - A_p \times \left(\frac{CL}{V_p}\right) - A_p \times \left(\frac{CL_d}{V_p}\right) + A_t \times \left(\frac{CL_d}{V_t}\right); \text{For IV bolus and IF}: A_p(0) = \frac{k_0}{k_e}$$

$$\frac{dA_p}{dt} = k_0 - A_p \times \left(\frac{CL}{V_p}\right) - Ap \times \left(\frac{CL_d}{Vp}\right) + A_t \times \left(\frac{CL_d}{V_t}\right) + \text{Input}; \text{For SC and IP}: A_p(0) = \frac{k_0}{k_e}$$

$$\frac{dA_t}{dt} = A_p \times \left(\frac{CL_d}{V_p}\right) - A_t \times \left(\frac{CL_d}{V_t}\right); A_t(0) = k_0 \times V_t / (k_e \times V_p)$$

$$\text{Input} = (1-\lambda) \times \text{Dose} \times (1-F_r) \times k \times F + \lambda \times \text{Dose} \times F_r \times \frac{F}{\tau}; \text{For SC and IP}$$

where:

A_p and A_t: GLP-1 amounts in central and peripheral compartments

V_p and V_t: central and peripheral distribution volumes, respectively

CL and CL_d: Systemic and distribution clearance, respectively

F: absorption bioavailability

F_r: fraction of dose absorbed by the zero-order process

k and k_e: first-order absorption and elimination rates, respectively

τ: duration of zero-order absorption (assumed to be first sampling time)

$\lambda = 1$ before time τ and 0 otherwise

Input: amount absorbed per min from the absorption compartment

k_0: GLP-1 endogenous synthesis rate

In this context, semi-mechanistic turnover models are widely used for characterizing data from animal disease models. For example, the PK and PD of rosiglitazone (a thiazolidinedione used in the treatment of type 2 diabetes) was characterized using semi-mechanistic models in diabetic rats [23] (Fig. 10.12).

The PK of the drug was defined using one-compartment equation:

$$C_{ROSY} = \frac{Dose \cdot F}{V \cdot (k_{el} - k_a)} \cdot \left(e^{-k_a \cdot t} - e^{-k_{el} \cdot t}\right)$$

Whereas, changes in glucose and insulin were modeled as two turnover compartments:

$$\frac{dG}{dt} = k_{inG} - k_{outG} \cdot G \cdot (1 + S_{Ins}[n] \cdot I) k_{pl} \cdot placebo \cdot G, \; G(0) = G_0$$

$$\frac{dI}{dt} = k_{inI} \cdot (1 + S_G \cdot G) - k_{out\_I} \cdot I, \; I(0) = I_0$$

The recognized side effect of the drug to inhibit weight loss was also incorporated using a turnover compartment model for weight change over time. Once the preclinical PK/PD relationship is established and a sufficient amount of confidence is achieved on the robustness of the model, the system and (semi-)mechanistic dose-response models can be used to make the first-in-human dose projections.

Clinical Stage Modelling

Clinical trials are intended to assure the safety and efficacy of novel drug candidates, to determine intrinsic and extrinsic factors affecting benefit and risk, and to inform the drug label. Quantitative analysis have become an essential part of the clinical drug development process as they enable the stepwise integration of knowledge on the drug's PK, its dose-response relationship, respective covariates, as well as on the impact of disease on

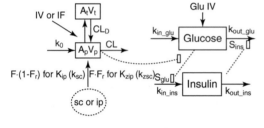

Fig. 10.11 Pharmacokinetic/pharmacodynamics (PK/PD) model for characterizing the time course of GLP-1 after several routes of dosing and dynamics of glucose-dependent insulinotropic acting process. *GLP-1* glucagon-like peptide, *Glu* glucose, *IV* intravenous, *IF* infusion, *sc* subcutaneous, *ip* intraperitoneal (With kind permission from Springer Science+Business Media: Cao et al. [22])

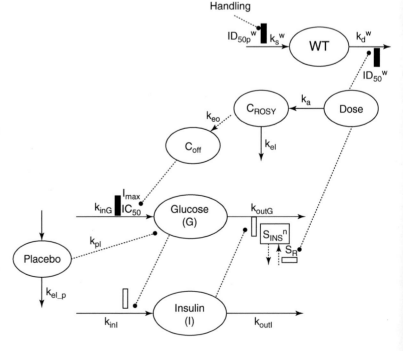

Fig. 10.12 Pharmacokinetic/pharmacodynamic (PK/PD) model for rosiglitazone. The drug effect was incorporated as inhibition of glucose production. Side effect of rosiglitazone was incorporated as inhibition of weight loss. *WT* weight, *ROSY* rosiglitazone, *C* concentration, ID_{50p} inhibition constant caused by animal handling, ID_{50w} inhibition constant of rosiglitazone for weight gain (Reprinted with permission from Gao et al. [23])

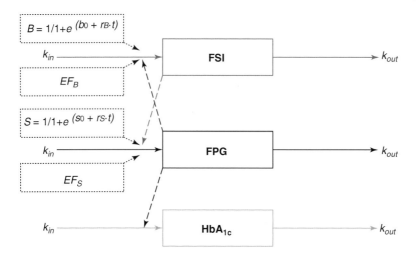

Fig. 10.13 de Winter et al. [24] model linking three clinical biomarkers using cascading turnover models. A feedback mechanism between fasting serum insulin (FSI) and fasting plasma glucose (FPG) and a feedforward mechanism between fasting plasma glucose and glycated haemoglobin (HbA$_{1c}$) were implemented. EF_B treatment effect on β-cell function, EF_S treatment effect on insulin sensitivity, B remaining fraction of β-cell function relative to healthy individuals, S remaining fraction of insulin sensitivity relative to healthy individuals (With kind permission from Springer Science+Business Media: de Winter et al. [24])

PK and/or PD as the drug traverses through the different clinical trial stages in healthy volunteers and patients. The model by de Winter et al. [24] was one of the first of its kind that allowed characterizing the mechanistic link between the different short- (fasting serum insulin, fasting plasma glucose) and long-term (HbA$_{1c}$) biomarker data on the basis of clinical data (Fig. 10.13). It further allowed to making inferences about the state of the disease by linking these biomarkers to β-cell function and insulin sensitivity:

$$\frac{dFSI}{dt} = EF_B \times B \times (FPG - 3.5) \times k_{in, insulin} - FSI \times k_{out, insulin}$$

$$\frac{dFPG}{dt} = \frac{k_{in, FPG}}{EF_S \times S \times FSI} - FPG \times k_{out, FPG}$$

$$\frac{dHbA1c}{dt} = FPG \times k_{in, HbA1c} - HbA1c \times k_{out, HbA1c}$$

where:
FSI: fasting serum insulin
FPG: fasting plasma glucose
EF_B and EF_S: treatment effect on β-cell function or insulin sensitivity, respectively

B and S: remaining fraction of β-cell function or insulin sensitivity, respectively, relative to healthy individuals

Interestingly, de Winter et al. also showed that the system has already lost much of its insulin sensitivity and β-cell function once clinically relevant changes in short- and long-term biomarkers occur. It is consequently important to expand this type of model with even earlier biomarkers or covariate information in order to be able to capture the onset of the disease and to intervene therapeutically as early as possible (intent to prevent vs. intent to treat).

In late clinical stages of drug development, the challenges to be addressed are largely related, but not limited to, benefit-to-risk assessment, labeling information, determining variability in patient-specific drug response and superiority/non-inferiority criteria. As such, the developed models are geared to be drug-centric in nature. The use of asymptotic time-course (ATC) drug-disease model to describe fasting plasma glucose and HbA$_{1c}$ profiles in patients with type 2 diabetes is a respective example for this type of model [25]:

$$\begin{aligned}HbA1c = {} & E0_{HbA1c} - EMAX_{HbA1c} \times (1+BL_{HbA1c} \times (E0_{HbA1c} - 8.2)) \times (1 - EXP(-KEFF_{HbA1c} \times TIME)) \\ & + DPSL_{HbA1c} \times TIME\end{aligned}$$

$$HbA1c_{obs} = HbA1c_{pred} \times (1 + ERR(1))$$

where:
- Baseline HbA_{1c} effect on E_{max} (linear), scaled at baseline HbA_{1c} of 8.2 %
- K_{EFF} = rate constant of HbA_{1c} change
- DPSL = disease progression slope
- Exponential intertrial variability (ITV), proportional residual error

Clinical Trial and Treatment Outcome Modelling

Several physiology-based modelling platforms, such as the Physiome Project [15] and Archimedes [26], were set up with the objective of developing an infrastructure that links models of biological structure and function across multiple spatial and temporal levels and, ultimately, to predict clinical outcomes [15, 27]. These models can be quite complex and integrate knowledge on genes to whole organisms and typically represent significant expansions. These examples include the homeostasis model assessment of β-cell (HOMA-B) function and homeostasis model assessment of insulin resistance (HOMA-IR) models [28], which enables clinical trial outcome modelling through the interactive adjustment of physiology and treatment effects (Fig. 10.14a–c).

As mentioned earlier, the Archimedes model is an encompassing model, spanning from biological aspects of the care processes, logistics, resources to the costs of healthcare systems (Fig. 10.15). It integrates a deep level of biological, clinical, and administrative detail. Biological variables that are continuous in reality are represented continuously in the model. It also includes multiple diseases simultaneously and

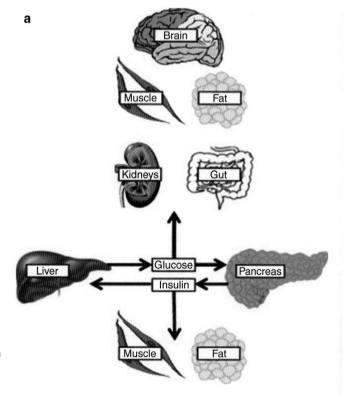

Fig. 10.14 (a) Interrelationship of various organs in the homeostasis of glucose; (b) profiles of glucose-insulin dynamics in the various organs; (c) mathematical modelling of the concentration-time profiles (From Hill et al. [28]. American Diabetes Association, Diabetes Care, 2013. Copyright and all rights reserved. Material from this publication has been used with the permission of American Diabetes Association)

b

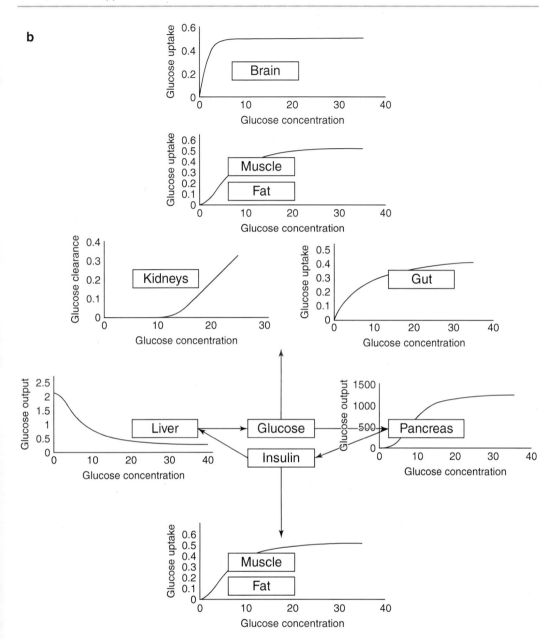

Fig. 10.14 (continued)

Fig. 10.14 (continued)

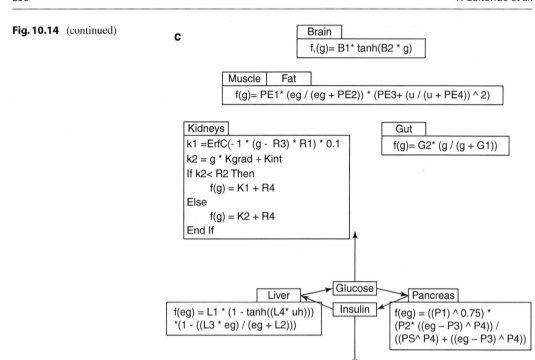

interactively in a single integrated physiology, enabling it to address comorbidities, syndromes, and treatments with multiple effects.

The average time and cost of bringing a drug to the market is more than 10 years and approximately US$1 billion, respectively. There is a huge and imminent need for highly robust, predictive, accurate, and precise quantitative solutions to reduce the time and costs. Considering that a major portion of the research and development budget is spent on clinical trials, a virtual patient population development and simulation would be an attractive proposition. Several research groups and companies are developing such tools. One example is the Entelos PhysioLab® platform. The metabolism platform is a multi-scale model representing whole-body nutrient metabolism with an emphasis on the physiological and metabolic systems involved in blood glucose regulation. This includes nutrient absorption and elimination, substrate metabolism, hormone regulation, and spatial configuration of organs. Substrate metabolism, for example is represented by simulation components that capture salient features of different organ systems, including the liver, muscle, adipose tissue, and the brain [29].

Model-Base Meta-Analysis

The nature of cardiometabolic diseases results in exposure of patients to multiple drug therapies, treating the various facets of the comorbidities often for many years. Adding layers of complexity, there are numerous classes of glucose-lowering agents available on the market, as well as a plethora under development. The heterogeneity in patient population worldwide can additionally influence

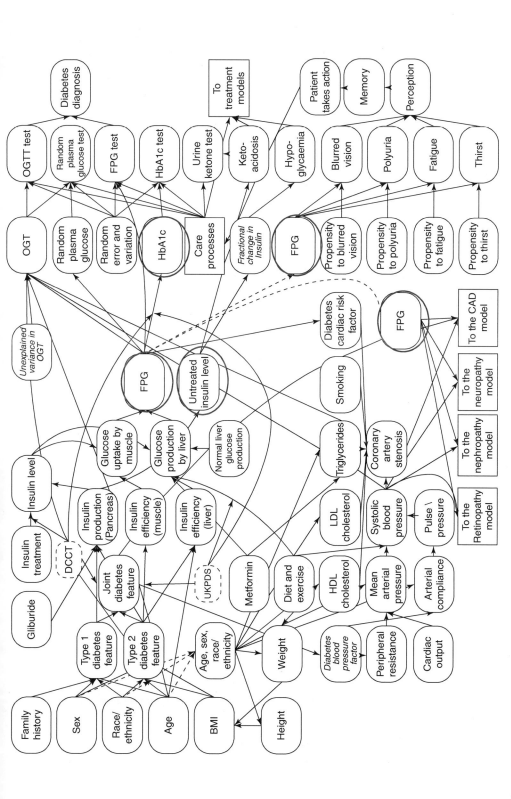

Fig. 10.15 Archimedes model with the three clinical biomarkers *circled* in *red*. *DCCT* The Diabetes Control and Complications Trial, *UKPDS* United Kingdom Prospective Diabetes Study, *HDL* high-density lipoprotein, *LDL* low-density lipoprotein (From Eddy and Schlessinger [26]. American Diabetes Association, Diabetes Care, 2003. Copyright and all rights reserved. Material from this publication has been used with the permission of American Diabetes Association)

Fig. 10.16 (a) Graphic representation of the components for study arms that include patients washing out their prior antihyperglycemic medication in the run-in period. (b) Components of the model for study arms that include patients who were treatment naïve or had completely washed out their prior antihyperglycemic medication before enrollment. The figure demonstrates the comparison between change in glycated haemoglobin (HbA$_{1c}$, X-axes) across different studies (Y-axes) for placebo, linagliptin, and sitagliptin. E efficacy of drug (Reproduced from Gross et al. [30], with permission from BMJ Publishing Group Ltd)

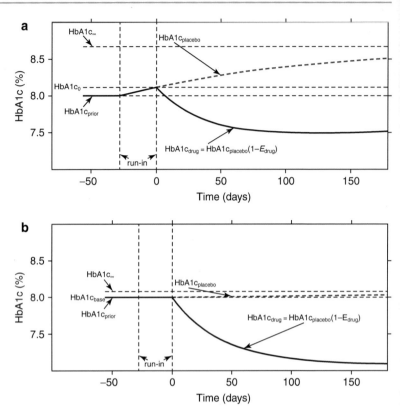

the treatment outcome. In such situations, model-based meta-analysis (MBMA) allows for indirect comparison with a competitor's drug and comparison between different demographic and across different studies/trials [30] (Fig. 10.16).

Future Opportunities and Path Toward Personalizing Medicine

With the completion of the human genome project, a substantial amount of research has been dedicated to the quest of improved disease diagnosis and prevention, as well as tailoring therapy based on a patient's genetic makeup, disease condition and comorbidities [31]. It is recognized that cardiometabolic diseases are associated with non-modifiable and modifiable risk factors. In contemporary predictive modelling situations, these risk factors would be included as covariates that influence the model outcome. However, to tailor drug therapy, one should also use information gained from the (i) identification of newer, reliable, and more informative biomarkers; (ii) genomic studies, e.g., genome-wide association studies (GWAS) and translation of the outcomes; and (iii) integration of the knowledge of epigenetics and epidemiological risk factors. Despite the number of known risk factors, the identification of individuals at increased risk for type 2 diabetes and/or cardiovascular disease remains an arduous undertaking [32]. The fundamental task in the context of risk prediction is not that of finding biomarkers associated with the incident disease but, rather, finding those that are sufficiently uncorrelated with established risk factors so that they can be used to better improve risk prediction over and above these established clinical risk factors. For example, the discovery of the adipocytokine adiponectin has proven to be of value in delineating the cardiometabolic consequences of obesity [33]. Some examples of other biomarkers of potential use in the prediction of type 2 diabetes and cardiovascular disease are listed in Table 10.2. Adiponectin, which is produced by white adipocytes and circulates in high concentrations, is readily quantitated using accessible methodologies. In contrast to all other adipose-derived circulating factors, adiponectin has the epidemiologically interesting but unexplained feature of circulating in lower concentrations in proportion to the degree of obesity. At present, it appears that factors that determine the overall concentration are distinct from the factors that reduce the concentration in relation to degree of obesity and metabolic dysfunction. Similarly, the relationships between plasma adiponectin levels and the risk of myocardial infarction were evaluated. Pischon and coworkers [34] conducted a case-control study involving 18,225 male participants of the Health Professionals Follow-up Study, aged 40–75 years and free of cardiovascular disease at baseline. During the 6 years of follow-up in the main cohort, 266 men developed fatal or nonfatal myocardial infarction. It was found that low adiponectin levels were associated with a higher risk of myocardial infarction. This increased risk remained significant even after adjusting for variables used in matching cases to controls, adjusting for family history of myocardial infarction, body mass index, alcohol use, physical activity, and history of diabetes or hypertension. In addition, even after adjusting for glycemic status, C-reactive protein and lipid parameters, i.e., low-density lipoprotein (LDL) cholesterol and high-density lipoprotein (HDL) cholesterol, the increased risk remained unaltered.

New multidisciplinary fields of public health genomics can help to translate gene discoveries into appropriate actions to reduce the burden of type 2 diabetes in the population [35]. Currently, there is limited ability to predict the risk of type 2 diabetes in the general population based on genetic profiles, especially when added to established nongenetic risk factors. This observation is consistent with recent findings with genetic factors from other common diseases such as prostate cancer and coronary heart disease. The ability to predict type 2 diabetes using genetic risk factors is likely to improve as more variants are discovered. This is particularly true if these variants have stronger effect sizes than the current ones utilized, if strong gene-gene and gene-environment interactions are found, or if biochemical or physiological biomarkers that are more proximal to the development of type 2 diabetes are discovered and validated. The probability of risk analysis is many a time described as odds ratio (OR). Odds are the probability of an event occurring divided by the probability of the event not occurring [36]. An OR is then considered as the odds of the event in one group, for example, those exposed to a drug, divided by the odds in another group not exposed [36]. An OR = 1 would mean that exposure does not affect odds of outcome, OR >1 suggests exposure associated with higher odds of outcome, and OR <1 indicates exposure associated with lower odds of outcome [37]. Currently most OR studies for prediction of type 2 diabetes resulted in an OR of below 2, suggesting absence of a strong correlation with risk factors [35]. Nevertheless, findings from GWAS have great implications in terms of understanding disease biology and pathogenesis and the future development of preventive and treatment interventions. Advances in human genetics are leading to a relatively new type of study aimed at understanding the disease mechanisms behind diabetes [38]. It is now possible to recruit research volunteers based on an interesting genetic variant they possess and perform in-depth physiological studies on the volunteers to understand how the gene variant functions.

Epigenetics is the study of changes in gene function that are mitotically and/or meiotically heritable and that do not entail a change in deoxyribonucleic acid (DNA) sequence [39]. In contrast, epidemiology is the study of the distribution and determinants of health-related states or events (including disease) and the application of this study to the control of diseases and other health problems. An epigenetic change might result in a perceptible alteration later in life such as cancer, coronary heart disease, stroke, or diabetes. Increased risks of heart disease, stroke, and diabetes are considered to be associated with malnutrition in utero and low birth weight [40]. Concurrently, various methods can be used to

Table 10.2 Biomarkers with potential relevance to prediction of type 2 diabetes and cardiovascular disease

Category	Biomarker
Genome	Single nucleotide polymorphisms
	Rare variants
	Copy-number variants
	Epigenetic modifications (e.g., methylation)
	Telomere length
Transcriptome	mRNA
	miRNA
Proteome	Peptides, proteins, and glycoproteins in peripheral blood and other body fluids
Metabolites	Lipids
	Sugars
	Nucleotides
	Organic acids
	Amino acids
Markers of subclinical disease	Triglyceride content in liver, muscle, pancreas, and heart (ectopic fat)
	Aotric plaque burden, aortic plaque phenotype (e.g., calcification), ankle-brachial index, intima-media thickness (arterial structure)
Metabolic end products	Urinary proteins and metabolites in urine
	Volatile organic compounds in exhaled breath
	Gut microbiota, bacterial strains in feces

Reprinted by permission from Macmillan Publishers Ltd: Herder et al. [32], copyright 2011

carry out epidemiological investigations; surveillance and descriptive studies can be used to study distribution; analytical studies are used to study determinants.

Dashboard systems as decision-making tools could be made available to a physician to prescribe optimal treatment for an individual patient [41]. A dashboard is a user interface that, like a dashboard in a car, organizes and presents information so that it is easy and quick to read and interpret. Given the vast amount of data available in the diabetes arena, such dashboard systems could also be developed and applied in the clinic setting to improve patient therapy and quality of life. It also would enable the flow of information garnered in the clinic to be channeled back to the research knowledge base (see Fig. 10.2) – in essence leading to a "bench-to-bedside and back" flow of knowledge and information. Throughout the translational stages of drug development, application of quantitative approaches should effectively result in a feedback closed loop of a learn-confirm-apply paradigm. This would lead to further scientific and rational refinement of the drug development process. Patient management dashboards might obtain information from electronic medical records, laboratories, clinician interviews, and patient input and present it from one unified source. An example of a dashboard system for type 2 diabetes was developed by the University of Missouri Health System (UMHS) family physicians in 2007 in collaboration with Cerner Corporation that would be automatically generated by the Electronic Health Records and summarize patient-level data important for diabetes care. More recently, Glooko Inc. received US Food and Drug Administration (FDA) clearance in 2013 for its diabetes management system including an iPhone application, MeterSync cables, and web dashboards for both patients and healthcare providers [42].

Historically, clinical trials have been conducted in adults and predominantly male subjects. However, with the enactment of the US Pediatric Research Equity Act (PREA) and Best Pharmaceuticals for Children Act (BPCA), there is a huge push toward developing translational tools to enable optimal treatment and care in children [43]. This had direct impact on cardiometabolic diseases, because even though they were typically diagnosed in adults, they are now being diagnosed in pediatrics. Type 2 diabetes and obesity are closely associated and growing epidemics among children. Sedentary lifestyle in children is linked to increased cardiometabolic risk [44]. To further complicate treatment, research is still evolving to fully elucidate the age-dependent changes in the maturation and function of drug metabolizing enzymes that can alter the PK/PD of many currently used glucose-lowering drugs in children. At the other end of the spectrum, there is further work to be done on optimizing therapy for the geriatric diabetes population, in which comorbidities and reduced life expectancy may modify the aims and intensity of diabetes pharmacotherapy [45]. Alongside, there also is the need to design an effective training program in translational research to offer the opportunity to master a combination of skills that are not taught together in traditional training programs.

References

1. Plutzky J. A cardiologist's perspective on cardiometabolic risk. Am J Cardiol. 2007;100(12A):3P–6. Epub 2007/12/25.
2. Go AS, Mozaffarian D, Roger VL, Benjamin EJ, Berry JD, Borden WB, et al. Heart disease and stroke statistics–2013 update: a report from the American Heart Association. Circulation. 2013;127(1):e6–245. Epub 2012/12/15.
3. Vlasakakis G, Pasqua OD. Cardiovascular disease: the other face of diabetes. CPT Pharmacometrics Syst Pharmacol. 2013;2:e81. Epub 2013/10/25.
4. Lesko LJ, Zheng S, Schmidt S. Systems approaches in risk assessment. Clin Pharmacol Ther. 2013;93(5):413–24. Epub 2013/03/28.
5. Rubio DM, Schoenbaum EE, Lee LS, Schteingart DE, Marantz PR, Anderson KE, et al. Defining translational research: implications for training. Acad Med. 2010;85(3):470–5. Epub 2010/02/26.
6. Woolf SH. The meaning of translational research and why it matters. JAMA. 2008;299(2):211–3. Epub 2008/01/10.
7. American Diabetes Association. Standards of medical care in diabetes–2014. Diabetes Care. 2014;37 Suppl 1:S14–80. Epub 2013/12/21.
8. Jain R, Chung SM, Jain L, Khurana M, Lau SW, Lee JE, et al. Implications of obesity for drug therapy: limitations and challenges. Clin Pharmacol Ther. 2011;90(1):77–89. Epub 2011/06/03.
9. Biomarkers Definitions Working Group. Biomarkers and surrogate endpoints: preferred definitions and conceptual framework. Clin Pharmacol Ther. 2001;69(3):89–95. Epub 2001/03/10.
10. Danhof M, Alvan G, Dahl SG, Kuhlmann J, Paintaud G. Mechanism-based pharmacokinetic-pharmacodynamic modeling-a new classification of biomarkers. Pharm Res. 2005;22(9):1432–7. Epub 2005/09/01.
11. Sorger PK, Allerheiligen SRB, Quantitative and Systems Pharmacology in the Post-genomic Era: New Approaches to Discovering Drugs and Understanding Therapeutic Mechanisms. An NIH White Paper by the QSP Workshop Group. 2011; http://www.nigms.nih.gov/NR/rdonlyres/8ECB1F7C-BE3B-431F-89E6-A43411811AB1/0/SystemsPharmaWPSorger2011.pdf.
12. Lalonde RL, Kowalski KG, Hutmacher MM, Ewy W, Nichols DJ, Milligan PA, et al. Model-based drug development. Clin Pharmacol Ther. 2007;82(1):21–32. Epub 2007/05/25.
13. Shafrir E. In: Shafrir E, editor. Animal models of diabetes, frontiers in research. 2nd ed. Boca Raton: CRC Press; 2007.
14. Shafrir E. Contribution of animal models to the research of the causes of diabetes. World J Diabetes. 2010;1(5):137–40.
15. Hunter P, Nielsen P. A strategy for integrative computational physiology. Physiology. 2005;20:316–25.
16. Ploeger BA, van der Graaf PH, Danhof M. Incorporating receptor theory in mechanism-based pharmacokinetic-pharmacodynamic (PK-PD) modeling. Drug Metab Pharmacokinet. 2009;24(1):3–15. Epub 2009/03/03.
17. Gallenberger M, Castell W, Hense BA, Kuttler C. Dynamics of glucose and insulin concentration connected to the β-cell cycle: model development and analysis. Theor Biol Med Model. 2012;9:46.
18. Luni C, Marth JD, Doyle 3rd FJ. Computational modeling of glucose transport in pancreatic beta-cells identifies metabolic thresholds and therapeutic targets in diabetes. PLoS One. 2012;7(12):e53130. Epub 2013/01/10.
19. Jauslin PM, Silber HE, Frey N, Gieschke R, Simonsson US, Jorga K, et al. An integrated glucose-insulin model to describe oral glucose tolerance test data in type 2 diabetics. J Clin Pharmacol. 2007;47(10):1244–55. Epub 2007/10/02.
20. Ajmera I, Swat M, Laibe C, Novere NL, Chelliah V. The impact of mathematical modeling on the understanding of diabetes and related complications. CPT Pharmacometrics Syst Pharmacol. 2013;2(7):e54.
21. Schaller S, Willmann S, Lippert J, Schaupp L, Pieber TR, Schuppert A, et al. A generic integrated physiologically based whole-body model of the glucose-insulin-glucagon regulatory system. CPT Pharmacometrics Syst Pharmacol. 2013;2(8):e65.
22. Cao Y, Gao W, Jusko WJ. Pharmacokinetic/pharmacodynamic modeling of GLP-1 in healthy rats. Pharm Res. 2012;29(4):1078–86. Epub 2011/12/20.
23. Gao W, Jusko WJ. Modeling disease progression and rosiglitazone intervention in type 2 diabetic Goto-Kakizaki rats. J Pharmacol Exp Ther. 2012;341(3):617–25. Epub 2012/03/02.
24. de Winter W, DeJongh J, Post T, Ploeger B, Urquhart R, Moules I, et al. A mechanism-based disease progression model for comparison of long-term effects of pioglitazone, metformin and gliclazide on disease processes underlying type 2 diabetes mellitus. J Pharmacokinet Pharmacodyn. 2006;33(3):313–43. Epub 2006/03/23.
25. Tay JC GP, Geiser JS, Chien JY, Sinha VP. Time course models for long-term treatment of Type II diabetes mellitus with oral medications. American Conference on Pharmacometrics (ACoP) meeting. 2011.
26. Eddy DM, Schlessinger L. Archimedes: a trial-validated model of diabetes. Diabetes Care. 2003;26(11):3093–101. Epub 2003/10/28.

27. Bassingthwaighte JB. Strategies for the physiome project. Ann Biomed Eng. 2000;28(8):1043–58. Epub 2001/01/06.
28. Hill NR, Levy JC, Matthews DR. Expansion of the homeostasis model assessment of beta-cell function and insulin resistance to enable clinical trial outcome modeling through the interactive adjustment of physiology and treatment effects: iHOMA2. Diabetes Care. 2013;36(8):2324–30. Epub 2013/04/09.
29. Klinke 2nd DJ. Integrating epidemiological data into a mechanistic model of type 2 diabetes: validating the prevalence of virtual patients. Ann Biomed Eng. 2008;36(2):321–34. Epub 2007/11/30.
30. Gross JL, Rogers J, Polhamus D, Gillespie W, Friedrich C, Gong Y, et al. A novel model-based meta-analysis to indirectly estimate the comparative efficacy of two medications: an example using DPP-4 inhibitors, sitagliptin and linagliptin, in treatment of type 2 diabetes mellitus. BMJ Open. 2013;3(3):e001844. Epub 2013/03/08.
31. (NIH)-Fact-Sheets NIoH. Research Portfolio Online Reporting Tools (RePORT) – Human Genome Project. 2013.
32. Herder C, Karakas M, Koenig W. Biomarkers for the prediction of type 2 diabetes and cardiovascular disease. Clin Pharmacol Ther. 2011;90(1):52–66. Epub 2011/06/10.
33. Mather KJ, Goldberg RB. Clinical use of adiponectin as a marker of metabolic dysregulation. Best Pract Res Clin Endocrinol Metab. 2014;28(1):107–17. Epub 2014/01/15.
34. Pischon T, Girman CJ, Hotamisligil GS, Rifai N, Hu FB, Rimm EB. Plasma adiponectin levels and risk of myocardial infarction in men. JAMA. 2004;291(14):1730–7. Epub 2004/04/15.
35. Khoury MJ, Valdez R, Albright A. Public health genomics approach to type 2 diabetes. Diabetes. 2008;57(11):2911–4. Epub 2008/10/31.
36. Grimes DA, Schulz KF. Making sense of odds and odds ratios. Obstet Gynecol. 2008;111(2 Pt 1):423–6. Epub 2008/02/02.
37. Szumilas M. Explaining odds ratios. J Can Acad Child Adolesc Psychiatry. 2010;19(3):227–9. Epub 2010/09/16.
38. Timothy F. The genetics behind type 2 diabetes – lessons from GWAS. Diabetes Voice. 2012;57(4):24.
39. Dupont C, Armant DR, Brenner CA. Epigenetics: definition, mechanisms and clinical perspective. Semin Reprod Med. 2009;27(5):351–7. Epub 2009/08/28.
40. Delisle H. Foetal programming of nutrition-related chronic diseases. Sante (Montrouge, France). 2002;12(1):56–63. Epub 2002/04/12. La programmation foetale des maladies chronique liees a la nutrition.
41. Mould DR, Lesko LJ. Personalized medicine – integrating individual exposure response information at the bedside. In: Schmidt S, Derendorf H, editors. Applied phamacometrics. New York: Springer; 2014.
42. FDA. Section 6: 510(k) summary (21 CFR 807.92(c)) – Glooko blood glucose meter and data management system. 2013.
43. Vanchieri. Addressing the barriers to pediatric drug development: workshop summary. Washington, DC: National Academy of Sciences; 2008.
44. Saunders TJ, Chaput JP, Goldfield GS, Colley RC, Kenny GP, Doucet E, et al. Prolonged sitting and markers of cardiometabolic disease risk in children and youth: a randomized crossover study. Metab Clin Exp. 2013;62(10):1423–8. Epub 2013/06/19.
45. Sue Kirkman M, Briscoe VJ, Clark N, Florez H, Haas LB, Halter JB, et al. Diabetes in older adults: a consensus report. J Am Geriatr Soc. 2012;60(12):2342–56. Epub 2012/10/31.

Computational Modelling of Energy Metabolism and Body Composition Dynamics

11

Kevin D. Hall

Abstract

Experimental investigation of human metabolism, nutrition, and body composition over the past century has produced a wealth of quantitative data on how the body dynamically adapts in response to diet changes. Our current physiological understanding is sufficiently detailed to develop mechanistic computational models that can quantitatively integrate past data, help identify important knowledge gaps, generate novel hypotheses, design key new experiments, and predict their results. This chapter provides an overview of our computational modeling efforts in the fields of nutrition and metabolism and their application to understanding and treating obesity from a variety of perspectives including pharmacological approaches.

Keywords

Mathematical model • Energy expenditure • Body composition • Energy balance • Energy partitioning • Macronutrient metabolism • Obesity

Introduction

The 1963 Nobel Prize in Physiology and Medicine recognized the landmark studies of Hodgkin and Huxley who established the primary exemplar of how computational modelling can be used to integrate and analyze experimental data, quantify assumptions about the system under investigation, and follow their logical consequences through numerical simulation of the mathematical model equations [1]. Interestingly, the Hodgkin and Huxley "computational" model of squid giant axon electrophysiology did not use a computer to solve the equations. Rather, numerical solutions were tediously calculated by hand, requiring more than a day of work to simulate less than 10 ms of electrical activity.

The work of Hodgkin and Huxley illustrated that systematic development of a physiologically realistic mathematical model can help identify important knowledge gaps, generate novel

K.D. Hall, PhD
Laboratory of Biological Modeling, National Institute of Diabetes and Digestive and Kidney Diseases, National Institutes of Health, Bethesda, MD, USA
e-mail: kevinh@niddk.nih.gov

hypotheses, design key new experiments, and predict their results which can then be quantitatively integrated within a unifying framework. The rise of "systems biology" in the past decade has promised the development of detailed computational models beyond the realm of electrophysiology, including gene regulation, signaling networks, metabolism, and the interactions between these systems [2].

Computational systems biology models often involve hundreds or thousands of variables and parameters and are typically targeted at the level of genes, molecules, and cells [3]. Detailed mathematical reconstructions of human cellular metabolism have recently been constructed, including representation of metabolism in various human cell types [4]. One could imagine extending such cellular level models to represent interacting tissues, organs, and ultimately whole-body human physiology. While such an endeavor may result in significant scientific progress, simulating whole-body human energy metabolism and the development and treatment of obesity would appear to be a very distant goal.

Fortunately, rather than modelling metabolism from the "bottom-up" including all known interactions, there is an alternative approach that involves targeting the complexity of a mathematical model to the physiological phenomena that the model is intended to address [5]. Recently, such mathematical models have become sufficiently sophisticated to provide important insights regarding whole-body human energy metabolism and body weight regulation. This chapter will provide an overview of our computational modelling efforts in this field and their application to understanding and treating obesity, including their potential role in obesity pharmacotherapy.

Energy Balance

At the whole-body level, models of human energy regulation and macronutrient metabolism are constrained by conservation principles and knowledge of the main metabolic pathways that contribute to metabolic imbalances and body composition changes. For example, most mathematical models of energy regulation make the assumption that weight change is determined by an imbalance between dietary energy intake and the energy expended by the body to maintain life and perform physical work. The theoretical underpinning of this energy balance concept is the first law of thermodynamics, and all valid models of whole-body metabolism are constrained to obey the energy balance equation:

$$\frac{d}{dt}(\rho BW) = EI - EE \qquad (11.1)$$

where the left side of the equation is the rate of change of body energy stores with BW being the body weight and ρ being an energy density converting between units of metabolizable energy and mass. The right side is the energy imbalance between the body's energy intake rate, EI, and the energy expenditure rate, EE. Any of the terms in the energy balance equation can depend on time, t, as well as other parameters. In particular, the three terms of the energy balance equation are highly interdependent [6]. In the following sections, I will describe the various components of the energy balance equation and some mathematical models that have been developed to represent each component.

Energy Storage and Body Composition

A simple translation between the energy imbalance and the rate of weight change in Eq. 11.1 occurs only if the energy density of the weight change, ρ, is a constant parameter. However, the body is composed of a variety of chemical constituents with widely varying energy densities. For example, fat has an energy density of about 9.4 kcal/g, whereas protein and carbohydrate have metabolizable energy densities of about 4.7 and 4 kcal/g, respectively [7]. Other major chemical constituents of the body (e.g., water and minerals) have energy densities of zero. Therefore, translating a given energy imbalance to a rate of weight change requires additional assumptions about the chemical composition of the weight change in terms of changes in body

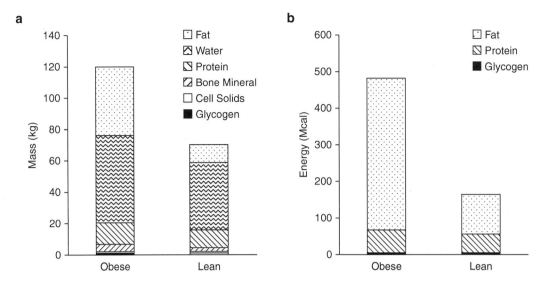

Fig. 11.1 Human body composition in example sedentary obese and lean men in terms of (**a**) their chemical composition and (**b**) their metabolizable energy storage

fat, protein, and glycogen along with associated fluid shifts.

Figure 11.1a illustrates the composition body in terms of body fat and fat-free mass in example obese and lean men. [Women generally have a higher body fat content for the same weight and height, and computational modelling also accounts for sex differences in body composition and metabolism.] Obesity is characterized by a greatly expanded body fat mass, but also an increased amount of fat-free mass. Figure 11.1a also illustrates the chemical composition of the fat-free mass with water being its greatest component. The absolute masses of body protein and bone mineral are also increased in obesity. Glycogen and cellular solids, such as potassium and nucleic acids, contribute a very small fraction of the fat-free mass.

Body fat, protein, and glycogen comprise the stored energy of the body and these stores must be mobilized when the diet is insufficient to meet the body's energy requirements. Figure 11.1b illustrates the composition of the body in terms of its energy content with fat stored in adipose tissue providing the overwhelming majority of the available stored energy, especially in obesity. Despite dietary carbohydrate typically providing the majority of the body's energy demands on a daily basis, glycogen represents a relatively insignificant store of energy (~2,000 kcal). Body protein represents a substantial amount of energy, but in humans it is not a storage pool in the same sense as adipose tissue triglyceride. Rather, body proteins are functionally important and cannot be depleted by a significant fraction without serious complications and death. In contrast, fat stores represent a considerable energy reserve and body fat can be depleted to very low levels without substantial functional impairments [8, 9].

Long-term changes in body fat are accompanied by changes in lean tissue mass whose metabolizable energy density is significantly less than that of body fat [10]. To model these longer-term body composition changes, Forbes hypothesized that the proportion of weight change resulting from lean versus fat tissue is a nonlinear function of body fat [11, 12]. The Forbes hypothesis has since been extended and validated to demonstrate that ρ is a nonlinear function of the body composition [13–15]. Nevertheless, for small changes of weight from an initial baseline, it is valid to approximate the nonlinear Forbes curve with a line, and the resulting slope gives a value for ρ. For moderately overweight and obese individuals, the $\rho = 3{,}500$ kcal/lb (or 7,700 kcal/kg) is a reasonable approximation, but this value significantly overstates ρ for lean individuals [10].

Energy Partitioning Models

The energy balance equation (Eq. 11.1) can be written as a pair of equations for the changes in both lean tissue, L, and body fat, F:

$$\rho_L \frac{dL}{dt} = P(EI - EE)$$
$$\rho_F \frac{dF}{dt} = (1-P)(EI - EE) \quad (11.2)$$

Depending on assumptions about the chemical composition of lean mass changes, the corresponding energy density, ρ_L, ranges between 1 and 1.8 kcal/g, and the energy density of fat, ρ_F, is about 9.4 kcal/g [10]. The energy partition ratio, P, ranges between 0 and 1 and determines the proportion of an energy imbalance directed to and from lean versus fat mass.

Applying the Forbes hypothesis to the energy partition model reveals that P is a nonlinear function of F: $P = C/(C+F)$ where $C = 10.4 \text{ kg} \times \rho_L/\rho_F$ [13, 16]. The initial value of P can be quite diverse for individuals with very different fat mass. However, the nonlinearity of the Forbes body composition curve suggests that P is not a fixed parameter since it depends continuously on the fat mass, which can change considerably with large weight changes.

Macronutrient Balance Models

While energy-partitioning models use the concept of energy balance and a partitioning rule to constrain their behavior, a more physiologically detailed perspective considers the source of dietary energy in the form of carbohydrate, fat, and protein. The human body uses these three dietary macronutrients to both fuel metabolism and provide substrates for body constituents. The typical diet derives about 50 % of the energy from carbohydrate, 35 % from fat, and 15 % from protein [17]. However, these average diet proportions can vary widely from person to person and also from day to day. Complex physiological mechanisms maintain normal functioning of the body despite marked fluctuations of diet quantity and composition.

A computational model has been developed that quantitatively tracks the metabolism of all three dietary macronutrients and simulates how diet changes result in adaptations of whole-body energy expenditure, metabolic fuel selection, and alterations in the major whole-body fluxes contributing to macronutrient balance [18, 19]. The macronutrient balance model is mathematically represented by the following equations describing changes in the body's energy stores of glycogen (G), fat (F), and protein (P):

$$\rho_C \frac{dG}{dt} = CI - DNL + GNG_p + GNG_f - G3P - CarbOx$$
$$\rho_F \frac{dF}{dt} = FI + \varepsilon_d DNL - KU_{excr} - (1-\varepsilon_k) KTG - FatOx \quad (11.3)$$
$$\rho_P \frac{dP}{dt} = PI - GNG_p - ProtOx$$

where ρ_C, ρ_F, and ρ_P are the energy densities of carbohydrate, fat, and protein, respectively. The macronutrient intake rates, CI, FI, and PI, refer to the metabolizable energy intake rates of dietary carbohydrate, fat, and protein, respectively. The rates of gluconeogenesis from amino acids and glycerol are indicated by GNG_p and GNG_f, respectively. The efficiencies of de novo lipogenesis, DNL, and ketogenesis, KTG, were represented by the parameters ε_d and ε_k, respectively. When the ketogenic rate increases, ketones are excreted in the urine at the rate KU_{excr}. Some flux of carbohydrates are provided for the production of glycerol 3-phosphate, $G3P$, that is used in the synthesis of triglyceride. The oxidation rates, $CarbOx$, $FatOx$, and $ProtOx$, sum to the energy expenditure rate, EE, less than the small amount of heat produced via flux through ketogenic and de novo lipogenic pathways. Turnover of glycogen, fat, and protein and the corresponding energy costs are also included in the model.

The main model assumptions are that changes of the body's energy stores are given by the sum of metabolic fluxes entering the pools minus the fluxes exiting the pools. Hence, the macronutrient metabolism model obeys the first law of thermodynamics, and the most recent version was developed using published human data from over 50 experimental studies and was validated by comparing model predictions with the results from several controlled feeding studies not used for model development [19]. To date, this is the only mathematical model of human metabolism to consider all three dietary macronutrients and accurately simulate the metabolic and body composition changes in response to diet and physical activity changes in a wide variety of subject groups.

The macronutrient imbalances between dietary intake and metabolic utilization underlie changes of stored fat, glycogen, and protein and result in changes in the chemical composition of the body [18, 19]. To account for body water shifts with diets that vary in both macronutrient and sodium content, the model also simulates intracellular and extracellular fluid changes. Thus, the macronutrient balance model leads to a detailed description of body composition dynamics, and the overall body weight change is just the sum of the individual changes in body constituents. Importantly, the macronutrient balance model does not rely on empirical relationships between body fat and lean tissue mass (such as the Forbes curve) and provides a more detailed molecular level description of body composition [20].

Energy Expenditure

For decades, weight-management professionals have used the energy balance equation (Eq. 11.1) to predict how body weight will change in response to a diet or physical activity intervention. Unfortunately, the vast majority of these calculations assumed that the energy expenditure rate, EE, was a static quantity and the resulting time course of weight change was therefore linear in time [21–23]. However, we now know that energy expenditure is a dynamic quantity that depends of a variety of factors and body weight predictions using the static assumption drastically overestimate weight change, especially over long time scales.

Improving body weight predictions requires a dynamic model of energy expenditure and its determinants. Figure 11.2 depicts the various components of energy expenditure in example sedentary lean and obese men. The obese man requires several hundred additional kcal/day to maintain his increased weight compared to the lean man. While this general dependence of weight on energy expenditure may be captured using a simple model of body weight alone, more realistic models have been developed that represent the dynamic changes in the various components of energy expenditure: the thermic effect of food, resting energy expenditure, and physical activity expenditure.

Thermic Effect of Food

The smallest component of the total energy expenditure rate in humans is the thermic effect of food (also sometimes called "diet-induced thermogenesis" or "specific dynamic action")

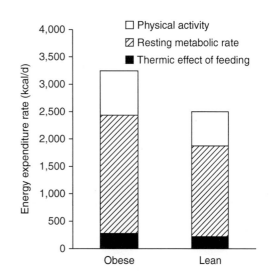

Fig. 11.2 Components of total energy expenditure in example sedentary obese and lean men

defined as the increase of metabolic rate observed for several hours following the ingestion of a meal. The thermic effect of food is believed to represent the energy cost of digestion and absorption as well as the storage and metabolic fate of dietary macronutrients [24]. While the precise mechanisms underlying the thermic effect of food are not fully understood, there is a clear dietary macronutrient hierarchy in the magnitude of the metabolic rate increase after feeding, with protein causing a greater increment than carbohydrate which is greater than that of fat. The computational model of macronutrient balance model accounts for this hierarchy [18, 19], but other energy balance and energy partition models ignore the macronutrient effect and assume that thermic effect of food is given by an overall proportion of energy intake, typically between 7 and 14 %.

Resting Energy Expenditure

The resting energy expenditure (REE) corresponds to the energy expended by the body when not performing physical work and is typically the largest contribution to the total energy expenditure rate. Contrary to popular belief, obese people generally have a higher absolute REE compared to lean people (see Fig. 11.2). Readily available clinical measures (e.g., sex, height, weight, and age) have been used along with REE measurements to generate empirical equations with REE being an increasing function of body weight, commonly a linear or a power law relationship. While several mathematical models of body weight dynamics have used this simplified approach to modelling REE [25–27], it has long been recognized that the main contributor to the REE is the fat-free mass since it comprises the metabolically active tissues of the body [28].

Fat-free mass is elevated in obesity along with the increased body fat mass (see Fig. 11.1) which also contributes a small amount to increased resting energy expenditure. The linear relationship between resting energy expenditure and fat-free mass is identical in obese and lean people [28, 29]. This means that the elevated resting energy expenditure in obesity is generally in line with what is expected for their body composition.

While fat-free mass, and to a lesser extent fat mass, are good predictors of REE, such models explain only about 70 % of interindividual REE variability such that for a given body composition the REE standard deviation is about 300 kcal/day [28, 29]. Since there is a large range of specific metabolic rates among various organs that contribute to the fat-free mass [30], some of this residual REE variability may be due to differences in organ masses. Magnetic resonance imaging methodologies have been used to quantify organ sizes, and using assumptions regarding the organ-specific metabolic rates, REE prediction equations that sum the individual metabolic rates of various organs explain about 80 % of the REE variability [31–33]. Thus, increasingly detailed knowledge of the body composition may improve REE predictions.

The computational model of macronutrient balance [19] incorporated how changes in the sizes of various organs affect REE, assuming linear relationships between changes of fat-free mass and various organ sizes based on cross-sectional data from 110 men and women with body mass index between 18 and 37 kg/m^2 (D. Gallagher, personal communication). Of course, longitudinal organ mass changes with weight gain and loss need not follow the cross-sectional relationships, and this possibility requires experimental investigation.

Another potentially important contributor to REE dynamics may involve flux changes through various energy-requiring metabolic pathways. The major macronutrient fluxes of gluconeogenesis, de novo lipogenesis, triglyceride synthesis, and protein turnover all affect energy expenditure, and these flux rates can be significantly influenced by both the energy content of the diet as well as the diet composition. For example, the breakdown and resynthesis of body fat requires 8 molecules of adenosine triphosphate [ATP] per molecule of triglyceride [34], and the flux through this pathway is strongly influenced by dietary carbohydrate via insulin's inhibition of lipolysis. Similarly, protein synthesis requires 4 ATP per peptide bond plus 1 ATP for amino acid transport

[35]. Such energy-requiring metabolic fluxes may explain the observed energy cost of tissue deposition that is especially important during growth and weight gain [36].

Physical Activity Expenditure

The physical activities of humans typically involve locomotion, and the energy costs are determined by the duration and intensity of physical activity in proportion to the overall body weight [37]. Thus, obese and lean people can have similar daily energy costs for physical activity despite obese people typically being less active. With weight loss, it costs less energy to perform most physical activities, and therefore, the physical activity expenditure typically decreases unless the quantity or intensity of physical activity increases to compensate.

Mathematical models of human energy expenditure include the body weight effect on physical activity expenditure. Some models further subdivide physical activity expenditure into volitional activities (e.g., exercise) and low intensity spontaneous physical activity or "non-exercise activity thermogenesis" (NEAT) [19, 26, 27].

Adaptive Thermogenesis and Metabolic Adaptation

During active weight loss, both REE and total energy expenditure have been observed to decrease to an extent greater than expected based on the measured body weight and composition changes [38–42]. Furthermore, this increased energy efficiency appears to persist once energy balance is established at a lower body weight [43], although the magnitude of this persistent effect is smaller than during active weight loss and its existence has been controversial [44, 45]. Conversely, overfeeding and weight gain can result in highly variable increases of energy expenditure that can be greater than expected based on the observed weight gain [46, 47]. Collectively, these phenomena have been called "adaptive thermogenesis" [41, 48] or "metabolic adaptation" [49, 50].

The energy partition models of Hall et al. incorporated adaptive thermogenesis as an additive term that was a linear function of the change in energy intake from baseline [14, 22, 51]. In these models, the value of the adaptive thermogenesis parameter was chosen to match changes in overall energy expenditure measured before and after approximately stable weight loss [14]. When active weight loss is followed by subsequent weight stabilization, the change in energy intake required for the weight loss phase is greater than that required for weight stabilization at the reduced weight. Thus, modelling adaptive thermogenesis as a function of energy intake change has the natural consequence of decreasing energy expenditure more during situations of active weight loss compared to maintaining a stable lower weight, in agreement with observations [44].

Experimental quantification of the adaptive thermogenesis magnitude depends on the definition of the "expected values" for REE and total energy expenditure. Typically, cross-sectional regression equations are used to calculate the expected values using for REE and energy expenditure measurements derived either from baseline body composition data in the same subjects [40, 42, 50] or from a separate group of similar subjects [38, 39]. But such expected values for REE and energy expenditure ignore the possible changes in organ size distribution as well as changes in fluxes through energy-requiring metabolic pathways during over- or underfeeding described above. Whether such considerations can explain the observed changes in energy efficiency is unclear.

The computational model of macronutrient balance that accounts for alterations of energy-requiring metabolic fluxes as well as organ mass changes also required a model of adaptive thermogenesis to explain the observed average decrease in both REE and total energy expenditure with weight loss [18, 19]. Adaptive thermogenesis was modeled as a linear function of the reduction in energy intake below baseline and was used to suppress the metabolic rate of all organs as well as reduce the energy expended in spontaneous physical activity. The mechanistic basis of such a metabolic adaptation is unclear but may be related to

Fig. 11.3 Computer simulations of the study by Leibel et al. [40] using the model of Hall [19] illustrating (**a**) dynamic changes in total energy expenditure (*TEE*) and resting energy expenditure (*REE*) during weight loss and (**b**) body weight and body fat dynamics. The *curves* are the model predictions and the data points represent the mean ± SD

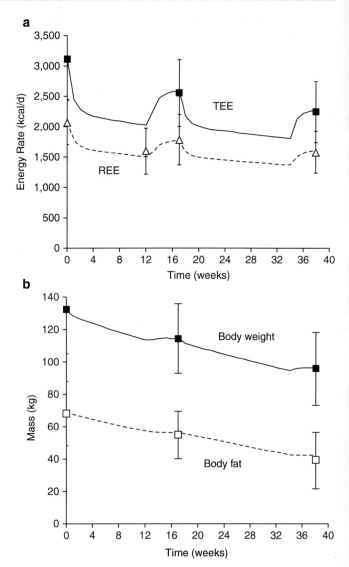

reduced sympathetic drive or blunted thyroid activity, possibly as a result of decreased circulating leptin [41, 49, 52–55].

Figure 11.3 shows the computational model simulation of the classic results of Leibel et al. [40] whose metabolic ward study provided obese subjects with an 800 kcal/day liquid formula diet until subjects had lost 10 % of their initial weight, after which the energy intake of the liquid formula was increased to achieve weight stability for at least 2 weeks. After measuring body composition and energy expenditure during weight maintenance at 10 % weight loss, subjects were returned to the 800 kcal/day diet until 20 % weight loss when the energy intake was again increased to stabilize body weight and make final measurements. Figure 11.3a illustrates the simulated dynamic changes in both total and resting energy expenditure in the solid and dashed curves, respectively. Without adjusting any model parameters (other than the initial conditions to match the baseline data), the model accurately reproduced the average energy expenditure data and demonstrated the highly dynamic nature of the metabolic adaptations. Both resting and total energy expenditure rapidly decreased following the onset of the reduced energy diet but increased after body weight stabilized at a lower level, albeit at a value that was significantly lower than the expenditure rate prior to weight loss. Figure 11.3b illustrates that the computational model also correctly simulated the observed body composition changes observed by Leibel et al. [40] based on the calculated macronutrient and water imbalances that accumulated over the course of the study.

Energy Intake

Human eating behavior is extraordinarily complex. Eating behavior is determined by dynamic interactions between homeostatic, hedonic, and cognitive processes. Our cognitive choices about when to eat are modulated by homeostatic hunger as well as the availability of food, the social context, our response to environmental food cues, and our habitual eating times. Food choice and how much we eat are also under cognitive control but strongly influenced by appetite, food variety, portion size, social context, habits, satiety, and the reward value of the food. Homeostatic hunger enhances, and satiety attenuates, both food and nonfood rewards and activation of hedonic circuits may override homeostatic satiety signals thereby facilitating eating in the absence of physiological hunger. We are only now beginning to understand this system, and quantitative mathematical models of these processes have not yet been developed in humans. A major barrier to the development of quantitative models of food intake is our current inability to make accurate measurements of this variable on the relevant time scale for addressing the question of obesity and its treatment [56].

Relevant Time Scale of Energy Intake

Human weight change and the development of obesity is a slow process. Mathematical modelling can be used to quantify the relevant time scale, and any model of human energy metabolism and body weight change can be linearized around a baseline body weight value, BW_0, to yield:

$$\frac{dBW}{dt} = \frac{\Delta EI}{\hat{p}} - \frac{(BW - BW_0)}{\tau} \qquad (11.4)$$

where ΔEI is the change in energy intake from an energy-balanced baseline, $\hat{p}$ is the effective energy density of the weight change, the time constant, $\tau = \hat{p}/\varepsilon$, sets the characteristic time scale of the system, and the parameter ε defines how energy expenditure depends on the weight change [22]. Using typical model parameter values, the characteristic time scale is approximately 1 year. This means that a step change in energy intake takes several years to fully play out and result in a new steady-state body weight. Furthermore, the long time scale implies that measuring short-term changes in energy intake in laboratory settings are of limited utility for understanding the natural development of obesity or its treatment.

Measuring Long-Term Energy Intake

Given the importance of long-term energy intake on determining body weight change in humans, it is unfortunate that this variable is so difficult to measure in free-living conditions [56–58]. While the doubly labeled water method is the gold standard for estimating the average rate of carbon dioxide production, this measurement is expensive and must be combined with assumptions about average metabolic fuel mix and measurements of body composition changes to calculate an estimate of average free-living energy intake [59]. Recently, dynamic mathematical models have begun to tackle the important problem of estimating changes in human free-living energy intake.

Jordan et al. demonstrated how a dynamic mathematical model can be used to quantitatively integrate longitudinal body composition data with repeated doubly labeled water measurements to calculate dynamic estimates of average free-living energy intake, energy expenditure, as well as the respiratory quotient [60].

Furthermore, the study demonstrated how variability in the experimental measurements [the model inputs] influenced the calculated time courses of energy intake, energy expenditure, and respiratory quotient [the model outputs]. While this model was applied to data from growing infants over their first 2 years of life [61, 62], the methodology is equally applicable to weight gain or loss data in adults.

In the absence of doubly labeled water or body composition data, Hall et al. proposed a method for calculating changes in adult energy intake using only repeated body weight measurements along with a dynamic mathematical model of adult energy metabolism and body composition change [19, 22, 51, 63]. Hall et al. have recently used such methods to help interpret the results of outpatient weight loss interventions [19, 22]. Such programs ubiquitously result in a period of weight loss that plateaus after about 6–8 months and often followed by slow weight regain [64, 65]. Using the longitudinal measurements of body weight, Hall et al. applied different mathematical models to estimate the changes of free-living energy intake underlying the typical weight loss, plateau, and regain trajectory. The conclusion was that the plateau was primarily due to a short-lived adherence to the diet intervention that was progressively relaxed to return to the pre-intervention level within the first year thereby leading to slow regain in subsequent years. Slowing of metabolic rate was found to play a secondary role in the weight plateau and regain trajectory. This interpretation differs markedly from the usual explanation that focuses on metabolic slowing as the prime culprit responsible for weight plateaus within the first year of an intervention [64, 66].

While calculating the free-living energy intake of groups over time is useful for data interpretation, predicting individual energy intake changes would be extremely valuable for assessing diet adherence during a weight loss program. Hall and Chow recently introduced a relatively simple methodology for using longitudinal weight measurements to estimate energy intake changes along with an explicit calculation of the confidence interval of the estimate, a useful metric for assessing individual diet adherence [63].

Computational Models of Mouse Metabolism and Body Weight Dynamics

Mouse models have proven to be particularly insightful for identifying molecular mechanisms of body weight regulation, and mouse models are routinely used in preclinical investigation of novel obesity therapeutics. But it is often unclear whether any observed body weight changes are the result of altered energy intake, expenditure, or both. While accurate and frequent measurements of food intake and weight change in mice can be performed over extended time periods, the same cannot be said of energy expenditure measurements. Rather, expensive indirect calorimetry systems are increasingly being used to measure energy expenditure and respiratory exchange over periods of a few days, but the mice are typically removed from their normal environment which can alter their behavior [67]. For example, the indirect calorimetry procedure can cause weight loss in mice that had previously been gaining weight in their home cages [68].

Guo et al. developed a mathematical method based on the law of energy conservation that used the measured body weight and food intake changes as model inputs to calculate the underlying energy balance and fuel selection dynamics [69]. The model predicted daily energy output, RQ, and net fat oxidation during the development of obesity and weight loss in male C57BL/6 mice consuming various ad libitum diets over several weeks while mice were housed in their home cages. Such methods will likely become increasingly important as the challenges of indirect calorimetry in mice are more widely recognized.

A mathematical model has recently been developed to predict the dynamics of body weight and fat mass in male C57BL/6 mice [70]. The model includes the cost of tissue turnover and deposition, physical activity, diet-induced thermogenesis, and the influence of body composition on metabolic rate. The model was calibrated using previously published data [71] and was validated by comparing its predictions to measurements from an independent validation study of five groups of male C57/BL6 mice provided ad libitum access to either chow or high-fat diets for varying time periods.

The model coefficients relating energy expenditure to body composition also agreed with previous independent estimates [72]. Metabolic fuel selection was predicted to depend on a complex interplay between diet composition, the degree of energy imbalance, and body composition.

Gennemark et al. recently adapted this model to help characterize the pharmacodynamics of compounds to treat obesity [73]. They implemented a pharmacokinetic model of an experimental compound which was connected to the computational model of mouse energy balance and body composition dynamics. The resulting model was used to quantitatively investigate the effects of the drug on mouse energy intake and expenditure dynamics along with the corresponding changes in body weight and composition. This study illustrates the potential use of computational modelling in preclinical investigations to quantitatively integrate the results of experimental studies and obtain a comprehensive picture of energy metabolism and body composition dynamics.

Implications of Computational Modelling for Obesity and Its Treatment

Modelling Populations and Policy Interventions

Mathematical models are also beginning to be used to predict the weight changes of entire populations. For example, Church et al. investigated the role of reduced occupational physical activity on the development of the US obesity epidemic [74]. This study used the dynamic mathematical model of Thomas et al. [26, 27] to simulate the changes in adult body weight corresponding to the calculated decreases in occupational physical activity over the past half century. Assuming that energy intake remained constant over this time period, the authors found that the observed increase in the average weight of men and women closely matched the model predictions.

The conclusion of Church et al. was that the US obesity epidemic was almost fully explained by the progressive decrease in occupational physical activity. However, this conclusion is complicated by the fact that the Thomas weight change model has not been validated for predicting the effects of altered physical activity. There is good reason to believe that the Thomas model overestimates the predicted weight change because it assumes that changes in any component of energy expenditure are positively correlated to changes in spontaneous physical activity or non-exercise activity expenditure [26, 27]. Hence, decreased occupational physical activity was assumed to lead to concomitant decreases in spontaneous physical activity – a property that is highly questionable and significantly limits the model's utility [75].

In another example of population modelling, Hall et al. employed a validated mathematical model of human weight change to address the question of whether changes in the US food supply could account for the increase in average US adult body weight since the 1970s [51]. The model calculated that an average progressive energy intake increase of about 250 kcal/day per person was required to generate the US adult obesity epidemic (assuming no changes in physical activity). This increment in food intake pales in comparison to the rate of increase in the per capita US food supply, which was about triple this amount over the same time period. Therefore, the authors calculated that per capita food waste has progressively increased by 50 % since the 1970s such that two-thirds of the increased food available was not eaten. This result was corroborated by independent data from the US Environmental Protection Agency who measured a parallel 50 % increase in per capita food waste in municipal landfills.

Using the dynamic simulation model of Hall et al. [22], Lin et al. estimated the impact of taxation policies for caloric sweetened beverages on the prevalence of overweight and obesity in the USA [76]. The authors compared the model-predicted changes in obesity prevalence to predictions obtained using the static 3,500 kcal per pound weight loss model that does not account for dynamic changes of energy expenditure. The dynamic model simulations predicted that proposed taxation policies will result in a modest decrease in overweight and obesity prevalence that is substantially less than the previously calculated values using the static model [77].

Unfortunately, economists and public health professionals have a long history of using the erroneous static weight loss rule when evaluating the potential efficacy of population-wide interventions for obesity. As emphasized in this chapter, such methods should be replaced by dynamic models that simulate the known changes in energy expenditure.

Clinical Obesity Management

Weight management professionals are often faced with providing concrete answers to questions like: How much weight will I lose if I start jogging and cut back on snacks? What diet and exercise program would be required to lose 20 lb [approximately 9 kg] in the next 6 months? How can I maintain my goal weight once it is reached? Reputable health and nutrition organizations around the world have attempted to address such questions by advising that a 500 kcal per day reduction of food intake or increase in exercise expenditure will lead to a steady rate of weight loss of about 1 lb (approximately 0.45 kg) per week [78–81]. This simple weight loss prediction overestimates the actual rate of weight loss primarily because it ignores the dynamic changes in energy expenditure discussed in the section "Energy Expenditure" [21, 22]. Furthermore, it provides no accounting for differences between individuals and no advice about maintenance of lost weight.

Dynamic models can be used to accurately predict how changes in diet and physical activity affect body weight and body composition over time. For example, building on a steady-state model of human weight change that was calibrated using data on long-term changes in body composition and energy expenditure [14], Hall et al. developed and validated a dynamic simulation model that calculates how factors such as diet and exercise can alter energy expenditure over time and thereby lead to dynamic changes of weight and body fat [22]. The model found that people with higher body fat can expect greater weight change with the same change in diet though it will take longer to reach a stable body weight than people with less body fat. Previous methods and tools used to estimate weight changes did not consider these important physiological differences between individuals.

A web-based implementation of the model [http://bwsimulator.niddk.nih.gov] provides accurate predictions of how long it will take for different people to reach their weight goals for a given change of diet or physical activity. This tool can be used to plan weight-management interventions, track progress, help people reevaluate their goals, and tailor the pace of weight loss. Most importantly, the tool offers a plan for the permanent lifestyle changes required to maintain weight loss and avoid weight regain. Recently, the model's applicability was investigated in a real-world setting of a medical weight loss clinic and was determined to provide accurate predictions in highly adherent patients as well as alert the clinician when weight loss veers outside the expected range [82].

Pharmacological Obesity Therapies

Most obesity drugs work in humans by decreasing metabolizable energy intake with minor effects on energy expenditure [83]. However, only recently have energy intake changes during long-term obesity pharmacotherapy been quantified [84]. Göbel et al. used repeated mean body weight measurements along with a validated mathematical model of human metabolism to calculate energy intake changes during long-term obesity pharmacotherapy with 14 different drugs or drug combinations from randomized, placebo-controlled trials. Despite the variety obesity pharmacotherapies investigated, Göbel et al. discovered a universal exponential time course with early large decreases in metabolizable energy intake followed by a slow waning of the drug effect to a much smaller persistent reduction in energy intake [84]. Different drugs could be characterized and compared with each other using three simple parameters describing the universal exponential pattern.

Table 11.1 Comparison of the energy intake change required for 5 % weight loss in 6 months to the permanent change in energy intake to maintain the lost weight

	Men		Women	
Initial BMI (kg/m²)	5 % weight loss in 6 months (kcal/day)	5 % weight loss maintenance (kcal/day)	5 % weight loss in 6 months (kcal/day)	5 % weight loss maintenance (kcal/day)
30	−300	−100	−260	−70
40	−420	−110	−350	−90
50	−550	−120	−480	−100

Does the exponential waning of the drug effect on energy intake during obesity pharmacotherapy imply that clinically significant weight loss cannot persist over the long term? Current regulatory guidance for the development of obesity therapeutics places an efficacy target at >5 % weight loss compared to placebo over a period of at least 1 year [85]. Fortunately, computational models of human energy metabolism demonstrate that the early reduction in energy intake required for short-term weight loss is substantially greater than that required to subsequently maintain lost weight [22]. Thus, the observed exponential waning of obesity pharmacotherapy on energy intake does not necessarily mean that weight regain is inevitable.

Table 11.1 illustrates model-predicted changes in energy intake required to achieve an efficacy target of 5 % weight loss in 6 months in comparison to the energy intake changes required to subsequently maintain this lost weight [22]. For example, an intervention delivered to an average obese woman with a body mass index of 40 kg/m² would need to result in an average decrease in calorie intake of about 350 kcal/day from her usual diet over the entire 6-month period to achieve a 5 % weight loss. In contrast, maintaining the lost weight after 6 months would require that the persistent effect of the intervention reduce energy intake by only 90 kcal/day below her baseline diet. This persistent reduction of energy intake is about what has been achieved with obesity pharmacotherapies investigated by Göbel et al. [84].

Mechanistic computational models can also be used to provide quantitative estimates of how hypothesized interventions affecting various components of macronutrient metabolism, energy expenditure, or food intake might lead to alterations in metabolism, body weight, and body composition over time. For example, the potential of activating or inducing brown adipose tissue has recently been considered as a possible obesity therapy [86]. Existing computational models of human metabolism could be adapted to simulate the effect on body composition of increased energy expenditure of brown adipose tissue as well as its impact on fat and carbohydrate oxidation over extended time periods. Such modelling could help follow the logical downstream consequences of various assumptions and quantitatively investigate hypotheses about how potential counter-regulatory increases in energy intake might limit changes in body weight and fat mass.

Childhood Obesity

Computational modelling of childhood energy metabolism and body composition dynamics is complicated by the processes of growth and development, with boys and girls having different patterns of body fat deposition as well as differing rates of growth. Recently, a validated mathematical model of childhood energy metabolism was developed that accounts for healthy growth in boys and girls, the development of childhood obesity, and makes quantitative predictions about weight-management interventions [87].

The computational model showed that the development of childhood obesity requires a much greater increase in energy intake compared to adults and was much greater than previous estimates that did not properly account for metabolic changes as children grow. The model also showed that there might be windows of therapeutic opportunity when children can outgrow obesity without necessarily losing weight. By timing a weight-management intervention over the course of a growth spurt, it may be possible to harness the power of growth to substantially reduce body fat while at the same time increasing muscle mass. If the child is not too overweight at the start of the intervention, he may be able to outgrow obesity without even losing weight. Because boys typically have a higher growth potential than girls, the model found that timing a weight-management intervention to occur during a growth spurt might be particularly effective in overweight boys. Nevertheless, overweight girls would also likely benefit from such a strategy but might have to lose some weight to normalize their body fat.

Conclusions and Future Directions

In the early twentieth century, Julian Huxley eloquently expressed the potential utility of mathematical modelling in biology, as well as the widespread resistance to this idea:

> ...there appears still to linger a distrust of the application of even such elementary mathematics to biological problems. The usual criticism is that the formulae arrived at may have a certain convenience, but can tell us nothing new, and nothing worth knowing of the biology of the phenomenon. This appears to me to be very ill-founded. In the first place, to have a quantitative expression in place of a vague idea of a general tendency is not merely a mild convenience. It may even be a very great convenience, and it may even be indispensable in making certain systematic and biological deductions. But further, it may suggest important ideas as to the underlying processes involved; ...there are certain hypotheses which square with the formula, others which do not: without the quantitative expression, we should be largely theorizing in the air [88].

More than 80 years after Huxley penned these lines, it is unfortunate that a distrust of mathematical and computational modelling as applied to biology remains somewhat prevalent. Nevertheless, there is an increasing acceptance that biology is now a quantitative discipline generating vast amounts of data and that computational models will be required to properly understand these complex systems [2, 89].

In this chapter, I have tried to illustrate how computational models of human energy metabolism can highlight knowledge gaps, integrate metabolic data within a broader context of knowledge, make testable predictions, and thereby help design new experiments that will both improve the models and our understanding of the overall system. In addition to helping obesity research, computational modeling has practical implications for clinical weight management as well as evaluating policies to address obesity at the population level and the development of pharmacological approaches to treating obesity.

Despite significant progress thus far, much work remains for improving and expanding the existing mathematical models of human energy regulation and body composition change. For example, even the most detailed computational models macronutrient metabolism implicitly represent the effect of hormones such as insulin, but an explicit representation of organ systems along with concentrations of hormones and metabolites would be desirable, especially on shorter time scales so that the response to individual meals could be simulated. The anatomical location of body fat, especially in visceral adipose tissue, has profound clinical importance, and mathematical models have only just begun to capture the relationship between body fat changes in various depots during weight loss and gain [90, 91]. Furthermore, current computational models do not yet address the potential role of brown adipose tissue or the gut microbiota in human energy metabolism. By addressing these issues through the iterative process of model development and experimental testing, computational modeling of human metabolism is likely to continue to make significant contributions to our understanding of the etiology of obesity and its treatment.

Acknowledgments This research was supported by the Intramural Research Program of the NIH, National Institute of Diabetes & Digestive & Kidney Diseases.

References

1. Hodgkin AL, Huxley AF. A quantitative description of membrane current and its application to conduction and excitation in nerve. J Physiol. 1952;117(4):500–44. PubMed PMID: 12991237, Pubmed Central PMCID: 1392413.
2. Di Ventura B, Lemerle C, Michalodimitrakis K, Serrano L. From in vivo to in silico biology and back. Nature. 2006;443(7111):527–33. PubMed PMID: 17024084. eng.
3. Karr JR, Sanghvi JC, Macklin DN, Gutschow MV, Jacobs JM, Bolival Jr B, et al. A whole-cell computational model predicts phenotype from genotype. Cell. 2012;150(2):389–401. PubMed PMID: 22817898, Pubmed Central PMCID: 3413483.
4. Thiele I, Swainston N, Fleming RM, Hoppe A, Sahoo S, Aurich MK, et al. A community-driven global reconstruction of human metabolism. Nat Biotechnol. 2013;31(5):419–25. PubMed PMID: 23455439.
5. de Graaf AA, Freidig AP, De Roos B, Jamshidi N, Heinemann M, Rullmann JA, et al. Nutritional systems biology modeling: from molecular mechanisms to physiology. PLoS Comput Biol. 2009;5(11):e1000554. PubMed PMID: 19956660, Pubmed Central PMCID: 2777333.
6. Hall KD, Heymsfield SB, Kemnitz JW, Klein S, Schoeller DA, Speakman JR. Energy balance and its components: implications for body weight regulation. Am J Clin Nutr. 2012;95(4):989–94. PubMed PMID: 22434603. eng.
7. Livesey G, Elia M. Estimation of energy expenditure, net carbohydrate utilization, and net fat oxidation and synthesis by indirect calorimetry: evaluation of errors with special reference to the detailed composition of fuels. Am J Clin Nutr. 1988;47(4):608–28. PubMed PMID: 3281434. eng.
8. Friedl KE, Moore RJ, Martinez-Lopez LE, Vogel JA, Askew EW, Marchitelli LJ, et al. Lower limit of body fat in healthy active men. J Appl Physiol. 1994;77(2):933–40. PubMed PMID: 8002550. eng.
9. Leiter LA, Marliss EB. Survival during fasting may depend on fat as well as protein stores. JAMA. 1982;248(18):2306–7. PubMed PMID: 7131684. eng.
10. Hall KD. What is the required energy deficit per unit weight loss? Int J Obes (Lond). 2008;32(3):573–6. PubMed PMID: 17848938. eng.
11. Forbes GB. Lean body mass-body fat interrelationships in humans. Nutr Rev. 1987;45(8):225–31. PubMed PMID: 3306482. eng.
12. Forbes GB. Body fat content influences the body composition response to nutrition and exercise. Ann N Y Acad Sci. 2000;904:359–65. PubMed PMID: 10865771. eng.
13. Hall KD. Body fat and fat-free mass inter-relationships: Forbes's theory revisited. Br J Nutr. 2007;97(6):1059–63. PubMed PMID: 17367567. eng.
14. Hall KD, Jordan PN. Modeling weight-loss maintenance to help prevent body weight regain. Am J Clin Nutr. 2008;88(6):1495–503. PubMed PMID: 19064508. eng.
15. Thomas D, Das SK, Levine JA, Martin CK, Mayer L, McDougall A, et al. New fat free mass – fat mass model for use in physiological energy balance equations. Nutr Metab (Lond). 2010;7(39). PubMed PMID: 20459692. eng.
16. Chow CC, Hall KD. The dynamics of human body weight change. PLoS Comput Biol. 2008;4(3):e1000045. PubMed PMID: 18369435. eng.
17. Austin GL, Ogden CL, Hill JO. Trends in carbohydrate, fat, and protein intakes and association with energy intake in normal-weight, overweight, and obese individuals: 1971–2006. Am J Clin Nutr. 2011;93(4):836–43.
18. Hall KD. Computational model of in vivo human energy metabolism during semistarvation and refeeding. Am J Physiol Endocrinol Metab. 2006;291(1):E23–37. PubMed PMID: 16449298. eng.
19. Hall KD. Predicting metabolic adaptation, body weight change, and energy intake in humans. Am J Physiol Endocrinol Metab. 2010;298(3):E449–66. PubMed PMID: 19934407. eng.
20. Heymsfield SB, Wang Z, Baumgartner RN, Ross R. Human body composition: advances in models and methods. Annu Rev Nutr. 1997;17:527–58. PubMed PMID: 9240939.
21. Hall KD, Chow CC. Why is the 3500 kcal per pound weight loss rule wrong? Int J Obes (Lond). 2013;37(12):1614. PubMed PMID: 23774459.
22. Hall KD, Sacks G, Chandramohan D, Chow CC, Wang YC, Gortmaker SL, et al. Quantification of the effect of energy imbalance on bodyweight. Lancet. 2011;378(9793):826–37. PubMed PMID: 21872751. eng.
23. Thomas DM, Martin CK, Lettieri S, Bredlau C, Kaiser K, Church T, et al. Can a weight loss of one pound a week be achieved with a 3500-kcal deficit? Commentary on a commonly accepted rule. Int J Obes (Lond). 2013;37(12):1611–3. PubMed PMID: 23628852.
24. Westerterp KR. Diet induced thermogenesis. Nutr Metab (Lond). 2004;1(1):5. PubMed PMID: 15507147.
25. Antonetti VW. The equations governing weight change in human beings. Am J Clin Nutr. 1973;26(1):64–71. PubMed PMID: 4682818. eng.
26. Thomas DM, Ciesla A, Levine JA, Stevens JG, Martin CK. A mathematical model of weight change with adaptation. Math Biosci Eng. 2009;6(4):873–87. PubMed PMID: 19835433. eng.
27. Thomas DM, Martin CK, Heymsfield S, Redman LM, Schoeller DA, Levine JA. A simple model predicting individual weight change in humans. J Biol Dyn. 2011;5(6):579–99.

28. Cunningham JJ. Body composition as a determinant of energy expenditure: a synthetic review and a proposed general prediction equation. Am J Clin Nutr. 1991;54(6):963–9. PubMed PMID: 1957828.
29. Weyer C, Snitker S, Rising R, Bogardus C, Ravussin E. Determinants of energy expenditure and fuel utilization in man: effects of body composition, age, sex, ethnicity and glucose tolerance in 916 subjects. Int J Obes Relat Metab Disord. 1999;23(7):715–22. PubMed PMID: 10454105.
30. Elia M. Organ and tissue contribution to metabolic rate. In: Kinney JM, Tucker HN, editors. Energy metabolism: tissue determinants and cellular corollaries. New York: Raven; 1992. p. 61–79.
31. Gallagher D, Belmonte D, Deurenberg P, Wang Z, Krasnow N, Pi-Sunyer FX, et al. Organ-tissue mass measurement allows modeling of REE and metabolically active tissue mass. Am J Physiol. 1998;275(2 Pt 1):E249–58. PubMed PMID: 9688626.
32. Muller MJ, Bosy-Westphal A, Kutzner D, Heller M. Metabolically active components of fat-free mass and resting energy expenditure in humans: recent lessons from imaging technologies. Obes Rev. 2002;3(2):113–22. PubMed PMID: 12120418.
33. Muller MJ, Bosy-Westphal A, Later W, Haas V, Heller M. Functional body composition: insights into the regulation of energy metabolism and some clinical applications. Eur J Clin Nutr. 2009;63(9):1045–56. PubMed PMID: 19623201. eng.
34. Elia M, Zed C, Neale G, Livesey G. The energy cost of triglyceride-fatty acid recycling in nonobese subjects after an overnight fast and four days of starvation. Metabolism. 1987;36(3):251–5. PubMed PMID: 3821505. eng.
35. Blaxter K. Energy metabolism in animals and man. Cambridge: Cambridge University Press; 1989.
36. Hall KD. Mathematical modelling of energy expenditure during tissue deposition. Br J Nutr. 2010;104(1):4–7. PubMed PMID: 20132585. eng.
37. van der Walt WH, Wyndham CH. An equation for prediction of energy expenditure of walking and running. J Appl Physiol. 1973;34(5):559–63. PubMed PMID: 4703728.
38. Doucet E, Imbeault P, St-Pierre S, Almeras N, Mauriege P, Despres JP, et al. Greater than predicted decrease in energy expenditure during exercise after body weight loss in obese men. Clin Sci (Lond). 2003;105(1):89–95. PubMed PMID: 12617720.
39. Doucet E, St-Pierre S, Almeras N, Despres JP, Bouchard C, Tremblay A. Evidence for the existence of adaptive thermogenesis during weight loss. Br J Nutr. 2001;85(6):715–23. PubMed PMID: 11430776.
40. Leibel RL, Rosenbaum M, Hirsch J. Changes in energy expenditure resulting from altered body weight. N Engl J Med. 1995;332(10):621–8. PubMed PMID: 7632212.
41. Rosenbaum M, Leibel RL. Adaptive thermogenesis in humans. Int J Obes (Lond). 2010;34 Suppl 1:S47–55. PubMed PMID: 20935667. eng.
42. Heilbronn LK, de Jonge L, Frisard MI, DeLany JP, Larson-Meyer DE, Rood J, et al. Effect of 6-month calorie restriction on biomarkers of longevity, metabolic adaptation, and oxidative stress in overweight individuals: a randomized controlled trial. JAMA. 2006;295(13):1539–48. PubMed PMID: 16595757.
43. Rosenbaum M, Hirsch J, Gallagher DA, Leibel RL. Long-term persistence of adaptive thermogenesis in subjects who have maintained a reduced body weight. Am J Clin Nutr. 2008;88(4):906–12. PubMed PMID: 18842775. eng.
44. Weinsier RL, Nagy TR, Hunter GR, Darnell BE, Hensrud DD, Weiss HL. Do adaptive changes in metabolic rate favor weight regain in weight-reduced individuals? An examination of the set-point theory. Am J Clin Nutr. 2000;72(5):1088–94. PubMed PMID: 11063433.
45. Flatt JP. Exaggerated claim about adaptive thermogenesis. Int J Obes (Lond). 2007;31(10):1626; author reply 7–8. PubMed PMID: 17533410. eng.
46. Levine JA, Eberhardt NL, Jensen MD. Role of nonexercise activity thermogenesis in resistance to fat gain in humans. Science. 1999;283(5399):212–4. PubMed PMID: 9880251.
47. Levine JA, Lanningham-Foster LM, McCrady SK, Krizan AC, Olson LR, Kane PH, et al. Interindividual variation in posture allocation: possible role in human obesity. Science. 2005;307(5709):584–6. PubMed PMID: 15681386.
48. Major GC, Doucet E, Trayhurn P, Astrup A, Tremblay A. Clinical significance of adaptive thermogenesis. Int J Obes (Lond). 2007;31(2):204–12. PubMed PMID: 17260010.
49. Lecoultre V, Ravussin E, Redman LM. The fall in leptin concentration is a major determinant of the metabolic adaptation induced by caloric restriction independently of the changes in leptin circadian rhythms. J Clin Endocrinol Metab. 2011;96(9):E1512–6. PubMed PMID: 21778216. eng.
50. Redman LM, Heilbronn LK, Martin CK, de Jonge L, Williamson DA, Delany JP, et al. Metabolic and behavioral compensations in response to caloric restriction: implications for the maintenance of weight loss. One. 2009;4(2):e4377. PubMed PMID: 19198647. eng.
51. Hall KD, Guo J, Dore M, Chow CC. The progressive increase of food waste in America and its environmental impact. PLoS One. 2009;4(11):e7940. PubMed PMID: 19946359. eng.
52. Rosenbaum M, Goldsmith R, Bloomfield D, Magnano A, Weimer L, Heymsfield S, et al. Low-dose leptin reverses skeletal muscle, autonomic, and neuroendocrine adaptations to maintenance of reduced weight. J Clin Invest. 2005;115(12):3579–86. PubMed PMID: 16322796.
53. Rosenbaum M, Murphy EM, Heymsfield SB, Matthews DE, Leibel RL. Low dose leptin administration reverses effects of sustained weight-reduction on energy expenditure and circulating concentrations of thyroid hormones. J Clin Endocrinol Metab. 2002;87(5):2391–4. PubMed PMID: 11994393. eng.

54. Rosenbaum M, Nicolson M, Hirsch J, Murphy E, Chu F, Leibel RL. Effects of weight change on plasma leptin concentrations and energy expenditure. J Clin Endocrinol Metab. 1997;82(11):3647–54. PubMed PMID: 9360521.
55. Weinsier RL, Hunter GR, Zuckerman PA, Redden DT, Darnell BE, Larson DE, et al. Energy expenditure and free-living physical activity in black and white women: comparison before and after weight loss. Am J Clin Nutr. 2000;71(5):1138–46. PubMed PMID: 10799376.
56. Winkler JT. The fundamental flaw in obesity research. Obes Rev. 2005;6(3):199–202. PubMed PMID: 16045634. eng.
57. Schoeller DA. How accurate is self-reported dietary energy intake? Nutr Rev. 1990;48(10):373–9. PubMed PMID: 2082216. eng.
58. Schoeller DA, Thomas D, Archer E, Heymsfield SB, Blair SN, Goran MI, et al. Self-report-based estimates of energy intake offer an inadequate basis for scientific conclusions. Am J Clin Nutr. 2013;97(6):1413–5. PubMed PMID: 23689494.
59. Racette SB, Das SK, Bhapkar M, Hadley EC, Roberts SB, Ravussin E, et al. Approaches for quantifying energy intake and %calorie restriction during calorie restriction interventions in humans: the multicenter CALERIE study. Am J Physiol Endocrinol Metab. 2012;302(4):E441–8. PubMed PMID: 22127229. eng.
60. Jordan PN, Hall KD. Dynamic coordination of macronutrient balance during infant growth: insights from a mathematical model. Am J Clin Nutr. 2008;87(3):692–703. PubMed PMID: 18326609. eng.
61. Butte NF, Hopkinson JM, Wong WW, Smith EO, Ellis KJ. Body composition during the first 2 years of life: an updated reference. Pediatr Res. 2000;47(5):578–85. PubMed PMID: 10813580. eng.
62. Butte NF, Wong WW, Hopkinson JM, Heinz CJ, Mehta NR, Smith EO. Energy requirements derived from total energy expenditure and energy deposition during the first 2 y of life. Am J Clin Nutr. 2000;72(6):1558–69. PubMed PMID: 11101486. eng.
63. Hall KD, Chow CC. Estimating changes in free-living energy intake and its confidence interval. Am J Clin Nutr. 2011;94(1):66–74. PubMed PMID: 21562087. eng.
64. Franz MJ, VanWormer JJ, Crain AL, Boucher JL, Histon T, Caplan W, et al. Weight-loss outcomes: a systematic review and meta-analysis of weight-loss clinical trials with a minimum 1-year follow-up. J Am Diet Assoc. 2007;107(10):1755–67. PubMed PMID: 17904936. eng.
65. Heymsfield SB, Harp JB, Reitman ML, Beetsch JW, Schoeller DA, Erondu N, et al. Why do obese patients not lose more weight when treated with low-calorie diets? A mechanistic perspective. Am J Clin Nutr. 2007;85(2):346–54. PubMed PMID: 17284728.
66. Franz MJ. The dilemma of weight loss in diabetes. Diabetes Spectr. 2007;20(3):133–6.
67. Guo J, Hall KD. Challenges of indirect calorimetry in mice. Am J Physiol Regul Integr Comp Physiol. 2011;300(3):R780; author reply R1-2. PubMed PMID: 21378217. eng.
68. Longo KA, Charoenthongtrakul S, Giuliana DJ, Govek EK, McDonagh T, Distefano PS, et al. The 24-hour respiratory quotient predicts energy intake and changes in body mass. Am J Physiol Regul Integr Comp Physiol. 2010;298(3):R747–54. PubMed PMID: 20018821. eng.
69. Guo J, Hall KD. Estimating the continuous-time dynamics of energy and fat metabolism in mice. PLoS Comput Biol. 2009;5(9):e1000511. PubMed PMID: 19763167. eng.
70. Guo J, Hall KD. Predicting changes of body weight, body fat, energy expenditure and metabolic fuel selection in C57BL/6 mice. PLoS One. 2011;6(1):e15961. PubMed PMID: 21246038. eng.
71. Guo J, Jou W, Gavrilova O, Hall KD. Persistent diet-induced obesity in male C57BL/6 mice resulting from temporary obesigenic diets. PLoS One. 2009;4(4):e5370. PubMed PMID: 19401758. eng.
72. Kaiyala KJ, Morton GJ, Leroux BG, Ogimoto K, Wisse B, Schwartz MW. Identification of body fat mass as a major determinant of metabolic rate in mice. Diabetes. 2010;59(7):1657–66. PubMed PMID: 20413511. eng.
73. Gennemark P, Jansson-Lofmark R, Hyberg G, Wigstrand M, Kakol-Palm D, Hakansson P, et al. A modeling approach for compounds affecting body composition. J Pharmacokinet Pharmacodyn. 2013;40(6):651–67. PubMed PMID: 24158456.
74. Church TS, Thomas DM, Tudor-Locke C, Katzmarzyk PT, Earnest CP, Rodarte RQ, et al. Trends over 5 decades in U.S. occupation-related physical activity and their associations with obesity. PLoS One. 2011;6(5):e19657. PubMed PMID: 21647427. eng.
75. Hall KD. Modeling metabolic adaptations and energy regulation in humans. Annu Rev Nutr. 2012;32:35–54.
76. Lin BH, Smith TA, Lee JY, Hall KD. Measuring weight outcomes for obesity intervention strategies: the case of a sugar-sweetened beverage tax. Econ Hum Biol. 2011;9(4):329–41. PubMed PMID: 21940223. eng.
77. Smith TA, Bing-Hwan L, Jong-Ying L. Taxing caloric sweetened beverages: potential effects on beverage consumption, calorie intake, and obesity. Washington D.C.: Economic Research Service, United States Department of Agriculture; 2010. Report No.: 100 Contract No.: ERR-100.
78. Duyff RL. American Dietetic Association complete food and nutrition guide. 3rd ed. Hoboken: Wiley; 2006.
79. NHLBI. Aim for a healthy weight. National Institutes of Health, National Heart, Lung and Blood Institute, 2005 Aug 2005. Report no.: 05-5213 contract no.: 05-5213.

80. NHLBI Obesity Education Initiative Expert Panel on the Identification E, and Treatment of Overweight and Obesity in Adults. The practical guide: identification, evaluation, and treatment of overweight and obesity in adults. National Heart, Lung, and Blood Institute, 2000 Contract no.: NIH publication number 00-4084.
81. NHS. Your weight your health: how to take control of your weight. London: National Health Service, Department of Health, 2006 Apr 2006. Report no.: 274537 Contract no.: 274537.
82. Brady I, Hall KD. Dispatch from the field: is mathematical modeling applicable to obesity treatment in the real world? Obesity. 2014;22(9):1939–41. PubMed PMID: 24895253.
83. Bray GA. Medications for weight reduction. Endocrinol Metab Clin North Am. 2008;37(4):923–42. PubMed PMID: 19026940.
84. Göbel B, Sanghvi A, Hall KD. Quantifying energy intake changes during obesity pharmacotherapy. Obesity (in press). 2014. PubMed PMID: 24961931.
85. Guidance for Industry Developing Products for Weight Management. U.S. Department of Health and Human Services, Food and Drug Administration, Center for Drug Evaluation and Research, 2007.
86. Harms M, Seale P. Brown and beige fat: development, function and therapeutic potential. Nat Med. 2013;19(10):1252–63. PubMed PMID: 24100998.
87. Hall KD, Butte NF, Swinburn BA, Chow CC. Dynamics of childhood growth and obesity: development and validation of a quantitative mathematical model. Lancet Diabetes Endocrinol. 2013;1:97–105.
88. Huxley J. Problems of relative growth. London: Methuen & Co. Ltd.; 1932. p. 276.
89. Pollard TD. The future of biomedical research: from the inventory of genes to understanding physiology and the molecular basis of disease. JAMA. 2002;287(13):1725–7. PubMed PMID: 11926899. eng.
90. Hall KD, Hallgreen CE. Increasing weight loss attenuates the preferential loss of visceral compared with subcutaneous fat: a predicted result of an allometric mode. Int J Obes (Lond). 2008;32(4):722. PubMed PMID: 18301391. eng.
91. Hallgreen CE, Hall KD. Allometric relationship between changes of visceral fat and total fat mass. Int J Obes (Lond). 2008;32(5):845–52. PubMed PMID: 18087265. eng.

Regulatory Considerations for Early Clinical Development of Drugs for Diabetes, Obesity, and Cardiometabolic Disorders

12

G. Alexander Fleming

Abstract

Advancing therapeutic discoveries through early clinical studies benefits from a working knowledge of regulatory history, practices, provisions, procedures, and controversies. This chapter aims to supplement readily available published and web-based resources that describe regulatory expectations and requirements. Though the Food and Drug Administration is emphasized, the importance of the European Medicines Agency (EMA) and other major authorities is acknowledged. Some relevant differences between EMA and the Food and Drug Administration (FDA) are discussed. With emphasis on early studies, selected regulatory considerations are presented for developing diabetes, anti-obesity, and lipid-lowering therapies toward existing therapeutic indications. Novel therapeutic indications that have reasonable prospects for approval are also described. Interpretations and preferences expressed reflect the author's experience as an endocrinologist and an FDA representative, educator, and reviewer responsible for approval of the first statin and insulin analog, metformin, and other metabolic products.

Keywords

European Medicines Agency (EMA) • Food and Drug Administration (FDA) • Good Clinical Practice (GCP) • International Conference on Harmonisation of Technical Requirements for Registration of Pharmaceuticals for Human Use (ICH) • Investigational New Drug (IND) • Institutional Review Boards (IRB) • Medical Dictionary for Regulatory Activities (MedDRA) • New Drug Application (NDA) • Orphan drug • Study design

G.A. Fleming, BS, MD
Kinexum Services LLC, Harpers Ferry, WV, USA
e-mail: zanfleming@kinexum.com

Introduction

Therapeutic development is appropriately among the most intensively regulated enterprises of any kind. A general knowledge of regulatory requirements and expectations is important for clinical investigators, scientists, and other professionals involved in early clinical research. Involving highly interdependent scientific disciplines, modern therapeutic regulation is at its heart a body of scientifically derived practices and methodologies defined and established by policies, regulations, and laws. Therapeutic regulation is therefore neither entirely prescriptive nor intuitive. It has a vocabulary and jargon unto itself, which must be learned and practiced as any other foreign language, to enable effective communication and operations.

The intent of this chapter is to equip those interested in the transition from therapeutic discovery and earlier phases of metabolic therapeutic development with sufficient knowledge of the subject for their participation in regulated research. Necessarily, the chapter's scope is limited, starting with a focus on the area of diabetic and cardiometabolic therapies—though much of the information provided applies to other therapeutic areas. On the other hand, this chapter will nominally cover the spectrum of therapeutic products aimed at the treatment of diabetes, prevention of diabetic complications, and reduction of cardiovascular risk. This includes conventional drugs (small molecules), smaller peptide products like insulin, and large, complex molecules like monoclonal antibodies.

As a regrettable compromise with pragmatism, this chapter will emphasize the US Food and Drug Administration (FDA) and only passingly cover the other major regulatory authorities. The European Medicines Agency (EMA) and other regional and national authorities have become peers of FDA in almost every respect. Early clinical development work is just as often conducted outside of the USA, and so even for US-based researchers, a familiarity with the major differences in global regulatory approaches is important.

Background

History

The history of drug regulation in the USA is interesting, sometimes quirky, and often marked by tragedy. The original Pure Food and Drug Act passed by Congress in 1906, the Federal Food, Drug, and Cosmetic (FDC) Act of 1938 (which required that new drugs be demonstrated to be safe before marketing), and other major FDA-related legislations were generally in response to disasters in which deaths resulted from toxic products sold as drugs. This provenance explains FDA's identity as the oldest comprehensive consumer protection agency in the USA, if not the world.

FDA's origin as a therapeutic regulatory agency can be traced back to the appointment in 1848 of Lewis Caleb Beck in the Patent Office to perform chemical analyses of agricultural products. This responsibility was transferred to the Department of Agriculture in 1862. Harvey Washington Wiley, Chief Chemist of the Bureau of Chemistry in the Department of Agriculture, was the driving force behind the 1906 Pure Food and Drugs Act. It was not until 1930 that the name of the Food, Drug, and Insecticide Administration was shortened to the Food and Drug Administration under an agricultural appropriations act. FDA was also then transferred from the US Department of Agriculture (USDA) to the Federal Security Agency, which later became the Department of Health, Education, and Welfare (HEW), and is today the Department of Health and Human Services. Nonetheless, to this day, FDA's budget is appropriated in Congress under the Agriculture Bill. Viewing FDA as a consumer protection agency is relevant and important today as a means of understanding its regulatory perspective in overseeing clinical investigation. Unlike the USDA, which traditionally has been more of a farm and industry advocate, FDA sees that its first responsibility is to protect the patient and the consumer.

It is appropriate to mention that the Insulin Amendment to the FD&C Act in 1941 required FDA to test and certify purity and potency of this newly discovered peptide drug product. Regulation of insulin products has continued under the Public Health Service Act of 1944, which came to cover biologic products—naturally occurring and, more recently, biosynthetic. In 1985, FDA approved human insulin as the first biosynthetically manufactured polypeptide therapeutic product. The FDA website contains a more detailed and fascinating historical record of FDA [1].

Other Important Regulatory Authorities

National therapeutic authorities in Europe and Japan evolved over the past century or longer according to models that differ from FDA [2]. In general, these authorities have relied on academic experts and other consultants to make recommendations to relatively small bureaus within the health ministry. As a result of the European Common Market movement and the formation of the European Union (EU), a centralized medicines regulatory authority was founded in 1995 as the European Agency for the Evaluation of Medicinal Products. Now called the European Medicines Agency (EMA), this organization was established with funding from the EU and the pharmaceutical industry. The EMA was established to harmonize, but not replace, existing national medicine regulatory bodies. To this day, the national authorities continue to operate both independently and as parties within the EMA. Medicinal products can be licensed through the individual national authorities or a centralized procedure that provides European-wide authorization. Other regions have come together to similarly harmonize regulatory requirements for their member states, i.e., the Gulf Co-Operative Countries (GCC) and the Association of South East Asian Nations (ASEAN) [3]. Several important differences between the European and US systems are relevant to early clinical investigation and therapeutic development. Early-phase clinical studies in Europe have traditionally been authorized by local review committees, which are similar to institutional review boards (IRB) in the USA. These committees are responsible for ethical review of protocols and clinical study conduct. However, unlike the IRB, the European review committees, for early studies, are vested with the overall legal responsibility of authorizing an experimental therapy to be tested in humans [4].

Another important difference is that, unlike FDA, European authorities do not have public advisory bodies. FDA advisory committees play a substantial role in the therapeutic product approval process [5]. These committees have accelerated some changes in policies at FDA. The most notable and relevant example is FDA's requirement for pre-approval cardiovascular safety trials of new therapies for type 2 diabetes. This requirement was put in place less than a year after an advisory committee was called to review evidence that rosiglitazone treatment was associated with an increased cardiovascular risk [6]. EMA and national authorities in Europe chose to take a case-by-case approach in whether to require prelicensing cardiovascular safety trials [8], and EMA has generally not required them. FDA's firm preapproval requirement of cardiovascular safety studies has had the important benefit of improving knowledge about a drug before it is marketed. However, the requirement has also had an enormous negative impact on the development of drugs for type 2 diabetes due to the resulting large increases in development time, costs, and overall risk of investment in this therapeutic class [7, 8].

Differences between FDA and the EU affect drug development planning and procedures. While FDA has been more conservative on the cardiovascular safety issue, it is more liberal than EU authorities in the encouragement of the participation of women in early clinical studies. Protection of patient confidentiality is a priority at FDA, but this protection is even more intense in the EU.

Global Regulatory Principles and Practices

ICH

One of the most important forces in the globalization of therapeutic development is the emergence of ICH—mercifully short for "The

International Conference on Harmonisation[1] of Technical Requirements for Registration of Pharmaceuticals for Human Use." The drug regulatory harmonization movement began in the EC in the 1980s to facilitate progress toward a single European market for pharmaceuticals [9]. This success encouraged bilateral discussions between the governments of Europe, Japan, and the USA on pursuing an international process. Representatives of the regulatory agencies and industry associations of Europe, Japan, and the USA formed ICH in 1990. Soon after, Canada, Switzerland, and other national representatives were added.

The major contribution of ICH has been a large body of guidelines that have become law in Europe and Japan and adopted as guidances at FDA[2]. This body of guidelines/guidances is called the Tripartite ICH Guidelines on Safety, Quality and Efficacy. Safety refers to nonclinical guidances that outline the requirements for in vitro and animal testing. Quality refers to manufacturing and analytical guidances that outline the requirements for demonstrating identity, level of purity, stability, and other properties of products to be used for clinical trials. Efficacy refers to clinical guidances that provide the standards and procedures by which the products will be evaluated for intended use, including the many guidances that are more related to clinical safety than efficacy. Draft and final versions of the 50+ guidances can be found on FDA, EMA, PMDA[3], and ICH websites. These ICH guidances are convenient references that summarize in readable form much of what is required or expected by FDA and other national authorities. These guidances do not replace the much larger body of FDA laws and regulations that have accumulated over many decades and are dispersed across many different documents. The FDA-adapted ICH guidances are consistent with these regulations and laws, but the latter apply when the ICH guidances are silent or not explicit on any given issue. The ICH guidances that are particularly important to early development include Good Clinical Practice (E6), Clinical Safety Data Management: Definitions and Standards for Expedited Reporting (E2A), Nonclinical Safety Studies for the Conduct of Human Clinical Trials, and Marketing Authorization for Pharmaceuticals [M3 (R2)].

ICH has contributed two other products important to both early- and later-phase studies: the MedDRA (Medical Dictionary for Regulatory Activities) and the CTD (Common Technical Document), which is discussed in the next section. MedDRA serves as the international standard for coding adverse events for purposes of reporting to all major regulatory authorities, including FDA. MedDRA replaces a number of older systems that are now obsolete.

Common Technical Document (CTD)

The CTD represents an achievement of one of the overarching goals of ICH: to establish a format and content of documents that are accepted by all regulatory authorities as an application for licensing or approval of a therapeutic product. In effect, the CTD format and content are necessary but insufficient to meet FDA's requirements for a New Drug Application (NDA). Figure 12.1 represents the sections of the CTD that are all that are necessary for European and Japanese submissions. The administrative section at the pinnacle of the diagram is not part of the CTD, and each country's regulatory authority has its own requirements for that section. FDA uniquely requires that the raw data from nonclinical and clinical studies also be submitted in the application so that independent statistical analyses can be performed by the agency. The CTD format has become relevant to early-phase research because FDA is now asking and will soon require investigational new drug applications (IND, which will be discussed below) to be submitted in this format. In addition to requiring the CTD format, FDA will soon require that the IND be submitted electronically in what is called eCTD format. ICH

---

[1] Ironically, the title could not be completely harmonized. The British/French spelling continues to be used in the official international title. FDA uses the American spelling.

[2] FDA adopted the ICH reports as guidances to avoid the much longer period of time that would have been required to make these laws or regulations.

[3] Pharmaceuticals and Medical Devices Agency of Japan

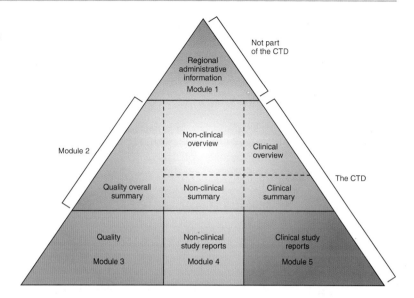

Fig. 12.1 The major components of the Common Technical Document (*CTD*)

has also supported electronic submissions by providing the guidance eCTD: Electronic Common Technical Document Specification (M2).

Recent History in the FDA Review Divisions

More recent history of the FDA reviews involved in cardiometabolic therapeutic regulation is relevant to early-phase investigation. This starts with understanding some evolutionary differences between what are now called the Division of Metabolism and Endocrinology Products (DMEP) and Division of Cardiovascular and Renal Products (DCaRP). DMEP maintains much of its heritage of approving drug products on the basis of reversing classic endocrine deficiency states or reducing abnormal metabolites such as blood glucose and cholesterol levels. DCaRP has always had more of a focus on clinical outcomes, but this was accentuated by its experience with the Cardiac Arrhythmic Suppression Trial (CAST) [10]. In short, a class of drugs for treating ventricular arrhythmias was approved based on reduction of premature ventricular contraction rates, a surrogate endpoint expected to predict clinical benefit. CAST was a post-approval outcome trial that demonstrated a substantial disadvantage of these drugs on survival. Almost all DCaRP approvals have since been based on outcome studies. The exception is approval of antihypertension agents, which continue to be based on reduction of blood pressure. DCaRP approved the first indication for treatment of diabetic nephropathy, the angiotensin-converting enzyme inhibitor (ACEI) captopril, on the basis of doubling of serum creatinine [11]. Compared to a simple treatment effect on creatinine clearance, creatinine doubling has been viewed by the expert community as a quasi-clinical outcome, proximate to end-stage renal failure [12]. Other ACEI and angiotensin receptor blockers (ARBs) have since been approved for this indication, and the indication has been extended to include patients with type 2 diabetes. The only other diabetic complication indication approvals have been for diabetic macular edema [13] despite over two decades of major effort to develop aldose reductase inhibitors for diabetic peripheral neuropathy and other diabetic complications [14].

DMEP continues to approve therapies for diabetes on the basis of glycemic control as reflected by haemoglobin A_{1c} (HbA_{1c}) and low-density lipoprotein (LDL) cholesterol-lowering agents on the basis of LDL cholesterol reduction [15, 16]. However, because of the controversy surrounding the increase of cardiovascular risks related to the thiazolidinedione agent rosiglitazone

(Avandia™) [17], DMEP has required data from cardiovascular outcome trials to rule out a defined level of risk for increasing major adverse cardiovascular events (MACE) before approval of drugs for type 2 diabetes [18]. In addition to accepting LDL-C reduction as the regulatory efficacy endpoint for cholesterol-lowering drugs, DMEP continues to accept reduction of very high levels (>500 mg/dL; >5.56 mmol/L) of triglyceride as a regulatory endpoint for reduction of high triglyceride levels (and specifically not for reduction of cardiovascular risk) [19]. However, all other non-LDL lipid-lowering indications aimed at cardiovascular risk reduction, including triglyceride-lowering agents, require outcome trials [20]. Even some doubt has been raised about LDL cholesterol as continuing to be a suitable regulatory endpoint [21].

Though these more recent issues pertain to late-stage and post-approval therapies, this understanding is relevant to early-stage investigation for several reasons. DMEP is busy, stressed, and perhaps more risk averse, which can have an impact on early IND review. Regulatory endpoints for assessment of efficacy in the metabolic space, such as HbA_{1c} and LDL cholesterol, are also increasingly debated. Even at the earliest phases of clinical investigation, sponsors are being pressured to show evidence of both safety and efficacy that is superior to currently marketed products [22]. Early-phase investigators benefit from understanding these dynamics since difficult benefit/risk judgments that must be made at the approval stage have an impact even on DMEP's review of initial in-human studies.

How Therapeutic Products Are Regulated at FDA

FDA is a vast organization with regulatory responsibility for more than $1 trillion worth of consumer goods, roughly a quarter of consumer expenditures in the USA. This includes $466 billion in food sales, $275 billion in drugs, $60 billion in cosmetics, and $18 billion in dietary supplements [23]. Unlike any other therapeutic regulatory authority in the world, FDA has an enormous staff of experts and specialists. Most of its work is done without the help of outside experts. FDA's budget in 2012 totaled $4.36 billion [24] and is expected to be about $4.7 billion in 2014 [25]. FDA is comprised of designated Centers with responsibility for regulating each of the major health product areas—drugs, biologics, and devices—as well as dietary supplements and food/nutrition.

Therapeutic Product Jurisdiction

The Center for Drug Evaluation and Research (CDER) is most likely to regulate the early clinical research of most readers, but the Center for Biologics Evaluation and Research (CBER), the Center for Food Safety and Nutrition (CFSAN), and the Center for Devices and Radiologic Health (CDRH) could also be involved. A product application will be assigned to the appropriate Center for review, but may be reviewed in some circumstances by more than one Center. For example, a dermal patch that delivers insulin would be reviewed by both CDER and CDRH. Some products may be more difficult to assign. For example, a gel that swells in the stomach to result in weight loss could be considered a medical device instead of a drug, but a nonabsorbed resin that binds cholesterol and bile acids would be considered a drug. Dietary supplements, regulated by CFSAN, are by definition used by consumers without physician supervision and can make no disease treatment claims. Supplements are required to have evidence of only safety and good manufacturing quality. Supporting data are not reviewed prior to marketing and may not ever be reviewed. A widely used dietary supplement becomes a drug under CDER review when it is being investigated for a disease treatment or prevention. However, parallel development of a product as a dietary supplement and drug product rarely occurs. Once a supplement is commercially available, there is less likelihood that any further investment will be made in studies for disease treatment or prevention. Typically, a strategic decision is made early in the developmental pathway to follow a supplement route or a drug route, since these routes are very different in both cost and time to market. The exception to this is omega-3 products derived from fish oil. Omega-3 products are available as dietary supplements [labeled as supporting heart, eye and bone health] and approved drug products [for treatment of severe hypertriglyceridemia]. Insulin and other smaller peptide hormones are considered drugs and approved by New Drug Applications (NDA). Monoclonal antibody products are now regulated by CDER, but are approved by Biologics Licensing Applications (BLAs). Some other products—cell and gene therapies and some therapeutic vaccines—are licensed by BLAs, but reviewed by CBER. Combinations of products, including drug-device, drug-drug, and drug-supplement, may be regulated by two or, conceivably, three FDA Centers. For example, a diabetic wound-healing drug that is applied in a synthetic matrix would be jointly reviewed by CDER and CDRH. The same drug in a cellular matrix would be regulated by CDER and CBER.

It is relevant here to mention perhaps the quirkiest regulatory pathway in all of FDA— that of the medical food, which is regulated by CFSAN. This route is often raised as an attractive commercialization approach since it does not involve an IND and premarket review and approval. Medical food products must have a food-like quality that addresses a nutritional deficiency or gastrointestinal condition. Specifically, FDA's definition is "a food which is formulated to be consumed or administered enterally under the supervision of a physician and which is intended for the specific dietary management of a disease or condition for which distinctive nutritional requirements, based on recognized scientific principles, are established by medical evaluation" [26]. These products can be studied without IND review [27], and they can have medical claims for treatment of disease. Ironically, the original law establishing the definition of medical food is the Orphan Drug Act, in part because some of the first medical foods were used for treatment of rare disease and inborn errors of metabolism. Recent modification to the FDA guidance for medical foods has made clear that a medical food is not a drug, nor need it be for an orphan indication. Furthermore, contrary to what has commonly been the case, a medical food label cannot bear an Rx symbol or "by prescription only" statement. Still, the product must be used under supervision of a physician [28]. This regulatory pathway is becoming more scrutinized by FDA as more dietary supplements and nonqualifying food products are sold as prescription products and/or for unaccepted indications.

The IND Review Process

The FD&C Act establishes that if an unapproved drug is used in the USA, it is considered misbranded and the marketer is therefore subject to prosecution. An exception to this requirement must be made for an experimental drug to be studied. FDA calls this an investigative new drug (IND) exemption. In common parlance, IND is used to refer to this exemption. FDA does not approve INDs or IND exemptions—it allows or issues them.

Pre-IND and Other Meetings with FDA

FDA's role in the development of a new drug begins when the drug's sponsor (an academic investigator, a manufacturer, or potential marketer) is preparing to conduct clinical studies in humans. CDER and CBER provide an option for a pre-IND meeting to provide advice in response to questions and preliminary data that the sponsor has compiled. CDRH provides a comparable pre-IDE (Investigation Device Exemption) meeting. Generally, for this meeting, the sponsor will present data to FDA that characterize efficacy and safety in animal models and that are sufficient to justify the anticipated initial exposure in humans. In some cases, the sponsor may have clinical data that have been produced in another country.

A request for a pre-IND meeting follows a standard outline and includes an initial draft of the questions that the sponsor wishes to have answered by FDA. In advance of the meeting, a briefing package of relevant data is submitted for review. If the meeting is granted, the divisions are generally required to provide preliminary written responses to the sponsor prior to the meeting or within about 30 days of submission of the briefing package. If the meeting is not granted, FDA will provided written comments. DMEP is among the busiest CDER review divisions and grants face-to-face pre-IND meetings less often, but does provide detailed written responses to submitted questions. The pre IND meeting as the first interaction between the FDA and the sponsor sets the tone for an ongoing working relationship. Therefore, careful and thoughtful preparation of questions, background material, and proposed product development plan is essential. After receiving final written responses or FDA meeting minutes, the sponsor may engage in some limited written exchanges.

The less well-known "End of Phase 2A (EOP2A)" meeting is now also provided by CDER, but infrequently held [29]. This meeting can be of value for early clinical programs to gain feedback from FDA on clinical pharmacology issues. As described in the FDA guidance,

> The overall purpose of an EOP2A meeting is to discuss options for trial designs, modeling strategies, and clinical trial simulation scenarios to improve the quantification of the exposure-response information from early drug development. The goal of these meetings is to optimize dose selection for subsequent trials to improve the efficiency of drug development. The exposure-response data discussed might be pertinent to evaluation of efficacy outcomes or adverse outcomes. In addition, the meetings would provide opportunities for discussions of complex issues pertaining to drug interactions, trials in special populations defined by genetic characteristics or other biomarkers, and other PK or PK/PD relationships.

In addition to the pre-IND meeting, FDA regulations provide two other formal meetings: the end of phase 2 (EOP2) meeting and the pre-NDA meeting. These are extremely important and valued landmark meetings for drug products in later-stage development, but are only mentioned here. The FDA guidance on formal meetings provides useful information [30].

The specific objectives of the EOP2A meeting are "to help select the dosing regimens for the next phase (typically phases 2 and 3) of drug development and to design informative dose-response trials that will inform later phase clinical trials by best incorporating prior quantitative knowledge."

In cases in which two or more treatment indications are sought by the sponsor, and these come under the purview of different divisions, the sponsor can request separate pre-IND meetings with more than one division. In other cases, representatives from another division can be requested to address a specific issue involving the consulting division's expertise. For example, a meeting involving a diabetes or obesity drug with potential for causing depression could benefit from participation from the Division of Psychiatry Products to discuss early evaluation of mood alteration as a safety issue.

Varieties of INDs

FDA provides two major categories of INDs and several less well-known specialized forms.

1. The investigator IND is submitted by a physician or a qualified nonphysician investigator with the participation of a responsible physician to conduct a clinical trial in humans. The physician conceives, designs, and conducts the investigation and is responsible for directing how the investigational drug is administered or dispensed. The physician sponsor is also ultimately responsible for meeting all IND requirements, including supervision of study personnel, handling and analysis of data, reporting of adverse events, and annual IND reports. These responsibilities may be delegated to others. Investigator-sponsored INDs are typically used to explore the potential of a new molecule or metabolite or to evaluate a hypothesis involving an approved drug for a different indication or new patient population. FDA has traditionally been more flexible in its review and requirements for investigator INDs, but there is no formal difference in requirements for investigator- and commercial-sponsored INDs.

2. A commercial IND is typically sponsored and owned by a company or research organization, though an individual (including, rarely, a physician investigator) could be the sponsor. The intent of the commercial IND is to develop a new molecule for approval or to develop an approved drug for a new indication, formulation, route of administration, patient population, and/or combination with another drug. All of the responsibilities described above and some others pertain to a commercial IND.

3. An emergency use IND involves the authorization of an experimental drug to be used in an emergency situation (life-threatening or severely debilitating disease) that does not

allow time for submission of a conventional IND. This provision is generally reserved for exceptional circumstances in which a very serious condition is involved and approved options have been exhausted.
4. The treatment IND is rarely used, particularly in the metabolic area. FDA provides this option for an experimental drug that shows significant efficacy in late-stage clinical trials. It enables a treatment of serious or immediately life-threatening condition to be used more widely prior to final FDA review and approval. The sponsor may also be allowed to charge for the product under the treatment IND prior to FDA clearance for marketing. This regulatory provision is an option only after pivotal phase 3 clinical trials have been started.
5. The exploratory IND [31] is a relatively recent provision aimed at streamlining the identification of lead molecules for further development. FDA describes in its guidance some additional flexibility and discretion in what is required to conduct a clinical study under an exploratory IND. Such a study is always conducted in phase 1, involves very limited human exposure, and has no therapeutic or diagnostic intent. The exploratory IND may be used to screen a number of related compounds or investigate the pharmacokinetics resulting from a "microdose" exposure. Because very small exposures are involved, FDA may waive or modify some of the nonclinical or product manufacturing requirements.

When an IND Is Not Needed

FDA has issued a guidance about when an IND is not required [32]. An IND is not required under two major circumstances—investigation of a marketed drug and bioequivalence studies of a marketed drug product and a generic version. A clinical study of a marketed drug is exempt from IND requirements if all of the following criteria are met:
- The drug product is lawfully marketed in the USA.
- The investigation is not intended to be reported to FDA as a well-controlled study in support of a new indication, and there is no intent to use it to support any other significant change in the labeling of the drug.
- The investigation is not intended to support a significant change in the advertising for the drug.
- The investigation does not involve a new route of administration, dose, patient population, or other factor that significantly increases the risk (or decreases the acceptability of the risk) associated with the use of the drug product.

When all of these criteria apply, not only is the IND requirement waived, but review divisions are also directed to decline such IND submissions even if the sponsor would like to have an IND.

Dietary supplements intended only to affect the structure or function of the body and not intended for a therapeutic purpose are not considered drugs by FDA. Products that are *not* drugs, such as foods or dietary supplements, do not require an IND. Exceptions include when a health claim is being sought for a food or a therapeutic or diagnostic use is being sought for a dietary supplement. For example, a study designed to evaluate whether vitamin D may reduce the risk of diabetes may require an IND since no health claim for this substance-disease relationship has been issued.

Content of the IND Submission

The required content of INDs is detailed in its rather old (but largely still current) guidance [33]. Additional details and updates are found in specialized guidances that have been more recently issued. One of the most significant recent changes to the IND has been in the format required for submission. As mentioned under the ICH section, the CTD (Common Technical Document) format is now being implemented as the required format for all IND submissions. In summary, the IND must contain information from the following three categories:
1. Nonclinical data, including animal pharmacology, toxicology, and in vitro studies. These are required to support the safety of human subjects in the initial proposed clinical study. In summary, two toxicology studies—one in a rodent and one in a non-rodent species—of

equal or greater duration to the proposed clinical study are required along with specialized animal safety studies. Animal studies that support the mechanism and targeted efficacy are desirable. In vitro studies include hERG, drug metabolism, and mutagenicity testing.
2. Manufacturing and analytical information, including descriptions of the manufacturing process, identity, strength, quality, and purity of the drug substance and drug product, analytical procedures and specification, stability, consistency among batches, and container systems. These requirements are detailed in a number of guidances, but enumerated in the description of Current Good Manufacturing Practice for Finished Pharmaceuticals under 21 CFR Part 211:
    (a) General Provisions
    (b) Organization and Personnel
    (c) Buildings and Facilities
    (d) Equipment
    (e) Control of Components and Drug Product Containers and Closures
    (f) Production and Process Controls
    (g) Packaging and Labeling Controls
    (h) Holding and Distribution
    (i) Laboratory Controls
    (j) Records and Reports
    (k) Returned and Salvaged Drug Products
3. Clinical protocols and investigator information, including one or more complete protocols, investigator brochure, any clinical data that may be available, qualifications of clinical investigators, and commitment to obtain informed consent from the research subjects, commitment to obtain review of the study by an institutional review board (IRB), and adherence to the investigational new drug regulations. The studies designed to be conducted in the following 12 months of the development plan should also be described so that FDA can offer suggestions or concerns that can be used to modify these plans.

IND Review Process

Once the IND is submitted, the sponsor must wait 30 calendar days before initiating the proposed clinical study. During this time, the primary chemistry, nonclinical, and clinical FDA reviewers will determine whether any substantial safety issues are involved. The reviewers usually provide concerns and recommendations, and they may also ask for further information from the sponsor. The primary goal of IND review is to assure that research subjects will not be exposed to unreasonable risk. This determination is based on having sufficient data and information from the three major review areas—nonclinical, CMC (chemistry, manufacturing, and controls), and clinical—aimed first at assessment of safety and second at achievement of other objectives.

If there are significant deficiencies and/or concerns about study participant safety, FDA can place a proposed or ongoing phase 1 clinical trial on full or partial clinical hold or, in extreme cases, even terminate the IND. A partial clinical hold means that a study may go forward or continue, but with some restrictions on the study design and execution. In some cases of IND review, one study may be allowed, while another is placed on clinical hold. A clinical hold is never issued lightly by FDA, and for phase 1 studies is only done for reasons of safety. FDA may place a phase 2 or 3 study on clinical hold for a substantial design or other non-safety issue, in addition to safety concerns. FDA is required to work with the sponsor to resolve the clinical hold on a timely basis. The sponsor can request a meeting if necessary to resolve the concern.

Once the IND review has been completed and the IND [exemption] allowed, the sponsor may submit subsequent protocols. FDA does not have a 30-day wait requirement for subsequent protocols submitted to the IND file, though it is prudent to wait for any FDA feedback on the protocol before beginning a study. Additional clinical studies may require supplementary nonclinical data and completion and analysis of data from a preceding clinical study. Communication from FDA may be very limited during the execution of the early-stage development plan until the EOP2 meeting.

The regulations allow for a stepwise process of accruing and refining CMC information. The amount of information and data needed will increase from phase 1 through phase 3 of the program, depending on the proposed duration of the investigation, the dosage form, and the amount of information otherwise available. For example, although stability data are required in all phases of the IND to demonstrate that the new drug substance and drug product are within acceptable chemical and physical limits for the planned duration of the proposed clinical investigation, if very short-term tests are proposed, the supporting stability data can be correspondingly limited for supporting short-term use and extended in parallel to support longer clinical studies.

Ethical Review

FDA has devolved primary responsibility for ethical review of clinical studies to institutional review boards (IRB). These boards are often chartered within an academic institution or hospital to provide local ethical review, but boards may also be independent and review studies remotely. The responsibilities of IRBs and investigators/sponsors have grown to include financial interest disclosure, verification of adequate research facilities, and others. Details for these responsibilities are found on the FDA website [34].

FDA clinical reviewers take into account ethical considerations as part of the evaluation of submitted studies. It is not required that informed consent documents be submitted to the IND file, but reviewers have the option of requesting the consent document. An ethical concern with a protocol can be a basis for a clinical hold.

Special Regulatory Programs

Early-phase investigators should be aware of special regulatory provisions and their potential relevance to studies that are done in phases 1 and 2.

Orphan Drug Program

The Orphan Drug Program at FDA has catalyzed the development and commercialization of high market value metabolic products including growth hormone and β-glucocerebrosidase (Cerezyme®), which is among the most expensive drug products now on the market [35]. The Orphan Drug Program was designed to encourage development of therapies aimed at small patient populations, which were originally neglected by the pharmaceutical community, but many orphan drugs have developed high market values after achieving FDA approval with relatively fewer clinical studies [36]. Market values for smaller Abundant information about the Orphan Drug Program is available on the FDA website [37–39]. When an orphan indication is targeted, the provisions of the Orphan Drug Act can provide a number of benefits, including grants for clinical investigation. Of relevance to the early investigator is the fact that today's reviewers at FDA's Office of Orphan Products are increasingly looking for more clinical evidence of a drug's promise for treating the orphan condition than has been the case in the past. Before, emphasis was primarily put on insuring that the prevalence of the condition was below 200,000 people in the USA. Results from an early PK/PD study could be decisive in winning an orphan designation [40]. As mentioned above, orphan therapies have been approved in the broader metabolic area. It should be borne in mind that even for common conditions like diabetes, an orphan indication could be developed for a rare form of diabetes that has a well-understood genetic basis, is identifiable, affects fewer than 200,000 people in the USA, and is responsive to the therapy.

Such an example is FDA's February 2014 approval of metreleptin (Myalept™, Bristol-Myers Squibb) as replacement therapy to treat the complications of leptin deficiency in patients with congenital generalized or acquired generalized lipodystrophy [41]. Metreleptin, a synthetic analog of the hormone leptin, had originally been envisioned as a therapy for obesity and type 2 diabetes. The drug's value in improving the metabolic control in patients with the orphan condition of congenital generalized or acquired generalized lipodystrophy was demonstrated in a 3-year study organized by the National Institute of Diabetes and Digestive and Kidney Diseases at the National Institutes of Health. Metreleptin treatment resulted in substantial improvements in both glycemic control and triglyceride levels [42].

Given the orphan indication, FDA's approval was based on a relatively very small clinical development program.

Europe has a comparable orphan disease program, and FDA and EMA have created a common format for applying for orphan status with both agencies [43].

Fast Track and Breakthrough Therapy Programs

FDA has created several programs for speeding the development of drug and biologics therapies. These are explained in more detail on the FDA website [44]. Fast Track status and Breakthrough Therapy Designation are both available to products that show promise for meeting serious unmet clinical need. Generally, some clinical efficacy data are required for consideration. The FDA review divisions vary significantly in their willingness to consider and grant Fast Track status. DMEP has been among the most parsimonious divisions in granting Fast Track status.

Key Regulatory-Related Considerations in the Design and Conduct of Early Metabolic Studies

Therapeutic Indications

When filing for an IND (investigator or commercial sponsored), it is necessary to specify a therapeutic indication. Specifying the indication is even more important for a commercial IND. The stated indication is used for assigning the IND to the appropriate division. For a conventional diabetes or lipid-lowering treatment indication, the review division selection is straightforward. All such indications go to the Division of Metabolism and Endocrinology Products (DMEP). Diabetic complication indications go instead to the division that focuses on the affected organ system. See Table 12.1 for these assignments. The table also provides descriptions of the wording of approved therapeutic indications, the primary efficacy endpoint currently accepted by FDA, and some examples of approved products.

As will be discussed below, the primary efficacy endpoint for regulatory approval is of importance to the earliest studies even if it cannot be measured until later studies. To a large extent, the approved therapies define minimal efficacy targets for newer therapies. Pressure is increasingly added to early studies to provide some efficacy data that will allow an estimate of the relative treatment effect on the regulatory endpoint.

Several novel metabolic indications are under consideration or being pursued, and all involved in the metabolic field should be aware of them (Table 12.2). Numerous attempts have been made at developing therapies for new-onset (within 6 months of diagnosis) type 1 diabetes, and one program is in the second of two phase 3 trials [45] though the data integrity of the first trial has just been called into question [46]. Regulatory and other considerations for early clinical studies are discussed elsewhere [46]. On the other hand, two decades of serious efforts to develop aldose reductase inhibitors for diabetic peripheral neuropathy and microvascular complications have ended. Tantalizing are the prospects for prevention of type 2 diabetes and metabolic syndrome treatment indications. FDA has provided attention in its diabetes drug guidance to these potential indications, including a general sense of what would be required for approval [47]. The growing recognition of nonalcoholic steatohepatitis (NASH) as a major cause of cirrhosis [48] is encouraging some sponsors with agents with efficacy in patients with type 2 diabetes to consider NASH as the lead indication [49–51]. This is largely driven by expectations that the regulatory pathway for a NASH indication could be reduced in time and cost compared to that for a type 2 diabetes indication because preapproval cardiovascular outcome data may not be required.

Important Early Study Considerations

Phase 1 Studies
Glucose-Lowering Products
Phase 1 studies for most oral metabolic therapies typically involve the classic rising single- and multiple-dose safety study design with blood

12 Regulatory Considerations for Early Clinical Development of Drugs

Table 12.1 Approved therapeutic indications and regulatory endpoints for metabolic diseases

Indication	Phrasing	Primary efficacy endpoint	Approved therapies	FDA review division
Type 2 diabetes treatment	Improve glycemic control in patients with type 2 diabetes	HbA_{1c}	Many oral and injected products	DMEP
Insulin products for type 1 and type 2 diabetes	Treatment of patients with diabetes mellitus for the control of hyperglycaemia	HbA_{1c}	Many injected products Inhaled insulin	DMEP
Weight loss	Chronic weight management in adults with an initial BMI of 30 kg/m² without and 27 kg/m² with the presence of at least one weight-related comorbidity	Body weight—continuous and categorical variables	Qsymia® (phentermine/topiramate) Belviq® (lorcaserin HCl) Contrave® (bupropion/naltrexone) Orlistat (Alli®) phentermine	DMEP
Lipid lowering—LDL cholesterol	To reduce elevated total-C, LDL-C, apo B, and TG levels and to increase HDL-C in patients with primary hypercholesterolemia	Serum LDL cholesterol levels	Many statins Ezetimibe Nicotinic acid Fenoglide® (fenofibrate)	DMEP
Lipid lowering—triglycerides	To reduce triglyceride (TG) levels in adult patients with severe (≥500 mg/dL) hypertriglyceridemia	Serum triglyceride levels	Lovaza® (DHA and EPA esters) Vascepa® (EPA ester) Epanova® (omega-3-carboxylic acids) Fenoglide® (fenofibrate)	DMEP
Nephropathy	Treatment of diabetic nephropathy with an elevated serum creatinine and proteinuria (urinary albumin to creatinine ratio ≥300 mg/g) in patients with type 2 diabetes	Reduction in creatinine doubling time	Many ACEI and ARBs	CaRD
Retinopathy	Treatment of diabetic macular edema	Chart reading visual function	Lucentis® (ranibizumab injection)	DTOP
Diabetic wound healing	Treatment of lower-extremity diabetic neuropathic ulcers that extend into the subcutaneous tissue. Bring up 'Diabetic gastroparesis' from table 2 and add as last rows in table 1. The approved therapy is: Reglan® (metoclopramide hydrochloride)	Complete wound closure	Regranex® (becaplermin)	DDDP

Abbreviations: *ACEI* angiotensin-converting enzyme inhibitor, *ARB* angiotensin receptor blocker, *DMEP* Division of Metabolism and Endocrinology Products, *DcaRP* Division of Cardiovascular and Renal Products, *DNP* Division of Neurology Products, *DTOP* Division of Transplant and Ophthalmology Products, *DGIE* Division of Gastroenterology and Inborn Errors Products, *DDDP* Division of Dermatology and Dental Products

sampling for pharmacokinetics as the important secondary objective. Phase 1 studies of insulin products require a means of preventing or controlling hypoglycemia, such as a glucose clamp procedure [47]. Phase 1 studies of insulin products may be undertaken in patients with type 1 or type 2 diabetes and/or healthy volunteers. Patients with type 1 diabetes provide the most straightforward way of eliminating endogenous insulin secretion as a confounder, but normal subjects are often used. The starting dose and dose range are largely dependent on the results of animal disease model and toxicology studies. Testing some immunotherapies with more substantial risks may not be appropriate in normal subjects.

Table 12.2 Potential therapeutic indications and regulatory endpoints for metabolic diseases

Indication	Phrasing	Speculated efficacy endpoint	Review division
Cardiovascular risk reduction in patient with diabetes	Decrease the rate of a combined endpoint of CV death, MI, or stroke	Major adverse cardiac events (MACE)	DCaRD or DMEP
New-onset type 1 diabetes	Preserve endogenous insulin secretion in newly diagnosed patients with type 1 diabetes	C peptide	DMEP
Prevention of type 1 diabetes	Decrease the rate of type 1 diabetes onset	Time to incident diagnosis of type 1 diabetes	DMEP
Prevention of type 2 diabetes	Decrease the rate of type 2 diabetes onset and reduce the rate of a combined endpoint of CV death, MI, or stroke	Co-primaries: (1) Time to onset of type 2 diabetes (2) MACE	DMEP
Metabolic syndrome	Improve the clinical components of metabolic syndrome and reduce the rate of a combined endpoint of CV death, MI, or stroke	Co-primaries: (1) Composite of MS components (2) MACE	DMEP
Nonalcoholic steatohepatitis (NASH)	Reduce the rate of fatty liver progression to hepatic fibrosis	Fibrosis and cirrhosis in biopsied liver specimens	DGIE
Cachexia/sarcopenia	Increase or preserve physical function and muscle mass	Composite or co-primaries lead by physical function and lean body mass	DMEP
Diabetic peripheral neuropathy	To improve signs, symptoms, and dysfunction of diabetic peripheral neuropathy	Composite of nerve conduction velocity and functional endpoints	DNP
Diabetic cardiac autonomic neuropathy	Reduce the rate of cardiac-related death	Composite of cardiac-associated death and loss of consciousness	DCaRD
Diabetic gastroparesis	Treatment of the symptoms of diabetic gastroparesis	Rate of vomiting and other symptoms	DGIE

Abbreviations: *DMEP* Division of Metabolism and Endocrinology Products, *DNP* Division of Neurology Products, *DGIE* Division of Gastroenterology and Inborn Errors Products

The FDA guidance implies a preference for using healthy normal subjects for initial phase 1 studies aimed at characterizing pharmacokinetic parameters of non-insulin therapeutics, and that pharmacokinetic studies also may "be appropriate in the intended patient population." It can be argued that PK assessment in normal subjects can be skipped and that the first in-human study can be done in patients. Normal subjects may provide somewhat less variability in drug handling than uncomplicated diabetic patients, but it is unlikely that presence of disease per se can significantly affect variability of drug levels, PK results, or safety assessment. FDA has allowed initial in-human studies to be done in patients, though I have seen DMEP reviewers discourage this in some cases. The rising multiple-dose study does provide an opportunity to measure glucodynamic responses. It is therefore reasonable to use patients in favor of normal subjects in this early study to provide a preliminary dose-response with respect to glucose-lowering activity. These data can help to select the dose range of the next study and in some cases provide an early estimate of glucose-lowering efficacy.

Food effects on pharmacokinetics of oral products should be evaluated early—perhaps as soon as the first in-human study. Single-dose administration of the new drug can readily be done under fed and fasting conditions. This early preliminary assessment and a more formal food effect study can be deferred if nonclinical studies have shown evidence of moderately high bioavailability under fasting conditions. A fasted dog study would generally be adequate, but rodent studies with chow-administered drug do not provide such assurance. Often the phase 1 program will not have the benefit of an optimized formulation. Ideally, the formal food effect study would be done with a reasonably advanced formulation. Other specialized clinical studies will be required at some point in phase 2, including drug-drug interactions, "thorough QT," and renal and hepatic impairment studies, but these are not generally performed without cause in phase 1.

Phase 1 studies of injected insulin products represent a special case (see Chap. 1). To avoid methodological and interpretational problems posed by endogenous insulin secretion in both normal subjects and patients with type 2 diabetes and insulin resistance in patients with type 2 diabetes, these studies are frequently done in subjects with type 1 diabetes, but certainly can be done in normal subjects with correction for endogenous insulin secretion. Glucose clamping reduces variability of the pharmacodynamic measures. Given the expense of these procedures and the crucial data that they provide, using patients with type 1 diabetes is sensible. Distinctions should be made between injected and alternately delivered insulin products. In most cases, oral, pulmonary, topical, and other delivery approaches have been conceived as an add-on therapy for patients with type 2 diabetes. Except for having to manage the hypoglycemic effects, these products can be approached similarly to standard oral product delivery. A carefully designed phase 1 study can serve to evaluate the possible advantages of this approach beyond time-action profile and convenience.

Weight-Loss (Anti-Obesity) Products

Phase 1 studies of weight-loss products entail generally straightforward single- and multiple-rising-dose studies. Unlike the case for glucose-lowering therapies, direct readouts on weight reduction are not feasible until phase 2. The shortest treatment duration to provide a reliable treatment effect on body weight reduction is about 8 weeks—in part to accommodate the menstrual-cycle-related variability of weight in women. Other approaches are realistic for a phase 1b/2 study to measure treatment effects on food intake, food preference, activity level, and respiratory quotient [52, 53].

Lipid-Lowering Drugs

Lipid-lowering studies are the easiest phase 1 studies to execute because of the large population of otherwise healthy people with lipid abnormalities. As discussed below, measurement of the regulatory endpoint—LDL cholesterol or triglycerides—is feasible in the first multiple-dose study. LDL cholesterol levels are generally stable and not substantially affected by meals or time of day. A small phase 1b study with adequate duration in hypercholesterolemic patients could therefore potentially provide reliable efficacy readouts. In contrast, triglycerides are much more variable from hour to hour and substantially affected by meals. Much more attention must therefore be given to dietary stabilization and timing of samplings of triglyceride measurements than is the case for LDL cholesterol. In addition, FDA has recommended that several baseline values be obtained to compensate for this greater variability.

Efficacy Endpoints

As discussed, there is a spectrum of feasibilities for measuring the regulatory primary and secondary endpoints for the respective metabolic indications in early-phase studies. Advice about the regulatory endpoints for weight-loss drugs is found at the FDA website [54]. Efficacy endpoints for lipid-lowering agents are undergoing rethinking among regulators and experts [22]. A few points about regulatory endpoints for diabetes drugs are worth mentioning here. It is well known that HbA_{1c} is currently accepted as the primary regulatory endpoint for assessment of all glucose-lowering therapies [47], though FDA has referred to this measure as a "surrogate measure." Superiority and/or non-inferiority HbA_{1c} treatment effect comparisons are ultimately required of any glucose-lowering therapy in registration trials. Approval of most therapies for type 2 diabetes primarily involves demonstrating an added glucose-lowering benefit compared to placebo. However, non-inferiority comparisons to an approved therapy are often needed and are frequently performed in early phase 2 studies. Because the HbA_{1c} effect is not reliably measured in early phase 2 studies, continuous glucose monitoring (CGM) has increased the ability to project changes in HbA_{1c}. CGM provides many more data points over a short period of time compared to the traditional multiple daily glucose measurements.

Therapies aimed at improving postprandial hyperglycaemia are disadvantaged by the ongoing debate regarding the clinical value or benefit to patients of this specific glucose-lowering effect [55], as well as by the fact that FDA continues to emphasize that postprandial glycemic control is not accepted as a primary efficacy endpoint. Therapies that primarily affect postprandial glycemic control are limited in the HbA_{1c}-lowering effect that they can provide since postprandial glycaemia contributes only about one-third to the HbA_{1c} effect [56, 57]. Nonetheless, evaluation of postprandial glycaemia with standardized meal tests is an important secondary endpoint and provides an early clinically meaningful evaluation of a glucose-lowering therapy.

Measurement of the regulatory endpoint—LDL cholesterol or triglycerides—can easily be done in the first multiple-dose study. Increasing attention is being given in both early and late studies to the characterization of lipoprotein fractions and other biomarkers [58]. These supportive data are considered secondary endpoints and are of interest to regulatory reviewers, but do not currently play a major role in regulatory benefit/risk estimates. As previously mentioned, greater attention has to be paid to the conditions and design approaches for triglyceride-lowering therapies.

Subject Population

The issue of using normal vs. diabetic subjects in phase 1 studies has been discussed above and is considered further in Chap. 9. Other important study population considerations include level of glycemic control and the use of treatment-naïve or untreated patients with type 2 diabetes vs. washing off or continuing background glucose-lowering therapy. These are actually more thorny issues for later-stage studies, but do impact early multiple-dose studies in which glucose efficacy is assessed. The ideal subject for these earlier studies is the treatment-naïve patient with inadequate (but not poor) glycemic control. However, treatment-naïve patients are difficult to find; therefore, a frequent compromise is to find patients who have not recently been on a glucose-lowering treatment or to actually withdraw the current treatment (typically metformin and often one other drug). Medication withdrawal has its own ethical and methodological disadvantages, including having to reestablish a metabolic baseline and greater risks of screen failures and dropouts due to patients exceeding maximum permitted fasting and random blood glucose levels (see the FDA diabetes guidance for these details). In phase 1b and 2 studies in which demonstration of an impressive glucose-lowering effect is sought, the temptation is to admit patients with very poor glycemic control to allow for a potentially greater absolute treatment effect. The danger of using poorly controlled patients is that they may prove to be less responsive and/or less reliable subjects in adherence to the study protocol. If their poor control involves glucose toxicity and/or substantial β-cell failure, their responsiveness to the investigative therapy may be reduced. Perhaps the largest threat is that such patients are likely to experience a strong study effect, which is the drug-independent improvement in glycemic control that results from participating in a more intensively encouraged and monitored environment (the Hawthorne effect [71]). I have seen a number of cases in which a strong study effect undermines the treatment effect and has jeopardized the entire development program. Thus, a balance should be struck in selecting patients on the basis of glycemic control.

Number of Subjects

Adequate statistical powering for efficacy endpoints is important for almost all later-phase studies, but phase 1 studies are usually not sized on the basis of formal statistical considerations. As efficacy evaluation becomes the focus, formal statistical powering based on the primary endpoint is expected. While not a direct concern of the early investigator, diabetes drug development programs now require on the order of 3,000 exposed patients for NDA approval, which is substantially greater than expected of other chronically administered drugs [59]. This number can easily double when a cardiovascular safety trial is required.

Study Designs

Usually, initial in-human studies of oral new molecular entities will involve stepwise, rising-dose designs. For safety reasons, each dose group is usually completed before the next higher dose is started. FDA in rare cases will ask that safety lab data from the first two or more dose groups be evaluated before going on to the higher doses. Some degree of delaying or staggering the start of successively higher-dose groups is typically used in phase 1 and 1b studies.

A crossover design is sometimes used in phase 1 studies, but more typically these are used in phase 2 when an active comparator and/or multiple treatment permutations are involved. Crossover designs are generally not appropriate for early multiple-dose safety studies since some subjects would be exposed to the high dose initially. However, a crossover design has the advantage of reducing imbalances in potentially confounding covariates since each patient serves as his/her own control. Crossover designs have some statistical power advantages over parallel designs. The disadvantages to the crossover design include the "order" effect, in which the treatment order may affect efficacy response, or bias in adverse event reporting. The "carryover effect" is another potential problem, particularly in studies involving products with prolonged biologic effects. Finally, the possible bias of a "learning effect" is not a problem for efficacy assessments involving objective laboratory tests, but for adverse event reporting and physical function tests such as treadmill performance, forced expiratory volume (FEV_1), and cognitive testing, the learning effect is likely to be significant.

Latin square or factorial designs are used to support the development of fixed-dose combination products of already approved products. Weight-loss products that consist of two additively or synergistically acting drugs approved for other indications provide a more interesting example of an early clinical study requiring the use of the factorial design [60, 61]. A factorial parallel design was required to show that the combination of two agents results in greater weight-loss activity than either alone. Once additivity of each component's efficacy and the optimal doses were established, the product could be developed in a fixed-dose ratio and compared as one or more strengths to placebo. Such an approach would be open to novel combinations of approved drugs that, together, would form an efficacious glucose-lowering therapy. In this case, the factorial design could be combined with a crossover design since the treatment periods could be short. The 6-week (or more) treatment period required for weight-loss evaluation is far too long for a crossover design.

Selection of Control Group, Randomization, and Blinding

Placebo comparisons are the rule in phase 1 metabolic studies of non-insulin therapies. Sometimes an active comparator group is included to provide an estimate of relative efficacy of the new agent. Active comparisons are the rule in injected insulin product studies. In some cases, the intent is to show similar PK and PD profiles, as would be the case for development of a "biosimilar"[4] version of an approved insulin product [62]. In other cases, the objective may be to contrast the time-action profile of the new insulin product to that of an approved human insulin product.

Randomization is expected of virtually all phase 1 trials as a fundamental means of reducing bias.

---

[4] Development of biosimilar insulins and other peptide therapies has been the subject of much interest and regulatory activity. More information is found at the FDA website. See reference.

Blinding, which tends to go hand in hand with randomization, is also expected at some level. Double blind is preferred over single blind, especially if a nonobjective efficacy measure is being used. Even when objective efficacy measures are involved, adverse event identification and reporting can be biased when the investigator knows the treatment assignment. Triple blinding (involving the sponsor) is preferable, though not required if appropriate safeguards are taken to prevent unblinding the investigator. Blinding is often very challenging for early studies. Placebo or active comparator dose forms identical to the active dose forms may be impractical to produce for initial studies.

Challenges with Early-Phase Metabolic Studies

With the exception of injected insulin products, there are few, if any, challenges unique to metabolic studies. Adequate documentation, subject recruitment difficulties, dropouts, and missing data are challenges faced across all therapeutic areas. Early in-human, single-, and multiple-dose studies for oral metabolic products are straightforward and usually can be completed in a single qualified centre. Challenges increase to the extent that early diabetes and obesity studies involve patients and objectives to assess efficacy. Larger and more ambitious early studies start to encounter the same issues that plague later-stage studies.

Documentation, data acquisition, and data management involved in the clinical trial process are going through a transition from paper to being electronically based. As mentioned, FDA submissions will soon be required to be in a highly structured electronic form [63]. The standards for electronic data and regulatory requirements for electronic data handling have been established [64]. These developments are putting pressure on early-stage companies, smaller investigation sites, and academic sites in which legacy paper systems are more cost-effective and work perfectly well. All these transitions to electronic systems will provide cost and time savings for FDA and the sponsor over time as the development program progresses and they are intended to improve overall results in the therapeutic development process. With the majority of development programs failing to advance beyond early-phase development, the electronic filing requirements impose a proportionately greater burden on early studies and their sites and sponsors.

Many early multiple-dose metabolic studies are on the cusp of requiring that multiple sites enroll adequate numbers of subjects and that this be completed in a reasonable amount of time. Multiple investigation sites drive up costs and variability. Organizations that specialize in phase 1 metabolic studies have frequently been associated with a large clinical specialty practice or have assembled a comparable means to facilitate patient recruitment. In all cases, care has to be taken regarding the suitability of subjects recruited for these studies. For obvious, multiple reasons, those patients who have had poor and/or inconsistent care for whatever reason, are generally not good subjects for investigation. They are most likely to fail to comply with the protocol and/or drop out of the study. Given the high per-subject cost of early clinical studies, dropouts must be minimized. Patients with poor glycemic control often present a higher risk of dropout and/or study effects.

Early weight-loss studies aimed at exploration of antiobesity effects entail special challenges in terms of demographics, logistics, facilities, and biologic limitations [65]. Women are clinical candidates for early trials on weight-loss drug therapy or other interventions, but the influence of the menstrual cycle on early efficacy indicators for antiobesity effects is an additional source of variability. Men can preferentially be utilized to reduce variability and increase statistical power to detect an early treatment effect, but the results may not be reflective of results in the general population, which for weight-loss drugs consist predominately of women. Obese subjects require compassionate and sensitive attention during the entire investigative process, starting with screening and baseline testing. Sites specialized for morbidly obese studies are well adapted to the requirements for venous blood access and large-size examination tables, blood pressure cuffs, and imaging equipment. Nonspecialized sites may not be adequately equipped. The greatest challenge to efficacy assessment of weight-loss therapies is the inherent biologic resistance to weight loss and the resulting small, slow rate of weight loss. This effect may be highly clinically meaningful if sustained, but is difficult to detect in smaller and shorter studies.

Weight-loss drugs have been a major contributor to the concern about dropouts and missing data in registration trials [66]. This general concern about registration trials has resulted in a guidance for handling missing data, which has been adopted by FDA [67]. This increased concern has pushed down into early clinical studies. Traditionally, early studies have not been closely scrutinized by FDA for trial execution and interpretation problems since it is the later trials that will be pivotal to approval. However, a high dropout rate in an early study will likely be noticed by FDA reviewers and perhaps reduce confidence in subsequent data.

In my experience, insufficient attention to the main contributors of a study effect bias has often led to misleading results of early and late studies. This is not so much an issue for small, in-house studies that involve rigorous protocol designs. However, when subjects are tested as outpatients, the study effect and dropouts become more confounding factors. Because glycemic control is sensitive to diet and exercise, a patient can unwittingly improve glycemic measures independent of assigned treatment (also see Chapter X). Patients are embarrassed by starting a study with poor metabolic control and naturally want to improve it. Some patients who claimed compliance with background metformin therapy may start to make good on that claim in the study or even add dietary supplements, forgetting that this is prohibited. Patients who are given glucose monitors or continue to use them in a study are somewhat unblinded and may consciously or unconsciously strive to improve glycemic control. The use of placebo run-in periods to reduce such effects is recommended by FDA, particularly for weight-loss studies. It is important even in early studies to avoid any major departure in the patient's care, while the patient is in a study, and to avoid subjects who will require major changes in their clinical care.

Finally, sloppiness and fraud should be mentioned as a threat across the entire spectrum of biomedical research. Examples of investigators who intentionally set out to commit fraud are very rare. More often, discovered cases of fraud that are documented on the FDA website [68] started down the slippery slope of cutting corners and taking on more studies than advisable. The increasing pressure on small studies to deliver more with less requires greater attention to trial monitoring and quality assurance.

The Overarching Goals of Early Metabolic Studies

It is clear that the overarching purpose of early-phase metabolic studies is to screen out further development of compounds that fail to achieve preliminary targets and to provide a solid foundation for performing later-phase and much more expensive studies [69]. The makeup of that foundation is more complicated. Timing of specialized studies to address important safety questions involves good judgment even with the availability of regulatory guidances and expert opinions. A compromise on every trial design element is to some extent always required. The choice is less often between the good and the perfect; it is more often between the acceptable and the good.

One example of a strategic compromise that is increasingly being made is to perform "proof of concept" (POC) trials as soon as possible for a new molecular entity that has gone through some preliminary vetting of safety and efficacy. For a diabetes product, a POC trial would typically involve 12 weeks' treatment in a patient population with one or two doses compared to placebo, and/or sometimes to an active comparator. With a positive POC study on the primary efficacy endpoint, a sponsor can then go back with more confidence to invest in the earlier studies that might have been delayed or abbreviated. This strategic approach has an impact on the "what" and the "how" of early clinical studies.

Looking Ahead to the Future of Early Metabolic Studies

Some challenges for early metabolic therapeutic investigation have been summarized. One conceivable challenge is a day when early clinical studies will be obviated by the technological advances in in silico, in vitro, and genetically modified animal testing. Such advances are likely to complement the clinical trial enterprise and accelerate overall success in meeting unmet clinical need and individualizing therapeutics. It is difficult to imagine that the need for early trial data will decline in any substantial way.

Truly exciting are the prospects for new metabolic indications, which can potentially avert metabolic diseases as we now know them and leverage major savings in lives and resources. Glucose lowering by itself is a palliative approach for managing a late-stage manifestation of a metabolic disorder that has reached the threshold for a diabetes diagnosis. Sponsors will no longer invest the roughly $1 billion required to develop a glucose-lowering therapy that does not have promise of providing major clinical outcome benefits [70]. Furthermore, we should not confine our focus to just diabetes, as we have become increasingly aware of the massive prediabetes population that closely underlies the disease. Advances in metabolic research have increased our understandings of the metabolic basis of cancer, dementia, and aging. We should lift our eyes to a horizon beyond that of conventional metabolic disease treatment and seek to address the significant unmet need for preventing metabolic diseases and their complications. Early clinical studies start to provide a means of identifying the promise of metabolic therapies. Promising metabolic compounds now have an expanding list of potential applications.

Translating Results into Clinical Practice

Early clinical studies are the first step in a long process that is intended to lead to two major achievements: a "safe" and "effective" treatment for a group of patients who need it and a user's manual for guiding the optimal use of the product. Results of early metabolic studies do end up in the user's manual—what FDA calls the "drug product label." Early studies are thus the first of many steps to translate observed results into clinical practice.

References

1. Significant Dates in U.S. Food and Drug Law History. http://www.fda.gov/AboutFDA/WhatWeDo/History/Milestones/ucm128305.htm. Accessed 12 Jan 2014.
2. European Medicines Agency: Human medicines regulatory information. http://www.ema.europa.eu/ema/index.jsp?curl=pages/regulation/landing/human_medicines_regulatory.jsp&mid=WC0b01ac058001ff89. Accessed 12 Jan 2014.
3. Rahalkar H. Historical overview of pharmaceutical industry and drug regulatory affairs. Pharmaceut Reg Aff. 2012;S11:002.
4. ICH Topic E6 (R1) Guideline for Good Clinical Practice. http://www.ema.europa.eu/docs/en_GB/document_library/Scientific_guideline/2009/09/WC500002874.pdf. Accessed 19 Sept 2014.
5. FDA Advisory Committees. http://www.fda.gov/AdvisoryCommittees/CommitteesMeetingMaterials/Drugs/default.htm. Accessed 18 May 2014.
6. Hiatt WR, Kaul S, Smith RJ. The cardiovascular safety of diabetes drugs—insights from the rosiglitazone experience. N Engl J Med. 2013;369:1285–128.
7. Marris E. Diabetes drugs under scrutiny in a post-Vioxx world. Nat Rev Drug Discov. 2007;6:505–6.
8. Roy ASA. Stifling new cures: the true cost of lengthy clinical drug trials. http://www.manhattan-institute.org/html/fda_05.htm. Accessed 20 Jan 2014.
9. About ICH: History. http://www.ich.org/about/history.html. Accessed 31 Jan 2014.
10. Echt DS, Liebson PR, Mitchell LB, Peters RW, Obias-Manno D, Barker AH, et al. Mortality and morbidity in patients receiving encainide, flecainide, or placebo. The cardiac arrhythmia suppression trial. N Engl J Med. 1991;324:781–8.
11. Brown NJ, Vaughan DE. Cardiovascular drugs: angiotensin-converting enzyme inhibitors. Circulation. 1998;97:1411–20.
12. Lambers Heerspink HJ, Perkovic V, de Zeeuw D. Is doubling of serum creatinine a valid clinical 'hard' endpoint in clinical nephrology trials? Nephron Clin Pract. 2011;119:c195–9.
13. Jiang S, Park C, Barner C. Ranibizumab, VEG-F inhibitor Ranibizumab for age-related macular degeneration: a meta-analysis of dose effects and comparison with no anti-VEGF treatment and bevacizumab. J Clin Pharm Ther. 2014;39:234–9.
14. Chalk C, Benstead TJ, Moore F. Aldose reductase inhibitors for the treatment of diabetic polyneuropathy. Cochrane Database Syst Rev. 2007. (4):CD004572. doi:10.1002/14651858.CD004572.pub2.

15. Guidance for Industry–Diabetes Mellitus: Developing Drugs and Therapeutic Biologics for Treatment and Prevention. http://www.fda.gov/downloads/Drugs/GuidanceComplianceRegulatoryInformation/Guidances/UCM071624.pdf. Accessed 20 May 2014.
16. Tardif J-C, Heinonen T, Orloff D, Libby P. Vascular biomarkers and surrogates in cardiovascular disease. Circulation. 2006;113:2936–42.
17. Rosen CJ. Revisiting the rosiglitazone story—lessons learned. N Engl J Med. 2010;363:803–6.
18. Guidance for Industry Diabetes Mellitus — Evaluating Cardiovascular Risk in New Antidiabetic Therapies to Treat Type 2 Diabetes. http://www.fda.gov/downloads/Drugs/GuidanceComplianceRegulatoryInformation/Guidances/UCM071627.pdf. Accessed 20 May 2014.
19. Alldredge BK, Corelli RL, Ernst ME, Guglielmo BJ, Jacobson PA, Kradjan WA, Williams BR. In: Koda-Kimble & young's applied therapeutics: the clinical use of drugs. Published 10th ed. Lippincott Williams & Wilkins; 2012. p. 252–67.
20. Psaty BM, Lumley T. Surrogate end points and FDA approval: a tale of 2 lipid-altering drugs. JAMA. 2008;299:1474–6.
21. Institute for Quality and Efficiency in Health Care (2011, September 14). Elevated cholesterol levels: no clear benefit of ezetimibe, report suggests. ScienceDaily. Retrieved 9 Jun 2014 from www.sciencedaily.com/releases/2011/09/110914110109.htm.
22. Hirshberg B, Raz I. Impact of the U.S. food and drug administration cardiovascular assessment requirements on the development of novel antidiabetes drugs. Diabetes Care. 2011;34:s101–6.
23. What does FDA regulate? http://www.fda.gov/AboutFDA/Transparency/Basics/ucm194879.htm. Accessed 10 Jun 2014.
24. FDA Fundamentals. http://www.fda.gov/AboutFDA/Transparency/Basics/ucm192695.htm. Accessed 20 May 2014.
25. 2014 FDA Budget Summary. http://www.fda.gov/AboutFDA/ReportsManualsForms/Reports/BudgetReports/ucm388251.htm. Accessed 20 May 2014.
26. Medical Foods Guidance Documents and Regulatory Information. http://www.fda.gov/Food/GuidanceRegulation/GuidanceDocumentsRegulatoryInformation/MedicalFoods/default.htm. Accessed 31 Jan 2014.
27. Degnan FH. The US food and drug administration and probiotics: regulatory categorization. Clin Infect Dis. 2008;46 Suppl 2:S133–6. doi:10.1086/523324.
28. Draft Guidance for Industry: Frequently Asked Questions About Medical Foods; Second Edition. http://www.fda.gov/Food/GuidanceRegulation/GuidanceDocumentsRegulatoryInformation/MedicalFoods/ucm054048.htm. Accessed 31 Jan 2014.
29. Guidance for Industry: End-of-Phase 2A Meetings. http://www.fda.gov/downloads/drugs/guidancecomplianceregulatoryinformation/guidances/ucm079690.pdf. Retrieved January 2014.
30. Guidance for Industry: Formal Meetings Between the FDA and Sponsors or Applicants. http://www.fda.gov/downloads/Drugs/GuidanceComplianceRegulatoryInformation/Guidances/UCM153222.pdf. Retrieved January 2014.
31. Guidance for Industry, Investigators, and Reviewers: Exploratory IND Studies. http://www.fda.gov/downloads/Drugs/GuidanceComplianceRegulatoryInformation/Guidances/UCM078933.pdf.
32. Guidance for Clinical Investigators, Sponsors, and IRBs: Investigational New Drug Applications (INDs)—Determining Whether Human Research Studies Can Be Conducted Without an IND. http://www.fda.gov/downloads/drugs/guidancecomplianceregulatoryinformation/guidances/ucm229175.pdf.
33. Guidance for Industry: Content and Format of Investigational New Drug Applications (INDs) for Phase 1 Studies of Drugs, Including Well-Characterized, Therapeutic, Biotechnology-derived Products. http://www.fda.gov/downloads/Drugs/GuidanceComplianceRegulatoryInformation/Guidances/UCM074980.pdf.
34. Code of Federal Regulations Title 21 Chapter I—Food and Drug Administration Department of Health And Human Services Subchapter A—General Part 56 Institutional Review Boards. http://www.accessdata.fda.gov/scripts/cdrh/cfdocs/cfcfr/CFRSearch.cfm?CFRPart=56.
35. Engelberg AB, Kesselheim AS, Avorn J. Balancing innovation, access, and profits – market exclusivity for biologics. N Engl J Med. 2009;361:1917–9.
36. Meekings KN, Williams CS, Arrowsmith JE. Orphan drug development: an economically viable strategy for biopharma R&D. Drug Discov Today. 2012;17(13–14):660–4.
37. Developing Products for Rare Diseases and Conditions. http://www.fda.gov/forindustry/DevelopingProductsforrareDiseasesConditions/default.htm.
38. Shani S, Yahalom Z. Legal and regulatory aspects of orphan drugs. Pediatr Endocrinol. 2013;11 Suppl 1:110–5.
39. Pastores GM, Gupta P. Orphan drug development. Pediatr Endocrinol. 2013;11 Suppl 1:64–7.
40. Wizemann T, Robinson S, and Giffin R. 7 strategies for facilitating clinical trials breakthrough business models: drug development for rare and neglected diseases and individualized therapies. Workshop Summary. 2008;82–97.
41. FDA approves Myalept to treat rare metabolic disease. http://www.fda.gov/newsevents/newsroom/pressannouncements/ucm387060.htm.
42. Chan JL, Lutz K, Cochran E, Huang W, Peters Y, Weyer C, Gorden P. Clinical effects of long-term metreleptin treatment in patients with lipodystrophy. Endocr Pract. 2011;17(6):922–32.
43. Designating an Orphan Product: Drugs and Biological Products. http://www.fda.gov/ForIndustry/DevelopingProductsforRareDiseasesConditions/Howtoapplyfororphanproductdesignation/default.htm.
44. Fast Track, Breakthrough Therapy, Accelerated Approval and Priority Review. http://www.fda.gov/forconsumers/byaudience/forpatientadvocates/speedingaccesstoimportantnewtherapies/ucm128291.htm.
45. Treatment of recent-onset type 1 diabetic patients with DiaPep277: results of a double-blind, placebo-

controlled, randomized phase 3 trial. Raz I, Ziegler AG, Linn T, Schernthaner G, Bonnici F, Distiller LA, Giordano C, Giorgino F, de Vries L, Mauricio D, Procházka V, Wainstein J, Elias D, Avron A, Tamir M, Eren R, Peled D, Dagan S, Cohen IR, Pozzilli P; DIA-AID 1 Writing Group. Diabetes Care. 2014;37:1392–400.
46. Fleming GA. Regulatory and policy issues for T1DM immunotherapy. Human Vaccines. 7:1, 1–6; January 2011. http://investors.hyperiontx.com/releases.cfm. Accessed 19 September 2014.
47. Guidance for Industry Diabetes Mellitus: Developing Drugs and Therapeutic Biologics for Treatment and Prevention. http://www.fda.gov/downloads/drugs/guidancecomplianceregulatoryinformation/guidances/ucm071624.pdf.
48. Sanyal AJ, Chalasani N, Kowdley KV, et al. Pioglitazone, vitamin E, or placebo for nonalcoholic steatohepatitis. N Engl J Med. 2010;362(18):1675–85.
49. Intercept Announces NASH Primary Endpoint Met: FLINT Trial Stopped Early for Efficacy Based on Highly Statistically Significant Improvement in Liver Histology. http://ir.interceptpharma.com/releasedetail.cfm?ReleaseID=818119. Accessed 20 May 2014.
50. Galmed Pharmaceuticals: Aramchol — A first-in-class drug for NASH. http://www.galmedpharma.com/products-2/aramchol/. Accessed 20 May 2014.
51. Isis Pharma: Metabolic Diseases. http://www.isispharm.com/Pipeline/Therapeutic-Areas/Metabolic-Disease.htm#ISIS-DGAT2Rx. Accessed 20 May 2014.
52. Fountaine RJ, Taylor AE, Mancuso JP, Greenway FL, Byerley LO, Smith SR, Most MM, Fryburg DA. Increased food intake and energy expenditure following administration of olanzapine to healthy men. Obesity (Silver Spring). 2010;18(8):1646–51.
53. Yanovski SZ, Yanovski JA. Long-term drug treatment for obesity: a systematic and clinical review. JAMA. 2014;311(1):74–86.
54. Guidance for Industry: Developing Products for Weight Management. http://www.fda.gov/downloads/Drugs/Guidances/ucm071612.pdf. Accessed 6 Jun 2014.
55. Ceriello A. Postprandial hyperglycemia and cardiovascular disease: is the HEART2D study the answer? Diabetes Care. 2009;32(3):521–2.
56. Monnier L, Lapinski H, Colette C. Contributions of fasting and postprandial plasma glucose increments to the overall diurnal hyperglycemia of type 2 diabetic patients: variations with increasing levels of HbA(1c). Diabetes Care. 2003;26(3):881–5.
57. Riddle M, Umpierrez G, DiGenio A, Zhou R, Rosenstock J. Contributions of basal and postprandial hyperglycemia over a wide range of A1c levels before and after treatment intensification in type 2 diabetes. Diabetes Care. 2011;34(12):2508–14.
58. Rosenson RS, Underberg JA. Systematic review: evaluating the effect of lipid-lowering therapy on lipoprotein and lipid values. Cardiovasc Drugs Ther. 2013;27:465–79.
59. Guideline for Industry: The Extent of Population Exposure to Assess Clinical Safety: For Drugs Intended for Longterm Treatment of Non-Life-Threatening Conditions. http://www.fda.gov/downloads/Drugs/GuidanceComplianceRegulatoryInformation/Guidances/ucm073083.pdf. Accessed 6 Jun 2014.
60. Cosentino G, Conrad AO, Uwaifo GI. Phentermine and topiramate for the management of obesity: a review. Drug Des Devel Ther. 2013;7:267–78.
61. Ornellas T, Chavez B. Naltrexone SR/bupropion SR (Contrave): a new approach to weight loss in obese adults. Proc Natl Acad Sci U S A. 2011;36:255–62.
62. Biosimilars http://www.fda.gov/Drugs/DevelopmentApprovalProcess/HowDrugsareDevelopedandApproved/ApprovalApplications/TherapeuticBiologicApplications/Biosimilars/default.htm.
63. Electronic Common Technical Document (eCTD). http://www.fda.gov/drugs/developmentapprovalprocess/formssubmissionrequirements/electronicsubmissions/ucm153574.htm. Accessed 6 Jun 2014.
64. CDER Data Standards Program. http://www.fda.gov/Drugs/DevelopmentApprovalProcess/FormsSubmissionRequirements/ElectronicSubmissions/ucm249979.htm.
65. Rodgers RJ, Tschöp MH, Wilding JP. Anti-obesity drugs: past, present and future. Dis Model Mech. 2012;5(5):621–6.
66. Colombo IO, Ferretti VV, Ferraris C, Trentani C, Vinai P, Villani S, Tagliabue A. Is drop-out from obesity treatment a predictable and preventable event? Nut J. 2014;13:13.
67. The prevention and treatment of missing data in clinical trials. National Research Council. (U.S.). Panel on handling missing data in clinical trials.; National Research Council (U.S.). Committee on National Statistics.; National Academies Press (U.S.). Washington, D.C.: National Academies Press; 2010. NLM ID: 101555711 [Book].
68. Guidance for Industry: Oversight of Clinical Investigations — A Risk-Based Approach to Monitoring CDER Data Standards Program. http://www.fda.gov/downloads/drugs/guidancecomplianceregulatoryinformation/guidances/ucm269919.pdf. Accessed 10 Jun 2014
69. Krentz AJ, Morrow L, Hompesch M. Developing new drugs for diabetes and cardiometabolic disorders: a changing paradigm. Drugs. 2012;72(13):1709–11.
70. Svensson A. Sponsors viewpoint – the T2DM regulatory guidances and implications for drug development presentation at development of type 2 diabetes mellitus drugs: state-of-the-art cardiovascular safety assessments. October 5–6, 2010 L'Enfant Plaza Hotel, Washington, DC, USA http://www.diahome.org/Tools/Content.aspx?type=eopdf&file=%2fproductfiles%2f23808%2f10035%2Epdf.
71. Braunholtz DA, Edwards SJ, Lilford RJ. Are randomized clinical trials good for us (in the short term)? Evidence for a "trial effect", J Clin Epidemiol. 2001:54:217–224.

Index

A
Activity-induced energy expenditure (AEE), 178–181
Adiponectin, 260–261
Adverse drug events (ADEs), 244
American Diabetes Association (ADA), 237, 246, 256
Angiotensin-converting enzyme inhibitor (ACEI), 287
Angiotensin receptor blockers (ARBs), 234, 287
Anti-obesity products, 297
Archimedes model, 256, 259
Arginine stimulation test, 61–62
Association of South East Asian Nations (ASEAN), 285
Asymptotic time-course (ATC), 255

B
Basal insulin secretion, 46
Basal metabolic rate (BMR), 175–177, 179–180
Best Pharmaceuticals for Children Act (BPCA), 262
Biomarkers
    Archimedes model, 259
    cardiovascular disease and, 262
    for diabetes, 247
    omics technologies, 192
    quantifiable and accurate, 246–247
    type 2 diabetes and, 261
Biomarkers Definitions Working Group (BDWG), 246
Biosimilar insulins, 33–34
Body composition assessment
    anthropometric measurements, 144
    bioimpedance analysis, 139
    clinical practice, 163
    computed tomography
        abdominal image, 150
        advantages, 151–153
        disadvantages, 153
        drug development, 153–154
        midthigh image, 150
        phantom image, 151–152
        spine and hip scan, 151, 153
        supine position and fluid distribution, 151
    dual-energy X-ray absorptiometry
        advantages, 147
        bone mineral density, 145
        disadvantages, 148
        drug development, 149
        GE lunar whole body, 146
        hemi-scan, 146–147
        Hologic whole body, 146
        hydration status, 146
        whole body phantom, 147–148
    dynamic contrast-enhanced-magnetic resonance imaging, 162
    fat fraction imaging, 159–160
    image acquisition, 140
    image analysis, 140–141
    magnetic resonance imaging
        advantages, 157
        axial image acquisition, 154
        diffusion, 162
        disadvantages, 157
        drug development, 157–158
        iron, 161
        phantom image, 156
        physical characteristics, 156
        proton magnetic interaction, 154
        relaxometry, 159
        sodium, 161–162
        whole body scan, 155
    MRE, 162
    obesity/diabetes pathophysiology, 141–143
    pharmacological agents, 143–144
    three-compartment model, 144
Body weight dynamics, 274–275
Brown fat
    adipose tissue type, 122
    age and sex, 126
    animal studies, 127
    autonomic regulation, 123
    body mass index, 122
    cold and warm environments, 126
    computed tomography
        anatomical tissue segmentation, 125
        cylindrical water phantom, 124
        vs. FDG-PET, 123
        Hounsfield unit ratings, 123–124
        sternocleidomastoid muscle, 124
        thorax, 124–125
        x-ray attenuation, 123

Brown fat (*cont.*)
   diabetes, 134
   drug action, energy expenditure, thermogenesis, 122–123
   FDG imaging, 125–126
   histopathological and genetic validation, 126–127
   Hounsfield unit values, 125, 129, 131–133
   image analysis, 127
   metabolism, 133–134
   obesity, 134
   tissue segmentation study
      clustering voxels, 129–130
      FDG quantification, 128
      insulin-resistant subjects, 127
      leg metabolic activity, 131
      R language, 130–131
      total fat volume and fat Hounsfield units, 130
      whole slice glucose metabolic rate, 128–129

C

Cardiac Arrhythmic Suppression Trial (CAST), 287
Cardiometabolic diseases
   insulin resistance, 7–8
   modifiable and non-modifiable, 244
   nature, 258
   risk factors, 244
Cardiovascular disease
   and biomarkers, 262
   diabetes mellitus, 232
   insulin sensitivity, 9–10
   QT/QTc study, 232
CBER. *See* Center for Biologics Evaluation and Research (CBER)
CDER. *See* Center for Drug Evaluation and Research (CDER)
CDRH. *See* Center for Devices and Radiologic Health (CDRH)
β-cell function
   basal insulin secretion, 46
   clinical research methods, 55
   dynamic tests
      CIGMA, 60–62
      intravenous glucose tolerance test, 59–60
      mixed meal tolerance test, 58–59
      oral glucose tolerance test, 57–58
   glucose-stimulated insulin secretion, 48–50
   hepatic clearance, 50–51
   incretin system, 49–50
   islet physiology, 48
   non-stimulated assessments
      fasting insulin/C-peptide, 55–56
      HOMA-B, 56–57
      proinsulin, 56
   pharmaceutical agents, 54–55
   stimulated insulin secretion, 46–47
   type 1 diabetes
      pathogenesis, 51
      treatment and prevention, 52–53
   type 2 diabetes
      pathogenesis, 51–52
      treatment and prevention, 53–54
Cellular insulin signalling, 6–8
Center for Biologics Evaluation and Research (CBER), 288, 289
Center for Devices and Radiologic Health (CDRH), 288, 289
Center for Drug Evaluation and Research (CDER), 288, 289
Center for Food Safety and Nutrition (CFSAN), 288
Clinical and Translational Science Institute (CTSI) Award program, 246
Common technical document (CTD)
   components, 287
   description, 286
   format, 286
Computed tomography (CT)
   body composition assessment
      abdominal image, 150
      advantages, 151–153
      disadvantages, 153
      drug development, 153–154
      midthigh image, 150
      phantom image, 151–152
      spine and hip scan, 151, 153
      supine position and fluid distribution, 151
   brown fat
      anatomical tissue segmentation, 125
      cylindrical water phantom, 124
      vs. FDG-PET, 123
      Hounsfield unit ratings, 123–124
      sternocleidomastoid muscle, 124
      thorax, 124–125
      x-ray attenuation, 123
   liver fat, 99, 103–104
Continuous glucose monitoring (CGM), 298
Continuous infusion of glucose with model assessment (CIGMA)
   arginine stimulation test, 61–62
   graded glucose infusion, 62
   hyperglycaemic clamp, 60–61
C-peptide, 55–56, 230
CTD. *See* Common technical document (CTD)

D

DCaRP. *See* Division of Cardiovascular and Renal Products (DCaRP)
De novo lipogenesis (DNL)
   clinical practice, 80–81
   lipid synthesis regulation, 76
   measurement
      ^{13}C-acetate, 79–80
      deuterated water, 77–79
   nonalcoholic fatty liver disease, 76
   obesity, 76
Deuterated water (^2H_2O), 75, 77–79

Diabetes mellitus
    cardiovascular disease, 232–233
    concomitant medications, 234–235
    diabetic nephropathy, 233–234
    fatty liver disease, 233
    glycaemic control, 231
    other comorbidities, 234
    type 1, 235–236
    type 2, 236–237
Diabetic nephropathy, 233–234
Diet-induced energy expenditure (DEE), 177–178
Diffusion magnetic resonance imaging, 162
Division of Cardiovascular and Renal Products
    (DCaRP), 287
Division of Metabolism and Endocrinology Products
    (DMEP), 287–288, 294
Dixon method. See Fat fraction imaging
DMEP. See Division of Metabolism and Endocrinology
    Products (DMEP)
Doubly labelled water technique, 173–174
Drug regulation, 284
Dual-echo technique, 110
Dual-energy X-ray absorptiometry (DXA)
    advantages, 147
    bone mineral density, 145
    disadvantages, 148
    drug development, 149
    GE lunar whole body, 146
    hemi-scan, 146–147
    Hologic whole body, 146
    hydration status, 146
    whole body phantom, 147–148
Dynamic contrast-enhanced-magnetic resonance
    imaging (DCE-MRI), 162
Dyslipidemia, 237

E
Early metabolic study, FDA
    anti-obesity products, 297
    blinding, 299–300
    challenges with, 300–301
    control group selection, 299–300
    crossover design, 299
    efficacy endpoints, 297–298
    future, 302
    glucose-lowering products, 294–297
    lipid-lowering studies, 297
    number of subjects, 298–299
    overarching goals, 301
    proof of concept trials, 301
    randomization, 299–300
    study designs, 299
    subject population, 298
    therapeutic indications, 294
    weight-loss products, 297
Early phase clinical trials
    children and adolescents, 238–239
    diabetes mellitus
        cardiovascular disease, 232–233
        concomitant medications, 234–235
        diabetic nephropathy, 233–234
        fatty liver disease, 233
        glycaemic control, 231
        type 1, 229, 235–236
        type 2, 229, 236–237
    first-in-human studies, 226–227
    impaired fasting glucose, 237–238
    impaired glucose tolerance, 237
    older adults, 238
    women of childbearing potential, 239
eCTD format, 286
Ectopic fat, 101
Efficacy endpoints, 297–298
EGRIFTA®, 163
EMA. See European Medicines Agency (EMA)
End of Phase 2A (EOP2A) meeting, 290
Endogenous glucose production (EGP), 81
Energy
    adaptive thermogenesis, 271–273
    balance, 266
    expenditure, 269
    intake, 273
        measuring long-term, 273–274
        men vs. women, 277
        relevant time scale, 273
    metabolic adaptation, 271–273
    partitioning models, 268
    physical activity expenditure, 271
    REE, 270–271
    thermic effect of food, 269–270
Energy expenditure measurement
    body weight regulation, 171
    chronic obstructive pulmonary disease, 184–185
    energy requirement, 170
    Harris and Benedict equation, 170
    heat loss method, 171
    indirect calorimetry
        activity-induced energy expenditure, 178–179
        diet-induced energy expenditure, 177–178
        doubly labelled water, 173–174
        mouthpiece/facemask, 172
        respiration chamber, 173, 175
        sleeping and basal metabolic rate, 175–177
        validation, 174–175
        ventilated hood, 172–173
    physical fitness, 170
    validation of alternative methods
        activity-induced energy expenditure, 180–181
        basal metabolic rate, 179–180
        food intake, 182–184
        total energy expenditure, 181–182
    weight-maintenance diets, 170
Weir equation, 171
work efficiency, 172
Entelos PhysioLab® platform, 258
EOP2A meeting. See End of Phase 2A (EOP2A)
    meeting

Epigenomics, 190
  allele-specific oligo, 200
  bisulphite-converted DNA, 200
  DNA methylation, 194
  epigenetic disease biomarker genes, 202
  EpiTYPER assay, 200
  methylation-specific PCR, 199
  MethylC-seq, 194–195
  oligonucleotide-tiling arrays, 200
  pyrosequencing, 199
  reduced representation bisulphite sequencing, 201
  restriction enzymes, 199
  ribonucleic acid, 194
  shotgun bisulphite sequencing, 201
  whole-genome bisulphite sequencing, 201
Euglycaemic glucose clamp, 26–27
European Medicines Agency (EMA), 26, 33, 233, 284–285

F
Fasting EGP, 82–83
  gluconeogenesis and glycogenolysis, 83
  hyperinsulinaemic euglycaemic clamp, 83–84
Fasting insulin, 55–56
Fat fraction imaging, 159–160
Fat-free mass
  obesity, 267, 270
  resting energy expenditure and, 270
Fatty liver disease, 233
FDA. *See* Food and Drug Administration (FDA)
FD&C Act, 284–285, 289
18F-deoxyglucose-positron-emission tomography (FDG-PET), 122
Federal Food, Drug, and Cosmetic (FDC), 284
FerriScan™, 163
First-in-human studies, 28, 226–227
Food and Drug Administration (FDA)
  advisory committees, 285
  DCaRP, 287
  DMEP, 287
  drug product label, 302
  early metabolic study
    anti-obesity products, 297
    blinding, 299–300
    challenges with, 300–301
    control group selection, 299–300
    crossover design, 299
    efficacy endpoints, 297–298
    glucose-lowering products, 294–297
    lipid-lowering studies, 297
    number of subjects, 298–299
    overarching goals, 301
    proof of concept trials, 301
    randomization, 299–300
    study designs, 299
    subject population, 298
    therapeutic indications, 294
    weight-loss products, 297
  ethical review, 293
  Fast Track and Breakthrough Therapy programs, 294
  investigative new drug
    pre-IND and other meetings with FDA, 289–290
    requirements, 291
    review process, 292–293
    submission content, 291–292
    varieties, 290–291
  Orphan Drug Program, 293–294
  review divisions, 287–288
  therapeutic product jurisdiction, 288–289
Food, thermic effect of, 269–270
Forbes hypothesis, 267, 268

G
Gas chromatography/mass spectroscopy (GC/MS), 75
Genomics, 190
  chip arrays, 197
  DCTN4 identification, 198
  ENCODE, 194
  iPLEX Assay, 196
  mass modified nucleotides, 196
  next-generation sequencing, 193, 197
  personal genome sequencing, 194
  polymerase chain reaction, 193
  real-time sequencing, 198
  Sanger capillary sequencing system, 197
  Sequenom iPLEX technolgy, 198
  single nucleotide polymorphisms, 193
  TaqMan System, 196–197
Gerritzen's test, 26
Gilbert's syndrome, 233
GLP-1 agonists, 252, 254
Gluconeogenesis, 83, 86, 268
Glucose-lowering drugs, 26
Glucose-lowering products, 294–297
Glucose metabolism, 72–73
  bile acid pathway measurement, 86–87
  clinical practice, 86–88
  dual tracer approach, 84–85
  endogenous glucose production, 81
  fasting EGP, 82–83
    gluconeogenesis and glycogenolysis, 83
    hyperinsulinaemic euglycaemic clamp, 83–84
  oral glucose load disposal, 85–86
  tissue glucose disposal, 81
  type 2 diabetes, 81
Glucose-stimulated insulin secretion, 48–50
Glycaemic control, 25, 31, 54, 56, 231
Glycogenolysis, 83, 87
Good Clinical Practice (GCP), 286
Gradient-recalled-echo (GRE) sequences, 103
Gulf Co-Operative Countries (GCC), 285

H
Harris-Benedict equation, 229
Healthy obese population, 227
Homeostasis model assessment (HOMA-IR), 228
Homeostasis model assessment of β-cell (HOMA-B), 56–58, 256
Hyperglycaemic glucose clamp, 19–20

Index

Hyperinsulinaemic euglycaemic clamp, 83–84
Hyperinsulinaemic-euglycaemic glucose clamp, 20
    drug development, 24
    insulin sensitivity, 23–24
Hypoglycaemia, 226
    glucose clamp technique, 19–20, 25
    nocturnal, 30, 31
    risk of, 11, 14, 231–232
Hy's law, 233

I

ICH guidances
    contribution, 286
    CTD, 286
    MedDRA, 286
Impaired fasting glucose (IFG), 237
Impaired glucose tolerance (IGT), 237
Incretin system, 49–50
IND. *See* Investigative new drug (IND)
Indirect calorimetry method
    activity-induced energy expenditure, 178–179
    diet-induced energy expenditure, 177–178
    doubly labelled water, 173–174
    mouthpiece/facemask, 172
    respiration chamber, 173, 175
    sleeping and basal metabolic rate, 175–177
    validation, 174–175
Insulin Amendment to the FD&C Act in 1941, 284
Insulin sensitivity
    assessment, 3
    biosimilar insulins, 33–34
    cardiovascular disease, 9–10
    cellular insulin signalling, 6–8
    closed-loop methods, 4, 13–14
    confounding factors, 12–13
    glucose clamp parameters, 29–30
    glucose clamp technique, 5–6
    insulin resistance
        cardiometabolic consequences, 7–8
        type 2 diabetes pathogenesis, 8–9
    intravenous glucose tolerance test, 14–15
    investigative techniques, 12
    ITT, 16–17
    long-acting insulin formulations, 30–33
    measurement, 11–12
    open-loop methods, 5
        choice of test, 25
        experimental conditions, 21–22
        hyperglycaemic/hypoglycaemic glucose clamp, 19–20
        hyperinsulinaemic-euglycaemic glucose clamp, 20, 23–24
        insulin-sensitivity clamp, 17–18
        insulin suppression test, 17
        islet cell clamp, 19
        manual *vs.* automated glucose clamp, 20–22
        two-step hyperinsulinaemic-euglycaemic glucose clamp, 18–19
    oral and mixed meal tolerance tests, 15–16
    pharmacodynamic properties, 5
    pharmacokinetics and pharmacodynamics, 26–29
    physiology and metabolic regulation, 6–7
    rapid-acting and ultra-rapid-acting insulins, 30
    therapy, 10–11
    time-action profile, 26
    type 1 diabetes, 11
    type 2 diabetes, 3, 9–11
    whole-body insulin resistance, 6
Insulin suppression test (IST), 17
Insulin tolerance test (ITT), 16–17
Intramyocellular lipid (IMCL), 102
Intravenous bolus method, 90
Intravenous glucose tolerance test (IVGTT), 14–15, 59–60
Investigative new drug (IND)
    categories, 290–291
    pre-IND and other meetings with FDA, 289–290
    requirements, 291
    review process, 292–293
    submission content, 291–292
    therapeutic indications, 294
    varieties of, 290–291
Iron magnetic resonance imaging, 161
Islet cell clamp, 19
Islet physiology, 48
Isotopic tracers
    de novo lipogenesis
        clinical practice, 80–81
        lipid synthesis regulation, 76
        measurement, 77–80
        nonalcoholic fatty liver disease, 76
        obesity, 76
    deuterated/heavy water, 75
    gas chromatography/mass spectroscopy, 75
    glucose metabolism, 72–73
        bile acid pathway measurement, 86–87
        clinical practice, 86–88
        dual tracer approach, 84–85
        endogenous glucose production, 81
        fasting endogenous glucose production, 82–83
        oral glucose load disposal, 85–86
        sources of fasting EGP, 83–84
        tissue glucose disposal, 81
        type 2 diabetes, 81
    isotope ratio mass spectrometry, 75
    lipid metabolism, 72
    lipoprotein and protein metabolism, 73
        bolus decay method, 89
        clinical practice, 93
        deuterated water labeling, 89, 91
        diabetes and cardiovascular disease, 88
        fasting apo-B metabolism, 89
        intravenous bolus method, 90
        LC-MS/MS, 91–92
        polyacrylamide gel electrophoresis, 89
        primed constant infusion, 90–91
        protein synthesis, 88
        sequential ultracentrifugation, 89
        tissue and whole-body protein synthesis, 92–93
    metabolic flux, 74
    stable isotopes, 71

L

Lipid-lowering studies, 297
Lipid metabolism, 72
Lipoprotein and protein metabolism, 73
   bolus decay method, 89
   clinical practice, 93
   deuterated water labeling, 89, 91
   diabetes and cardiovascular disease, 88
   fasting apo-B metabolism, 89
   intravenous bolus method, 90
   LC-MS/MS, 91–92
   polyacrylamide gel electrophoresis, 89
   primed constant infusion, 90–91
   protein synthesis, 88
   sequential ultracentrifugation, 89
   tissue and whole-body protein synthesis, 92–93
Liquid chromatography-tandem mass spectrometry (LC-MS/MS), 75
Long-acting insulin formulations, 30–33
Long-term energy intake, 273–274

M

Macronutrient balance models, 268–269
Magnetic resonance elastography (MRE), 162
Magnetic resonance imaging (MRI), 103
   advanced, 100, 111–113
   advantages, 157
   axial image acquisition, 154
   conventional, 100, 109–111
   disadvantages, 157
   drug development, 157–158
   and MRS, 104–107
   phantom image, 156
   physical characteristics, 156
   proton magnetic interaction, 154
   whole body scan, 155
Magnetic resonance spectroscopy (MRS)
   drug development, 99
   liver fat measurement techniques
      fat fraction signal, 109
      MR scanners, 109
      multi-TE acquisition, 108
      point resolved spectroscopy, 107
      spectral analysis, 108
      stimulated echo acquisition mode, 107
      T2 decay equation, 108
      in vivo adipose spectrum, 105, 107
      voxel selection, 107
   and MRI, 104–107
   single-center exploratory study, 100
   skeletal intramyocellular lipid, 101
   skeletal muscle fat measurement technique, 113–115
Mathematical models
   body weight, 270, 274–275, 277
   energy expenditure, 271
   energy regulation, 266
   mouse models, 274–275
   relevant time scale, 273

Maturity-onset diabetes of the young (MODY), 52, 230
Mechanism-centric modeling, quantitative approaches, 252–254
Medical Dictionary for Regulatory Activities (MedDRA), 286
Metabolic adaptation, and adaptive thermogenesis, 271–273
Metabolic diseases, 294–296
Metabolomics, 191, 196
   angiotensin-converting enzyme, 209
   annotated metabolite concentration, 207
   biomedical applications, 208
   chemical shift, 206
   environmental and lifestyle factors, 208
   epidemiological population-based cohorts, 206
   health-care and nutrition strategy, 210
   heritability contribution, 209
   nontargeted, 207
   phenotypes, 208
   solute carrier family 16 member 9, 209
   standard operating procedures, 209
Mixed meal tolerance test (MMTT), 58–59
Model-base meta-analysis (MBMA), 258–260
Modification of Diet in Renal Disease (MDRD), 234
Mouse models metabolism, 274–275
MRI. *See* Magnetic resonance imaging (MRI)
MRS. *See* Magnetic resonance spectroscopy (MRS)

N

National Institutes of Health (NIH), 245
Nonalcoholic fatty liver disease (NAFLD), 76, 101–102
Nonalcoholic steatohepatitis (NASH), 294
Noninvasive imaging assessment
   liver fat
      computed tomography, 99, 103–104
      MRI, 100, 109–113
      MRS, 99–100, 107–109
      ultrasound, 99, 103
   skeletal intramyocellular lipid, 101, 113–115

O

Obesity
   brown fat, 134
   characterization, 267
   childhood, 277–278
   clinical management, 276
   disease populations, 227–229
   DNL, 76
   fat-free mass in, 270
   modeling populations, 275–276
   pharmaceutical product, 247
   pharmacological therapies, 276–277
   policy interventions, 275–276
Omics technologies
   biomarkers, 192
   clinical practice
      diagnostics, 210–211
      personalized medicine, 213–214

pharmacogenomics, 212–213
prediction, 211–212
systems approach, 214
therapeutic targets, 212
epigenomics, 190
  allele-specific oligo, 200
  bisulphite-converted DNA, 200
  DNA methylation, 194
  epigenetic disease biomarker genes, 202
  EpiTYPER assay, 200
  methylation-specific PCR, 199
  MethylC-seq, 194–195
  oligonucleotide-tiling arrays, 200
  pyrosequencing, 199
  reduced representation bisulphite sequencing, 201
  restriction enzymes, 199
  ribonucleic acid, 194
  shotgun bisulphite sequencing, 201
  whole-genome bisulphite sequencing, 201
genetic variants, 192
genomics, 190
  chip arrays, 197
  DCTN4 identification, 198
  ENCODE, 194
  iPLEX Assay, 196
  mass modified nucleotides, 196
  next-generation sequencing, 193, 197
  personal genome sequencing, 194
  polymerase chain reaction, 193
  real-time sequencing, 198
  Sanger capillary sequencing system, 197
  Sequenom iPLEX techonolgy, 198
  single nucleotide polymorphisms, 193
  TaqMan System, 196–197
metabolomics, 191, 196
  angiotensin-converting enzyme, 209
  annotated metabolite concentration, 207
  biomedical applications, 208
  chemical shift, 206
  environmental and lifestyle factors, 208
  epidemiological population-based cohorts, 206
  health-care and nutrition strategy, 210
  heritability contribution, 209
  nontargeted, 207
  phenotypes, 208
  solute carrier family 16 member 9, 209
  standard operating procedures, 209
proteomics, 190–191
  antibody-based protein identification, 195
  click chemistry, 196
  2D fluorescence difference gel electrophoresis, 204
  disease relevant proteins/pathways, 206
  Islet Human Diabetes Proteome Project, 206
  peptide-based, 205
  posttranslationally modified protein isoforms, 204
  pre-fractionation methods, 205
  protein capture-agent aptamer chips, 196
  selected reaction monitoring, 195, 205
  two-dimensional gel electrophoresis, 204

systems epidemiology, 192
transcriptomics, 190, 195
  complementary DNA, 202
  massively parallel signature sequencing, 202
  quantitative PCR, 203
  RNA hydrolysis/nebulization, 204
  RNA–RNA ligation, 204
  RNA sequencing, 203
Oral and mixed meal tolerance tests, 15–16
Oral glucose tolerance test (OGTT), 57–58, 85
Orphan Drug Act, 289, 293
Orphan Drug Program, 293–294
Over-the-counter (OTC), 228

P
Pharmacodynamics (PD)
  GLP-1 agonists, 252, 254
  rosiglitazone, 253, 254
Pharmacogenomics, 197, 212–213
Pharmacokinetics (PK)
  GLP-1 agonists, 252, 254
  rosiglitazone, 253, 254
Primed constant infusion, 90–91
Proinsulin, 56
Proteomics, 190–191
  antibody-based protein identification, 195
  click chemistry, 196
  2D fluorescence difference gel electrophoresis, 204
  disease relevant proteins/pathways, 206
  Islet Human Diabetes Proteome Project, 206
  peptide-based, 205
  posttranslationally modified protein isoforms, 204
  pre-fractionation methods, 205
  protein capture-agent aptamer chips, 196
  selected reaction monitoring, 195, 205
  two-dimensional gel electrophoresis, 204
Proton density fat fraction (PDFF)
  hepatic, 114, 115
  MRI, 103, 111–113
  MRS, 107–109
Public Health Service Act, 285
Pure Food and Drug Act, 284

Q
Quantitative approaches
  bench to bedside, 246, 262
  bottom-up approaches, 244–245
  drug development stages
    clinical stage modeling, 254–256
    clinical trial modeling, 256–258
    description, 248–249
    mechanism-centric modeling, 252–254
    model-base meta-analysis, 258–260
    system-centric modeling, 249–252
    treatment outcome modeling, 256–258
  opportunities, 260–263
  personalizing medicine, 260–263
  top-down approaches, 244–245
  translational research, 245–246

R
Radio-labelled insulin, 26
Rapid-acting and ultra-rapid-acting insulins, 30
Relevant time scale, energy intake, 273
Resting energy expenditure (REE), 270–271
Rosiglitazone, 253, 254

S
Sleeping metabolic rate (SMR), 176–177
Sodium magnetic resonance imaging, 161–162
System-centric modeling, quantitative approaches, 249–252
Systems biology, 266

T
Tetramethylsilane (TMS), 105
Thermogenesis, 122
    adaptive, 271–273
    brown fat, 123
Tissue and whole-body protein synthesis, 92–93
Total energy expenditure (TEE), 181–182
Transcriptomics, 190, 195
    complementary DNA, 202
    massively parallel signature sequencing, 202
    quantitative PCR, 203
    RNA hydrolysis/nebulization, 204
    RNA–RNA ligation, 204
    RNA sequencing, 203
Translational research
    overview, 245–246
    quantitative approaches
        bench to bedside, 246, 262
        bottom-up approaches, 244–245
        clinical stage modeling, 254–256
        clinical trial modeling, 256–258
        description, 248–249
        mechanism-centric modeling, 252–254
        model-base meta-analysis, 258–260
        opportunities, 260–262
        personalizing medicine, 260–263
        system-centric modeling, 249–252
        top-down approaches, 244–245
        treatment outcome modeling, 256–258
Tripartite ICH Guidelines, 286
Two-step hyperinsulinaemic-euglycaemic glucose clamp, 18–19
Type 1 diabetes
    β-cell function, 51–53
    early phase clinical trials, 229, 235–236
    insulin sensitivity, 11
Type 2 diabetes
    β-cell function, 51–54
    and biomarkers, 262
    early phase clinical trials, 229, 236–237
    glucose metabolism, 81
    insulin sensitivity, 3, 8–11

U
Ultrasound, 99, 103
US Pediatric Research Equity Act (PREA), 262

V
Very low-density lipoprotein (VLDL), 77, 79–80, 90–91

W
Weight-loss products, 297
Whole slice glucose metabolic rate, 128–129

Printed by Printforce, the Netherlands